Optical Coherence Tomography - Applications in Ophthalmology

Edited by Xiaogang Wang, Zhengwei Zhang and Liang Zhou

Published in London, United Kingdom

Optical Coherence Tomography - Applications in Ophthalmology
http://dx.doi.org/10.5772/intechopen.1003463
Edited by Xiaogang Wang, Zhengwei Zhang and Liang Zhou

Contributors
Ankit Butola, Ceren Durmaz Engin, Emine Tinkir Kayitmazbatir, Erick Quiroz-Gonzalez, Eva Maria Sobas Abad, Feiyan Chai, Francisco Javier Valentín-Bravo, Han Saem Cho, Jinhai Huang, José Carlos Pastor Jimeno, Kexin Li, Miguel A. Quiroz-Gonzalez, Miguel Angel Quiroz-Reyes, Miguel Busquets, Milagros Mateos-Olivares, Muki Rapp, Nikita Dash, Nishant Mohan, Ricardo Usategui Martín, Sae Chae Jeoung, Salvador Pastor-Idoate, Santiago Mejía-Freire, Xiaogang Wang, Xinning Yang, Yiran Wang, Yun Sik Yang

First published in London, United Kingdom, 2025 by IntechOpen
IntechOpen is the global imprint of INTECHOPEN LIMITED, registered in England and Wales, registration number: 11086078, 167-169 Great Portland Street, London, W1W 5PF, United Kingdom

For EU product safety concerns: IN TECH d.o.o., Prolaz Marije Krucifikse Kozulić 3, 51000 Rijeka, Croatia, info@intechopen.com or visit our website at intechopen.com.

British Library Cataloguing-in-Publication Data
A catalogue record for this book is available from the British Library

Optical Coherence Tomography - Applications in Ophthalmology
Edited by Xiaogang Wang, Zhengwei Zhang and Liang Zhou
p. cm.
Print ISBN 978-0-85466-365-1
Online ISBN 978-0-85466-364-4
eBook (PDF) ISBN 978-0-85466-366-8

Meet the editors

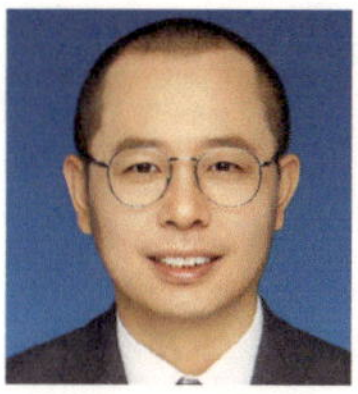

Dr. Xiaogang Wang is a faculty member of Shanxi Eye Hospital Affiliated to Shanxi Medical University, where he specializes in the treatment of cataracts and retinal diseases. He also serves as a tutor for postgraduate students at Shanxi Medical University. From October 2012 to November 2013, Dr. Wang studied in the COOL Lab as an international fellowship under the supervision of Dr. David Huang. He earned his MD from Shanxi Medical University and his Ph. D. from Shanghai Jiao Tong University. Dr. Wang has been awarded two research project grants focused on multimodal optical coherence tomography imaging and deep learning applications in cataracts and retinal diseases, funded by the National Natural Science Foundation of China. He has published approximately 60 peer-reviewed journal articles and six book chapters, in addition to co-editing four books.

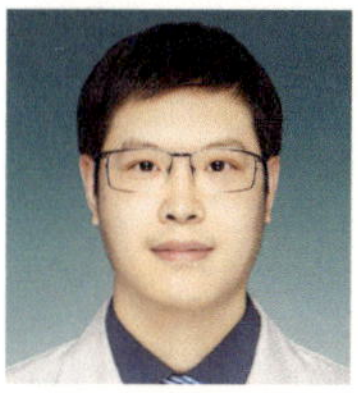

Dr. Zhengwei Zhang is a faculty member at Jiangnan University Medical Centre, specializing in choroidal and retinal diseases. He also tutors postgraduate students at Jiangnan University. From November 2023 to May 2024, Dr. Zhang was a visiting scholar in Yannis' Lab at the Kellogg Eye Centre, University of Michigan. He earned his MD from Nanjing Medical University and his MMed from Shanghai Jiao Tong University. Dr. Zhang has received two research grants for projects on multimodal optical coherence tomography imaging and deep learning applications in retinal diseases, funded by the Jiangsu Provincial Department of Science and Technology and the Wuxi Commission of Health. He has published around 30 peer-reviewed journal articles and two book chapters.

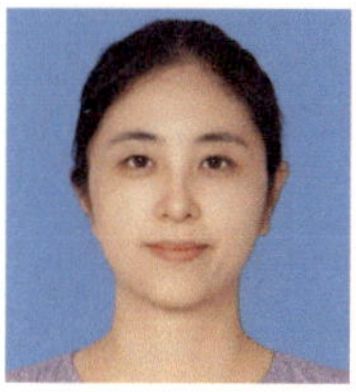

Dr. Liang Zhou is an Associate Professor of Surgical and Medical Retina in the Department of Ophthalmology at The Second Xiangya Hospital, Central South University. She specializes in the diagnosis and treatment of retinal diseases. Dr. Zhou earned her MD from Xiangya Medical School, Central South University, and jointly completed her Ph.D. in Ophthalmology at The Second Xiangya Hospital and the University of Louisville. Since 2024, she has been conducting research at the COOL Lab at Oregon Health & Science University, focusing on imaging analysis of retinal diseases. Supported by grants from the National Natural Science Foundation of China and the Natural Science Foundation of Hunan Province, her research targets retinal disease pathology and advanced imaging techniques. Dr. Zhou has published over 20 peer-reviewed articles.

Contents

Preface

The eye, as one of the vital organs in the human body, plays an essential role in the acquisition and analysis of a vast array of visual information. Clinically, the eye is divided into two primary sections based on anatomical location: the anterior segment and the posterior segment. The anterior segment primarily comprises structures such as the cornea, iridocorneal angle, iris, and lens, while the posterior segment includes the vitreous body, retina, and choroid. Consequently, the content of this book is organized around the themes of the entire eye, the anterior segment, and the posterior segment to enhance the reading experience for the audience.

With technological advancements, ophthalmic imaging techniques have achieved micron-level imaging, providing increasingly objective and significant evidence for the precise diagnosis and mechanistic exploration of some ocular diseases. Among the various imaging technologies, the advent of Optical Coherence Tomography (OCT) has considerably transformed the diagnostic and therapeutic processes for ophthalmologists. Early OCT imaging technology, such as time-domain OCT, encountered limitations due to the scanning speed of the light source, which resulted in prolonged capture times, sensitivity to eye movement, and various artifacts that were more pronounced in influencing results.

With the introduction of high-speed swept-source OCT (SS-OCT), the imaging range and scanning speed have dramatically improved, transforming the display of ocular structures from two-dimensional to three-dimensional imaging while progressively mitigating some of the artifacts that affected earlier results.

Similarly, SS-OCT enables panoramic imaging of the anterior segment, allowing for corneal imaging and data extraction and imaging of the iris, lens, and Berger's Space. This advancement provides surgeons with better evidence to assess surgical outcomes. The integration of OCT imaging with surgical microscopes further aids surgeons in adjusting and optimizing surgical strategies based on real-time conditions during surgical procedures, providing significant support for avoiding reoperations and reducing surgical complications.

The exploration of diseases by physicians does not solely concentrate on structural changes; functional alterations, such as changes in the microcirculation of the retina, may prove more sensitive for diagnosing certain conditions. Therefore, the emergence of Optical Coherence Tomography Angiography (OCTA), which utilizes different algorithms for obtaining retinal and choroidal vascular imaging, has brought about a paradigm shift in clinicians' approaches to diagnosing and treating retinal diseases. Unlike traditional Fluorescein Angiography (FA) and Indocyanine Green Angiography (ICGA), OCTA presents the vascular architecture of the retina and choroid in a non-invasive manner without the necessity for contrast agents. This capability particularly excels in identifying neovascularization, enabling physicians to observe the morphological characteristics of abnormal new blood vessels and develop more personalized treatment plans. However, it is essential to recognize that the current imaging range and depth of OCTA still possess certain limitations, which are areas that require further breakthroughs in future technological advancements.

The application and development of innovative medical technology, such as portable at-home OCT devices and real-time blood oxygen saturation monitoring OCT devices, necessitate continuous optimization and enhancement through collaboration between physicians and engineers. Thus, the collaborative partnership between medicine and engineering represents a vital direction for future development. Concurrently, integrating methods such as deep learning will be critical for achieving more detailed extraction and computation of feature data, aiming for more precise quantitative analyses.

The publication of this book reflects the collective wisdom of numerous ophthalmologists worldwide. I want to express my sincere gratitude to all the chapter authors for their contributions, as their knowledge-sharing has significantly enhanced their understanding of the importance of OCT. Additionally, I extend my thanks to Professors Zhengwei Zhang and Liang Zhou. Although their busy schedules did not permit them to review each chapter individually, their assistance in reviewing portions of the book has been invaluable.

Knowledge is continually evolving and updating. While each author has endeavored to summarize and share the most recent cases and information from their institutions, the content of this book may still fall short of perfection due to objective conditions such as regional limitations. I hope readers will extend their understanding and support in this regard.

Ultimately, this book aims to inspire and support ophthalmologists. I hope that in future editions, more authors will participate, facilitating the sharing of updated knowledge within the global ophthalmology community. Once again, I appreciate the diligent efforts of all the authors. Thank you.

Xiaogang Wang
Shanxi Eye Hospital Affiliated to Shanxi Medical University,
Taiyuan, China

Zhengwei Zhang
Jiangnan University Medical Centre,
Wuxi, China

Liang Zhou
Second Xiangya Hospital,
Central South University,
Changsha, China

Section 1

The Importance of OCT

Chapter 1

Introductory Chapter: OCT Enhances Precision Diagnosis and Treatment of Ocular Diseases

Xiaogang Wang

1. Introduction

The eye is the core of the visual system, and any ocular disease can potentially affect vision, thereby impacting quality of life. Common eye diseases include myopia, hyperopia, cataracts, glaucoma, macular degeneration, and diabetic retinopathy. Imaging technologies play a crucial role in ophthalmology. Traditional ophthalmic examinations primarily relied on visual acuity testing and fundus examination. However, with technological advancements, modern imaging techniques such as Optical Coherence Tomography (OCT) and OCT Angiography (OCTA) have greatly improved diagnostic accuracy and efficiency [1, 2].

OCT technology provides high-resolution cross-sectional images of ocular tissues, allowing clinicians to gain an in-depth understanding of the microstructures of the retina, optic nerve head, and associated pathologies. This noninvasive imaging modality enables doctors to obtain detailed pathological information without compromising patient comfort [3]. OCTA further enhances the ability to observe vascular structures and blood flow status, which is particularly important for diagnosing diabetic retinopathy and macular disorders [2].

Through imaging technologies, clinicians can not only identify ocular diseases earlier and more accurately but also monitor disease progression and treatment efficacy. This provides crucial evidence for personalized treatment and management, helping patients achieve better visual outcomes. In the future, as imaging technologies continue to advance, ophthalmic diagnosis and treatment will become more precise, bringing greater benefits to patients.

2. Overview of OCT

2.1 OCT and working principle

OCT, as an advanced imaging technology, is primarily used to obtain high-resolution cross-sectional images of biological tissues. The principle of OCT is based on low-coherence interferometry, which uses the phenomenon of light interference to provide information about the microscopic structure within tissues [3].

An OCT device typically consists of a laser light source, an interferometer, and a detector. First, the light source emits a broad-spectrum beam of light that illuminates the tissue being examined. Some of this light is reflected by the tissue, while some penetrates and is reflected by deeper structures. The reflected light combines with light from the reference arm, forming an interference pattern. By analyzing the phase and intensity of this interference pattern, depth information of the reflected signals can be obtained, allowing the reconstruction of cross-sectional images of the tissue.

2.2 Noninvasive and high-resolution imaging advantages of OCT

The noninvasive nature of OCT makes it an essential tool in ophthalmology. Unlike traditional biopsies or other invasive imaging techniques, OCT does not require direct contact with the tissue, meaning patients feel comfortable and safe during examination. This technique not only eliminates the risk of bleeding and infection but also reduces patient anxiety, making it an ideal choice for regular screening and monitoring disease progression.

The high-resolution imaging capability of OCT is another major advantage. By capturing details of microstructures, OCT can identify diseases at an early stage. For example, OCT can clearly display changes in retinal layers, timely detecting conditions such as macular degeneration and diabetic retinopathy. This ability for early diagnosis significantly improves the success rate of treatment.

3. History of OCT development

The development of OCT can be traced back to the 1990s, with the initial concept proposed by Professor David Huang and his team in 1991 [3]. The original OCT technology was primarily based on time-domain imaging principles, utilizing low-coherence interferometry to obtain cross-sectional images of biological tissues. This groundbreaking research marked the beginning of significant applications of optical imaging technology in ophthalmology.

With continuous technological advancements, Time-Domain OCT (TD-OCT) achieved its first clinical application in 1996. Although TD-OCT provided relatively high-resolution, its imaging speed was comparatively slow, limiting its widespread in clinics [4]. Entering the twenty-first century, the emergence of Fourier-Domain OCT (FD-OCT) represented a major breakthrough in OCT technology. FD-OCT significantly improved imaging speed and image quality by simultaneously acquiring signals from multiple depths. This technology enabled clinicians to obtain high-quality images in less time, thereby enhancing clinical diagnosis efficiency [5].

Subsequently, Swept-Source OCT (SS-OCT) emerged as a novel imaging technology, further enhancing OCT performance. SS-OCT utilizes tunable lasers to image across a wider range of wavelengths, providing information from deeper tissue layers. It has shown unique advantages, particularly in imaging the cornea, retina, and anterior chamber [6].

Today, modern OCT technology has not only improved in resolution and speed but also incorporated advanced technologies such as artificial intelligence, further enhancing image analysis and pathology recognition capabilities [7]. Through continuous exploration and innovation, OCT will continue to play a crucial role in future medical research.

4. Examples of OCT applications in ophthalmology

OCT, as a noninvasive, high-resolution imaging technology, not only provides detailed images of ocular anatomical structures but also effectively assists in early disease diagnosis and treatment evaluation. The following are specific examples of OCT applications in several common ophthalmic conditions.

1. *Diabetic retinopathy (DR):* OCT enables clinicians to observe detailed changes in retinal thickness and microvascular damage (**Figure 1**). By evaluating structural changes in the macular region, OCT can also assess the severity of diabetic macular edema. OCTA can reflect abnormalities in retinal microcirculation to varying degrees, providing a basis for interventional treatment [8, 9].

2. *Glaucoma:* OCT can precisely measure the thickness of the retinal nerve fiber layer (RNFL) and assess structural changes in the optic nerve head, such as the degree of cupping. Additionally, OCTA can visualize the blood supply to the optic nerve head, thereby further evaluating the risk of glaucoma (**Figure 2**) [10].

3. *Cataract:* Anterior segment OCT can provide detailed imaging of the lens, assisting ophthalmologists in identifying the degree and location of lens opacification (**Figure 3**). This is crucial for assessment and treatment planning. Furthermore, postoperative OCT examinations can be used to monitor the occurrence of postoperative complications such as inflammatory reactions, corneal edema, and posterior capsule opacification [11].

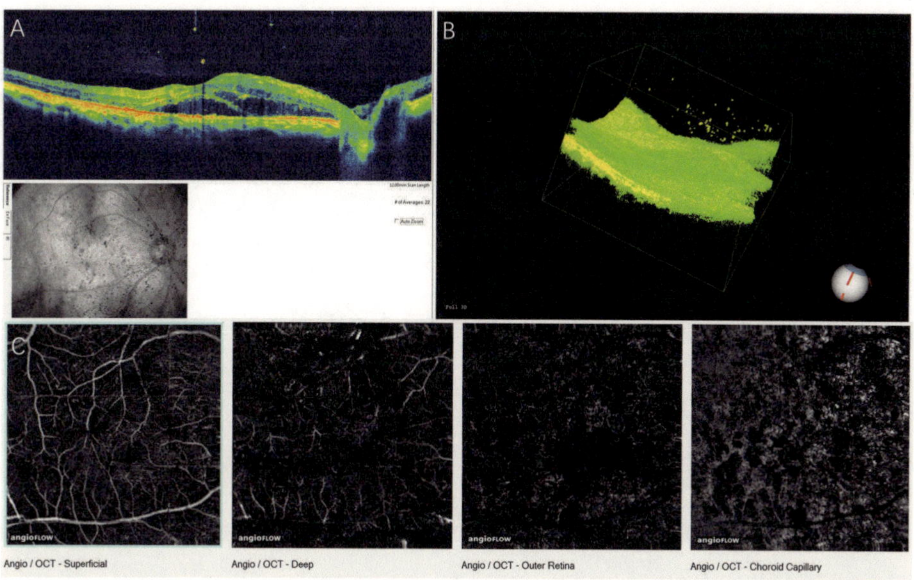

Figure 1.
OCT examination results of the right eye in a patient with diabetic retinopathy (DR). Panel A: Abnormal hyperreflective signals are visible in the vitreous cavity, along with intraretinal exudates and edema. Panel B: Three-dimensional reconstruction of structural OCT reveals distinct hyperreflective signal clusters in the vitreous cavity and morphological changes associated with retinal edema. Panel C: OCTA examination of a 6 mm x 6 mm macular area demonstrates significant perfusion abnormalities across all layers, from the superficial retina to the choriocapillaris.

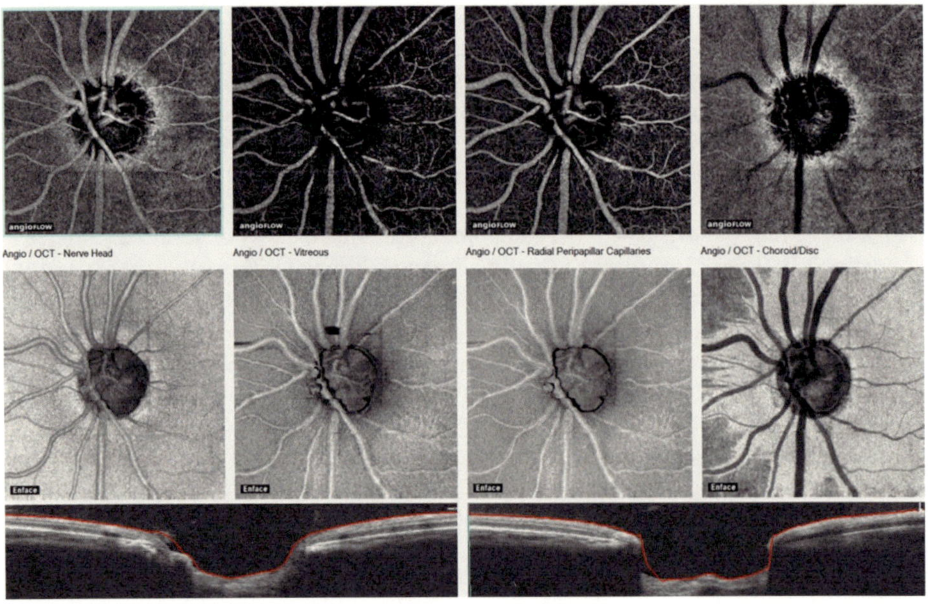

Figure 2.
OCTA scan results of a 4.5 x 4.5 mm optic disk area in the left eye of a glaucoma patient. First row: OCTA examination reveals only large vessel information remaining in the optic disk area. Due to long-term elevated intraocular pressure, the microvascular circulation is significantly compromised. Second row: Corresponding en-face images at various levels demonstrate marked enlargement of the optic cup. Third row: OCT cross-sectional images show deep excavation of the optic disk with significant expansion of the cup margins.

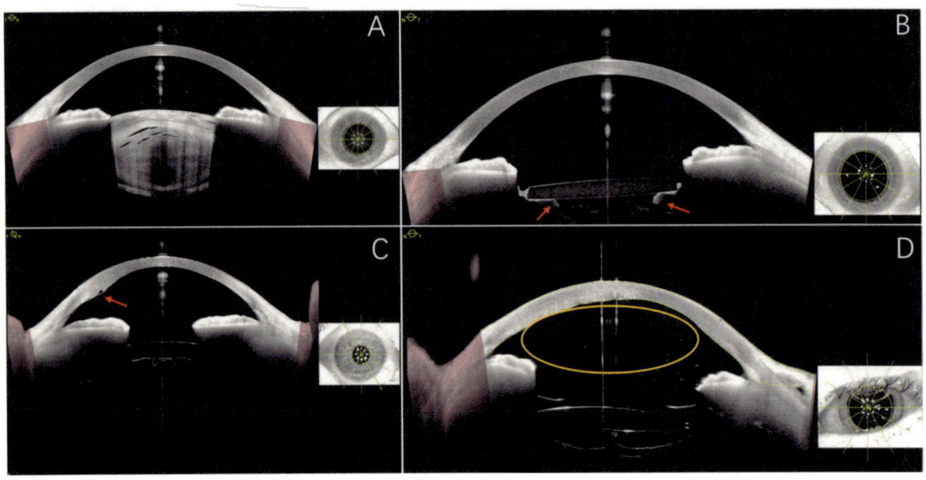

Figure 3.
Various OCT images related to cataract surgery. Panel A: Preoperative cataract OCT image showing a significant lens opacity. Panel B: Post-laser treatment for posterior capsular opacification (PCO), demonstrating discontinuity of the posterior lens capsule. The curling of the capsule edges is visible at both ends of the opening (red arrows). Panel C: Postoperative OCT image showing wound gaping and Descemet's membrane detachment at the main incision site (red arrow). Panel D: Postoperative OCT image revealing varying degrees of corneal edema and anterior chamber inflammatory reaction (yellow circle).

5. Future prospects

The widespread application of OCT technology in ophthalmology has made significant progress, but its future development still holds great potential, primarily in the integration with new imaging technologies, the application of artificial intelligence, and its potential in personalized medicine and treatment monitoring.

5.1 Integration with new imaging technologies

In recent years, OCT Angiography (OCTA) has emerged as a novel imaging technique that has been successfully integrated with OCT. OCTA enables noninvasive observation of ocular vascular structure and function, providing crucial reference information for diagnosing ophthalmic diseases such as diabetic retinopathy and wet age-related macular degeneration [9, 12]. The combination of OCT with other imaging technologies (e.g., fluorescein angiography and ultrasonography) will allow clinicians to obtain more comprehensive information about ocular health. This multimodal imaging strategy can not only improve early disease detection rates but also support the development of personalized treatment plans.

5.2 Application of artificial intelligence in OCT image analysis

The rapid development of AI has brought revolutionary changes to OCT image analysis. Through deep learning algorithms, AI can automatically identify and classify lesions in OCT images, improving the speed and accuracy of image analysis [13]. In the future, the application of AI is expected to reduce subjective bias in the diagnostic process, providing more objective assessments. Furthermore, AI can help researchers identify new biomarkers through the analysis of large-scale OCT datasets, promoting the development of novel treatment methods.

5.3 Potential of OCT in personalized medicine and treatment monitoring

With the rise of personalized medicine, the prospects for OCT in treatment monitoring and disease management are becoming increasingly broad. OCT can provide real-time information on the ocular structure and function, offering a basis for clinicians to formulate personalized treatment plans. Through regular OCT examinations, doctors can dynamically monitor changes in a patient's condition and adjust treatment plans in a timely manner. Additionally, with the development of telemedicine and mobile smart health technologies, OCT technology is expected to integrate with these emerging technologies to achieve more convenient patient management. Patients may be able to conduct preliminary screenings at home, with OCT images transmitted to doctors for analysis via cloud platforms, thereby improving the accessibility of medical services [14].

6. Summary

This book will compile the various aspects mentioned above, selecting key anterior segment and fundus diseases to delve into the application and analysis of OCT imaging technology in specific disease contexts. It emphasizes the importance of OCT in early diagnosis, treatment monitoring, and evaluation. Additionally, the book will focus on the application of artificial intelligence (AI) in the analysis of OCT images, exploring how to enhance the speed and accuracy of image processing and analysis, thereby aiding physicians in making more precise diagnoses. The introduction of AI will transform the traditional methods of ophthalmic diagnosis, making them more objective and intelligent.

We hope that readers will absorb the necessary knowledge from the chapters of this book, enabling them to contribute to global eye health from a perspective of wisdom and precision. By combining the latest advancements in OCT technology with AI, we anticipate that this book will provide valuable references and insights for ophthalmologists, researchers, and readers interested in ocular health, promoting further development and innovation in the field of ophthalmology. The ultimate goal is to improve the early detection rates and treatment outcomes of ocular diseases, thereby enhancing overall patient health and quality of life.

Author details

Xiaogang Wang
Shanxi Eye Hospital Affiliated to Shanxi Medical University,
Taiyuan, Shanxi Province, China

*Address all correspondence to: movie6521@163.com

References

[1] Kashani AH, Chen CL, Gahm JK, Zheng F, Richter GM, Rosenfeld PJ, et al. Optical coherence tomography angiography: A comprehensive review of current methods and clinical applications. Progress in Retinal and Eye Research. 2017;**60**:66-100. DOI: 10.1016/j.preteyeres.2017.07.002

[2] Pandya BU, Grinton M, Mandelcorn ED, Felfeli T. Retinal optical coherence tomography imaging biomarkers: A review of the literature. Retina. 2024;**44**(3):369-380. DOI: 10.1097/IAE.0000000000003974

[3] Huang D, Swanson EA, Lin CP, Schuman JS, Stinson WG, Chang W, et al. Optical coherence tomography. Science. 1991;**254**(5035):1178-1181. DOI: 10.1126/science.1957169

[4] Tsang SH, Sharma T. Optical coherence tomography. Advances in Experimental Medicine and Biology. 2018;**1085**:11-13. DOI: 10.1007/978-3-319-95046-4_3

[5] Bouma BE, Yun SH, Vakoc BJ, Suter MJ, Tearney GJ. Fourier-domain optical coherence tomography: Recent advances toward clinical utility. Current Opinion in Biotechnology. 2009;**20**(1):111-118. DOI: 10.1016/j.copbio.2009.02.007

[6] Mirzayev I, Gündüz AK, Aydın Ellialtıoğlu P, Gündüz ÖÖ. Clinical applications of anterior segment swept-source optical coherence tomography: A systematic review. Photodiagnosis and Photodynamic Therapy. 2023;**42**:103334. DOI: 10.1016/j.pdpdt.2023.103334

[7] Kapoor R, Whigham BT, Al-Aswad LA. Artificial intelligence and optical coherence tomography imaging. Asia-Pacific Journal of Ophthalmology. 2019;**8**(2):187-194. DOI: 10.22608/APO.201904

[8] Waheed NK, Rosen RB, Jia Y, Munk MR, Huang D, Fawzi A, et al. Optical coherence tomography angiography in diabetic retinopathy. Progress in Retinal and Eye Research. 2023;**97**:101206. DOI: 10.1016/j.preteyeres.2023.101206

[9] Szeto SK, Lai TY, Vujosevic S, Sun JK, Sadda SR, Tan G, et al. Optical coherence tomography in the management of diabetic macular oedema. Progress in Retinal and Eye Research. 2024;**98**:101220. DOI: 10.1016/j.preteyeres.2023.101220

[10] Geevarghese A, Wollstein G, Ishikawa H, Schuman JS. Optical coherence tomography and glaucoma. Annual Review of Vision Science. 2021;**7**:693-726. DOI: 10.1146/annurev-vision-100419-111350

[11] Ahmed TM, Siddiqui MAR, Hussain B. Optical coherence tomography as a diagnostic intervention before cataract surgery-a review. Eye (London, England). 2023;**37**(11):2176-2182. DOI: 10.1038/s41433-022-02320-y

[12] Vidal-Oliver L, Montolío-Marzo E, Gallego-Pinazo R, Dolz-Marco R. Optical coherence tomography biomarkers in early and intermediate age-related macular degeneration: A clinical guide. Clinical and Experimental Ophthalmology. 2024;**52**(2):207-219. DOI: 10.1111/ceo.14337

[13] Li D, Ran AR, Cheung CY, Prince JL. Deep learning in optical coherence tomography: Where are the gaps? Clinical and Experimental

Ophthalmology. 2023;**51**(8):853-863. DOI: 10.1111/ceo.14258

[14] Willis ET, Kim JE, Schneider EW. Home optical coherence tomography monitoring for Neovascular age-related macular degeneration: Transformative technology or cool toy? Ophthalmology and Therapy. 2024;**13**(6):1407-1416. DOI: 10.1007/s40123-024-00953-8

Chapter 2

Home Based Optical Coherence Tomography

Miguel Busquets, Muki Rapp and Nishant Mohan

Abstract

Home OCT allows for individualized management of patients with exudative disease. Fluid dynamic heterogeneity demands the use of artificial intelligence to track data. This is accomplished with the Unet encoder-decoder segmentation network. Clinical trials have shown that home OCT demonstrates excellent adherence, self-imaging, automated fluid quantification with high sensitivity and specificity, and disease management refinement. AI and human grader correlation for the technology ranges between 91.6–100%. Decision-making data shows a potential impact on disease management, with a possible doubling of the average treatment interval (8–15.3 weeks), and recommended sooner treatment in 57% of patients. Two thirds of patients treated sooner required treatment within one week. Home OCT-derived analytics shows that patients treated within 7 days of disease reactivation had lower fluid volume at treatment, resolution time and fluid AUC (area under the curve).

Keywords: artificial intelligence, AMD, home OCT, anti-VEGF, treat and extend management

1. Introduction

Optical coherence tomography (OCT) has found its first and most widespread clinical application in ophthalmology. This technology is particularly crucial in the treatment of retinal diseases such as age-related macular degeneration, diabetic retinopathy, and retinal vein occlusion. The acute nature of these conditions, characterized by rapid anatomical changes, demands immediate therapeutic interventions to prevent vision loss. This urgency, coupled with the significant burden of near monthly treatments, has driven the development of strategies for extending treatment intervals and creating longer-acting therapies. OCT has been demonstrated to be of such importance that data has supported its use at the exclusion of dilated fundus examinations [1]. Additionally, these challenges have spurred the innovation of home monitoring solutions based on OCT, aimed at providing high-frequency data to better manage these acute retinal conditions.

2. Age-related macular degeneration

Age-related macular degeneration (AMD) is a progressive disease and the leading cause of blindness in adults aged 50 and older [2]. In its early and intermediate stages, AMD is marked by the presence of retinal drusen and pigmentary changes visible in fundus images, typically without severe vision loss. However, 10–15% of patients progress to the advanced stage, known as neovascular AMD (nAMD) [3]. This advanced stage involves the growth of new blood vessels (neovascularization) and fluid accumulation in the retinal space, leading to rapid and severe vision loss if untreated.

The primary treatment for nAMD involves injecting anti-vascular endothelial growth factor (VEGF) drugs -now sometimes coupled with anti-angiopoietin 2 moieties - into the eye's vitreous cavity. These drugs inhibit blood vessel growth and help resolve retinal fluid, as evidenced by OCT images. Most nAMD patients require ongoing treatment for the rest of their lives. There are two common approaches to scheduling these treatments.

The first, and most widely used, is the treat-and-extend (TAE) method [4]. In this approach, an OCT scan is performed during each office visit, and the patient receives an anti-VEGF injection. If fluid is detected on the OCT scan, the next appointment is generally scheduled sooner than the previous interval, with a minimum gap of four weeks. If no fluid is detected, the interval before the next treatment is extended. The goal is to find the optimal interval to prevent disease recurrence.

A second approach is the pro re nata (PRN), or as-needed, method. Patients visit the clinic monthly and receive treatment only if fluid is present in the OCT scan. Both methods have limitations: TAE can lead to excessive treatments as intervals are gradually extended, and it cannot account for fluid recurrence sooner than the set interval. Conversely, PRN imposes a significant burden on patients and caregivers due to the frequent monthly visits. The PRN approach resembles the "set-interval" treatment models, although the former imposes the same burden on patients while incurring significantly higher direct and indirect healthcare costs.

These limitations are largely due to the infrequent data collection compared to the rapid progression of the disease. To address this, high-frequency OCT data acquisition and fluid characteristic analysis are needed to develop optimal management strategies. For elderly patients with nAMD, this could be achieved by providing them with home-based OCT devices, enabling more frequent monitoring, better disease management, and cost control.

3. Home monitoring

Home monitoring is increasingly critical in disease management across various fields, including endocrinology and cardiology [5, 6]. It enables interventions based on physiological parameters rather than fixed appointment schedules. However, transitioning monitoring from expert-guided clinics to patients' homes presents several challenges that must be overcome before such solutions become practical. Home monitoring solutions generally fall into two categories: passive and active monitoring.

Passive monitoring typically involves an implanted device that collects data and automatically transmits it for analysis and review. In contrast, active monitoring requires patient engagement in the data acquisition or transfer process. Currently, most remote ophthalmic monitoring systems are active. However, there are some fundamental requirements to make these monitoring systems practical.

Patient adherence is essential in active monitoring programs. Compliance is a significant challenge in healthcare, affecting medication adherence and routine clinical check-ups. It's even more crucial in remote monitoring for managing acute and irreversible diseases. All home monitoring programs should include strategies to ensure patient adherence. Various approaches have been tried, such as using patient care coaches [7] and digital health apps for reminders [8]. One approach for managing the progression from intermediate to wet AMD involved a dedicated monitoring center. This center, a digital healthcare provider, supports logistical needs like insurance verification, device provision, patient training, and technical support. Crucially, it aids in patient adherence and engagement. This method showed average patient adherence rates of 5.2 tests per week, surpassing the minimum required level for an ophthalmic home monitoring program. These rates were maintained over a 10-year retrospective study (**Figure 1**) [9].

Another critical aspect of home-based monitoring is data transfer and storage. Many remote monitoring techniques store data on localized devices, requiring manual transfer to the health system. However, advancements in broadband internet connectivity and cloud storage now allow automatic data transfer to cloud systems, making it accessible to physicians [10]. It's important to note that patients' personal health information requires robust data security beyond what consumer systems offer. Therefore, while connected networks are highly beneficial for remote monitoring, appropriate cybersecurity safeguards must be implemented in line with health authority regulations.

Home monitoring inherently generates significantly more data than in-clinic monitoring and diagnostics. This creates a natural challenge of needing automation to analyze and curate data for appropriate physician review. Recent advancements in machine learning and deep learning algorithms have enabled automated analysis, presenting condensed information to physicians for review and decision-making.

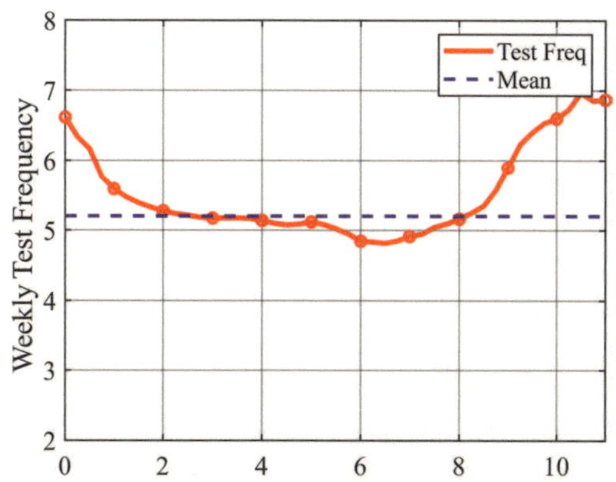

Figure 1.
Testing frequency of patients with intermediate AMD supported by a monitoring center to help with adherence to program as a function of time on the program.

4. Home OCT

Home (OCT) refers to a home-based system that is capable of acquiring OCT images. Its first use has been evaluated in retinal diseases, particularly AMD for the reasons discussed above.

OCT images of the retina are acquired by directing the beam to the retina through the pupil of the eye. The system uses the optics of the eye to project light on the retina. The reflected light goes through low coherence interference to form the OCT image as discussed in the earlier chapters. A typical OCT system used in the office operates with the help of a trained technician. The technician positions the OCT probe that emits the beam in appropriate position while the patient stays steady using a head and chin rest. This allows the appropriate position of the eye and probe in all 3 dimensions. Several modern systems do use automation to bring the probes in the correct position automatically, however a technician presence and intervention is still often needed. The patient is guided to fixate on a specific target, this allows the appropriate portion of the posterior segment of the eye to be in the field of view of the OCT.

A home OCT system must be fully self-operated with no presence of trained technician required. In addition, self-operation should be convenient for a patient suffering from visual disorders. For instance, it is known that in real-world only around 34% of nAMD patients have functional vision of 20/40 [11] at the time of diagnosis, the requirement for driving in most states in the United States. The average nAMD patient had a vision of 20/80. Self-operation requires few critical elements. The device configuration should be straightforward to start scanning without specialized knowledge. The device shall contain descriptive instructions that the patient can review at their convenience. The device shall bring the patient's eye into appropriate alignment to perform the scan. This includes bringing the pupil and the OCT beam into appropriate transverse alignment for beam to pass through without obfuscation. In addition, the axial position of the pupil and the beam scanning point should align to ensure the maximum field of view can be reached. The system shall also provide the ability for a patient with low vision to fixate during the process of the scanning to ensure scan can be completed without severe motion artifacts.

Another critical requirement for making home OCT systems practical for individual use is low manufacturing costs. The cost reduction from in-office to home-use devices is primarily achieved through use of components that are widely used in consumer goods. The high-volume production of such components allows them to be available at lower costs. The growth in semiconductor technologies has also allowed reduction in cost of several components in the OCT systems. The requirement of a large number of home OCT devices for patients suffering with nAMD supports economy of scales and further cost reductions.

The choice of modality of OCT used for the home version of such devices is an important consideration. OCT systems are categorized by the mode of interferometric method used to obtain axial localization during the image formation. The three most common methods are time domain, spectral domain and swept source OCT that use varying methods for axial localization. The systems are further classified based on methods used for transverse localization. These include point scanning, line scanning and full-field systems.

Home OCT systems are typically based on point-scanning spectral domain OCT and full-field time domain OCT. The point-scanning spectral domain systems are technologically equivalent to the most commonly used in-office OCT systems.

These systems are proven to allow adequate imaging of the retinal tissue as needed for observing disorders like AMD.

The full-field time-domain OCT systems are promising technology particularly due to simplicity and low cost. Such systems allow use of area scan cameras and do not require complex beam scanning mechanisms. The parallel nature of acquisition also allows for easier access to phase information in the OCT signal, allowing possibility of obtaining further information than available with standard OCT systems. However, such systems do suffer from transverse crosstalk between the pixels resulting in degradation of interferometric signal and hence system sensitivity. So far, full-field time-domain has not been used for clinical disease management on a regular basis.

5. Artificial intelligence and estimation of key biomarkers

Retinal fluid is the key physiological biomarker in management of nAMD. The presence of fluid as seen in OCT images is the key physiological biomarker in management of nAMD. The presence of fluid as seen in OCT image is one of the primary factors in determining the effectiveness and frequency of anti-VEGF therapies to manage nAMD. The retinal fluid when present anterior to the photoreceptor layer is called intraretinal fluid (**Figure 2(a)**). The fluid present between the photoreceptors and the retinal epithelial pigment (RPE) layer is called subretinal fluid (**Figure 2(b)**). The fluid present posterior to RPE is called sub-RPE fluid (**Figure 2(c)**).

The fluid is depicted in the retinal OCT images as hyporeflective space (HRS), as fluid-filled area in general reflects or scatters less light than the retinal tissue area. While the fluid is a physiological biomarker, HRS is an imaging biomarker. HRS is a more accurate description of appearance on the image without inferring the underlying physiology. In clinical terms it becomes important as presence of degenerative cysts, outer retinal tubulation and a few other structures can cause a hyporeflective appearance, however such spaces are not expected to change with anti-VEGF therapy. The HRS when present anterior to the photoreceptors is called intraretinal hyporeflective (IRO) space, and when present between the photoreceptors and the RPE is called subretinal hyporeflective (SRO) space. The sum of intraretinal and subretinal hyporeflective space is total retinal hyporeflective (TRO) space. The importance of these biomarkers in the retina for disease management has led to the development of multiple algorithms for automatic segmentation and quantification.

Multiple algorithms have been developed for segmentation of such biomarkers, the most common approaches currently include use of machine learning and deep learning-based methods. These methods require annotation or labeling of the images

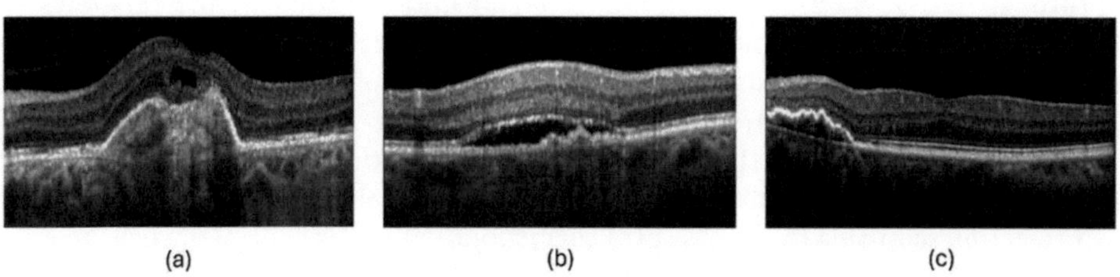

Figure 2.
Examples of: (a) Intraretinal, (b) Subretinal, and (c) Sub-retinal pigment epithelial (RPE) fluid.

by the expert graders. The algorithm is then trained on these annotations [12]. The algorithm first detects the retinal space through segmentation of inner limiting membrane (ILM) and retinal epithelial pigment (RPE). The retinal space is then segmented into pixels that are considered to represent HRS. The core segmentation in NOA is based on deep learning U-net architecture Ref. [13]. The U-net architecture in general consists of what are called contracting and expansive paths. The contracting path consists of repeated convolutions layers, rectified linear units and pooling operation with down sampling. The expansive path has a similar structure while using up-sampling instead of down-sampling. At the final stage each component vector is mapped to the desired features. Hyperparameters are then tuned to optimize the segmentation scheme.

The segmented regions are further classified into subretinal or intraretinal spaces by the algorithm. The TRO space volume is then estimated by summing up all pixels classified as HRS and multiplying them by the volume of each pixel. The estimates are expressed in volume units (VU). Physically 1 VU is equivalent to 1 nanoliter of volume. In addition to the quantification, the NOA generates annotated B-scans, with areas of HRS are shown color-coded according to the type (IRO or SRO), en-face maps of fluid projections) and ranking of B-scans by order of largest to smallest HRS areas. NOA is the first deep-learning based algorithm to receive clearance from the United States Food and Drug Administration (FDA), for segmentation of OCT images.

6. Home OCT data

Data acquisition at home allows for much higher resolution of the temporal information compared to the information available through only in-office data collection. This requires an enhanced approach for review and interpretation of the home OCT data. It should be noted that any feature and biomarker can be reviewed for more temporal detail. These features can be image based and be described as hypo-reflective areas in the image, or they can be interpreted and described as specific physiologic parameters like retinal fluid.

7. Home OCT data elements

Individual home OCT scans are similar to those obtained through standard in-office OCT devices used for retinal images. Multiple layers in retinal and subretinal regions can be observed through varying contrast corresponding to variation in amplitude of the scattered light. The full acquired volume can be reviewed by scrolling through individual B-scans. The OCT imaging data acquired on different days can be compared by simultaneous review of the scans. The regions of hyporeflective spaces in the OCT B-scans automatically detected by the AI-based algorithms can be annotated by an overlay color **Figure 3(a)**.

The next data element is the spatial location of the retinal biomarkers. For instance, the segmented intraretinal (IRO) and subretinal (SRO) spaces can be shown as a projection map on a transverse grid corresponding to the central of fixation. **Figure 3(b)** shows such projection maps. The transverse location of HRS area can be of important clinical significance. The ability to acquire data at high frequency allows us to create spatiotemporal maps for such biomarkers.

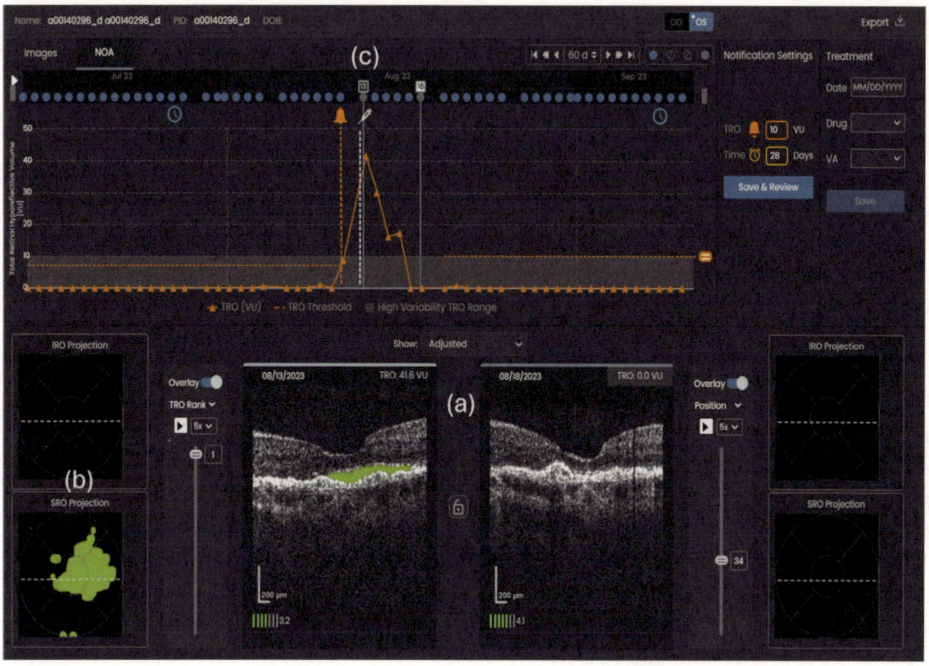

Figure 3.
(a) Demonstrates examples of OCT B-scans at near foveal position for OCT scans acquired on different days using home OCT with an overlay of hyporeflective spaces, (b) shows corresponding projections maps obtained after automated HRS detection and projection on a transverse area, and (c) shows the corresponding TRO space volume trajectory with the alerts marked by the bell icon, and the treatment dates marked by syringes icon.

Data acquisition at home allows very high temporal resolution. Hence the changes in the biomarkers like HRS can be observed at an unprecedented level. Home OCT data hence also has an important 1-d temporal element. **Figure 3(c)** shows 1-d temporal data from home OCT can be observed in the form of changing TRO space volume levels over time.

8. Home OCT clinical studies

The utility of any home monitoring technology requires validation that data can be acquired by the target disease population and that it can be done in their home setting repetitively over an extended period. Multiple studies have been conducted to understand the feasibility of home OCT in this regard. We will discuss several of them here.

Kim et al. [14] reported on prospective and cross-sectional study using two versions of Notal Vision Home OCT (NVHO). The two versions had a different form factor, however, used the same OCT electro-optical engine and provided the same user experience. The goal of the study was to determine feasibility of self-imaging using home OCT device in a clinic setting and comparing detection of retinal fluid on home OCT device versus the commercial OCT device available at the study sites.

The enrollment criterion for the study included presence nAMD in at least one eye and required patients to have visual acuity of at least 20/400. The enrolled patient performed self-imaging on a home OCT device present in the clinic. The patients also received regular in-office exam including measurement of best corrected visual acuity (BCVA) and commercial in-office OCT scanning using either the Cirrus-HD OCT (Carl Zeiss Meditec, Dublin, CA, USA) or the Spectralis OCT (Heidelberg Engineering, Heidelberg, Germany). The Cirrus OCT scans consisted of 128 B-scans using a central wavelength of 840 nm, while the Spectralis system used 40 B-scans or more operating at a central wavelength 870-nm.

The enrolled subject images on the home OCT device without any additional support from the staff. The subject watches a 2-minute video tutorial and is only guided to place their forehead on the device to perform self-scans. The device performs an automatic calibration at the first use to customize the optical path for a given patients refraction and eye length.

A total of 560 eyes of 301 subjects were enrolled in the study to perform home OCT based imaging. A total of 531 eyes that attempted self-imaging, at success rate of 88% (469/531). The mean (SD) age of subjects was 78.8 (8.8) with 58% of participants being female and the median VA of the participants was 20/40. The study found that subjects were able to successfully image when the VA of the testing eye was 20/320 or better, however subjects with a worse VA failed to scan in nearly 50% of the cases.

In regard to the quality of the images 464 out of 469 eyes produced images gradable by a reading ophthalmologist. In comparison, 468 out of 469 (99.8%) of images acquired by commercial OCT were gradable in a similar manner. The positive percent agreement (PPA) and negative percent agreement (NPA) were calculated for comparing the visualization of fluid in home and in-office OCT. A total 463 eyes of 264 subjects that had gradable images from both the devices were included in the calculation. The PPA and NPA for detecting presence of any fluid was 98% and 96% respectively. The accuracy of visualization was not found to be dependent on VA levels.

Overall, this cross-sectional study showed a significant portion of patients can scan on the NVHO device with only a self-tutorial and no additional help. The imaging rates were significantly high for the patients with vision better than 20/320. There was a high degree of correlation in detection of fluid between NVHO and commercial in-office OCT.

While cross-sectional studies in office and laboratory settings provide validation of self-imaging, the utility of home OCT cannot be realized without demonstrating extended and adherent use at home by the patient population of interest.

Blinder et al. [15] reported a clinical study to demonstrate use of home OCT by nAMD patients over a six-month period. It was a prospective observational study. The participants had at least one with previously untreated nAMD, also known as treatment naïve, and visual acuity between 20/20 and 20/320.

The participants who consented to the study received Notal Vision Home OCT (NVHO). The device and the user guide were shipped to the patient's home. The participants set up the device themselves or with the help of a caregiver, and watched an interactive, on-device tutorial video, followed by practice and calibration scans. The participants had the option of receiving telephone support from Notal Vision Monitoring Center (NVMC). Participants were instructed to perform self-imaging of both eyes daily for approximately 6 months. The standard of care data was collected during in-office visits. The collected OCT scans were uploaded, and a reading center reviewed the scans for presence or absence of fluid.

Fourteen participants completed the study. The participants had a median age of 74 years, and 57% were male. The median visual acuity at the time of enrollment was 20/63. Thirteen participants obtained scans eligible for fluid quantification upon the first attempt and one did so after 6 attempts. Participants perform a mean of 6.3 scans per week and 27.5 scans per month. The mean scans per week were relatively constant over time. It took patients a mean time of 47 seconds to acquire the OCT scans per eye. The presence of fluid as detected on home OCT scans was compared with the presence of fluid on in-office OCT scans. For fluid levels >10 nL home OCT and in-office OCT agreed 100% of the time.

The high rate of patient adherence, imaging success rates and agreement between home OCT and in-office OCT demonstrated potential usefulness of home OCT.

8.1 Studies demonstrating impact of home OCT on clinical decision making

The above studies demonstrated feasibility of acquiring high temporal frequency data by the patients at their home. Additional research has been conducted to understand impact of this high frequency data on clinical management of the patients.

Holekamp et al. [16] conducted a prospective clinical trial to understand the impact of home OCT on patient management. The treatment experienced nAMD patients were switched to home OCT-based management. This process involved providing patients with the home OCT monitoring service, where their daily artificial intelligence-analyzed OCT data was available to the investigators. The investigators set notifications thresholds based on time and disease activity to review the remote data. The patients were invited for treatments only based on the home OCT data. In-office diagnostics were performed to determine the need for the treatment.

The investigators found that the number of treatments were on an average significantly reduced for the patients once managed with home OCT compared to their earlier management. The mean retreatment interval before switching to home OCT management for patients was 8.0 weeks/treatment, that increased to 15.3 weeks/treatment after switching to home OCT based management. There was no statistically significant change in visual acuity (VA) before and during home OCT based management. This was largely attributed to reduced need of treating patients in a proactive manner to prevent future disease reactivation.

Another study was conducted by Heier et al. [17] to understand the impact of home OCT data on the physician decision making. They conducted a retrospective data review study, that used home OCT data from the patients that were managed by standard of care. Fifteen retina specialists (RS) in the United States participated. The home OCT data over a segment of time including the preceding treatment information was presented to the participating RS. They were asked to indicate if they would treat the patient during the presented time and if so on what date. A total of 150 such segments were presented. The patients were treated in each case on the last day of the presented segment, this information was masked from the retina specialist.

The RS decided not to treat patients in 42.7% of cases when they were treated in actual care. In the remaining 57.3% of cases when the retina specialist did decide to treat the patients, they recommended treating at least one week before the treatment was given in the actual care. The study demonstrated a strong impact of home OCT data on the physician decision making. It showed number of treatments and patient visits can be significantly reduced that would reduce burden both on the patients and the healthcare system. On the other it also showed numerous patients are potentially undertreated and should receive their treatments sooner than being in actual care.

An additional consecutive series of studies evolved from the first ever at home study of four participants that self-imaged for one month [18], followed by a study of 15 participants that monitored for three months [19].

9. Home OCT future and challenges

Home OCT is a novel monitoring tool, with the first regulatory approval for clinical use being received in May of 2024. It paves the way for several such diagnostics that allow patients to be more closely involved in management of their disease [20, 21]. We expect with the increased burden on healthcare providers the use of automated tools for acquiring diagnostic information in remote settings including home will continue to become more commonplace. This shall be beneficial for the patients, providers and the healthcare system in general.

This promise comes with its own challenges to overcome. The remote monitoring technologies will have keep increasing in reliability while lowering the cost on the system to become mainstream. The distributed acquisition of diagnostic information requires lower cost of hardware that is not always easily achievable. The remote acquisition also brings serious challenges to data safety and privacy, the growing threat of cyber-attacks are heightened when data is acquired remotely. It will be essential for those providing such services to ensure patient data is appropriately protected to maintain patient trust. Finally, all such new paradigms need to demonstrate increased health outcomes over extended period of time. The novel paradigms, while exciting still have to prove themselves as beneficial to patients in the long run.

10. Summary

The advancement in digital technologies has allowed capture of data outside the traditional care settings. Artificial intelligence has in turn allowed for the processing of innumerable data points in this context. This coupling enables data acquisition on a much larger scale than what is possible in a diagnostic clinic setting and promises a much deeper understanding of disease dynamics which could in turn lead to potentially better clinical decision-making, treatments, and outcomes for patients. OCT is a primary diagnostic tool in ophthalmic setting. The ability to perform patient self-operated OCT scans at home promises a more granular understanding of disease dynamics, particularly for conditions with rapidly changing anatomical features. Research efforts to date have demonstrated the feasibility of home OCT system use with scans performed over an extended period of time by patients with neovascular AMD. Future studies may support the feasibility of such use in other exudative conditions, such as diabetic macular edema and retinal vein occlusions.

Conflict of interest

Miguel Busquets is a consultant for Notal Vision. Muki Rapp and Nishant Mohan are employed by Notal Vision.

Author details

Miguel Busquets[1]*, Muki Rapp[2] and Nishant Mohan[3]

1 Chairman Medical Executive Board Technology and Innovation Committee, Lexington, KY, USA

2 Notal Vision Ltd., Israel

3 Notal Vision Inc., USA

*Address all correspondence to: mabbusquets@gmail.com

References

[1] Patel Y, Miller DM, Fung AE, Hill LF, Rosenfeld PJ. Are dilated fundus examinations needed for OCT-guided retreatment of exudative age-related macular degeneration? Ophthalmology Retina. 2020;**4**:141-147

[2] Fleckenstein M et al. Age-related macular degeneration. Nature Reviews. Disease Primers. 2021;**7**:31

[3] Ferris FL et al. Clinical classification of age-related macular degeneration. Ophthalmology. 2013;**120**:844-851

[4] Gupta OP et al. A treat and extend regimen using ranibizumab for neovascular age-related macular degeneration clinical and economic impact. Ophthalmology. 2010;**117**:2134-2140

[5] Cappon G, Vettoretti M, Sparacino G, Facchinetti A. Continuous glucose monitoring sensors for diabetes management: A review of technologies and applications. Diabetes and Metabolism Journal. 2019;**43**:383-397

[6] Kitsiou S, Paré G, Jaana M. Effects of home telemonitoring interventions on patients with chronic heart failure: An overview of systematic reviews. Journal of Medical Internet Research. 2015;**17**:1-30

[7] Thom DH et al. The impact of health coaching on medication adherence in patients with poorly controlled diabetes, hypertension, and/or hyperlipidemia: A randomized controlled trial. Journal of American Board of Family Medicine. 2015;**28**:38-45

[8] Santo K et al. Mobile phone apps to improve medication adherence: A systematic stepwise process to identify high-quality apps. JMIR mHealth and uHealth. 2016;**4**:1-11

[9] Mathai M et al. Analysis of the long-term visual outcomes of foresee home remote Telemonitoring: The ALOFT study. Ophthalmology Retina. 2022;**6**:922-929

[10] The State of US Broadband in 2022: Reassessing the Whole Picture|ITIF. Available from: https://itif.org/publications/2022/12/05/state-of-us-broadband-in-2022-reassessing-the-whole-picture/

[11] Ho AC et al. Baseline visual acuity at wet amd diagnosis predicts long-term vision outcomes: An analysis of the iris registry. Ophthalmic Surgery, Lasers & Imaging Retina. 2020;**51**:633-639

[12] Elman MJ, Schechet S. Performance of AI-based Notal OCT Analyzer (NOA) in retinal fluid volume quantification from repeated self-imaging with home OCT in eyes with neovascular age-related macular degeneration (nAMD). Investigative Ophthalmology & Visual Science. 2022;**63**:187-F0034-187-F0034

[13] Weng W, Zhu X. U-net: Convolutional networks for biomedical image segmentation. IEEE Access. 2015;**9**:16591-16603

[14] Kim JE et al. Evaluation of a self-imaging SD-OCT system designed for remote home monitoring. BMC Ophthalmology. 2022;**22**:1-13

[15] Blinder KJ et al. Home OCT imaging for newly diagnosed Neovascular age-related macular degeneration: A feasibility study. Ophthalmology Retina. 2024;**8**(4):376-387. DOI: 10.1016/j.oret.2023.10.012

[16] Holekamp NM et al. Prospective trial of Home OCT guided management of treatment experienced nAMD patients. Retina. Oct 2024;**44**(10):1714-1731

[17] Heier JS et al. Clinical use of home OCT data to manage neovascular age-related macular degeneration. Journal of VitreoRetinal Diseases. 2024. DOI: 10.1177/24741264241302858

[18] Keenan TDL et al. Prospective, longitudinal pilot study. Ophthalmology Science. 2021;**1**:100034

[19] Liu Y, Holekamp NM, Heier JS. Prospective, longitudinal study: Daily self-imaging with home OCT for Neovascular age-related macular degeneration. Ophthalmology Retina. 2022;**6**(7):575-585

[20] Keenan TDL, Loewenstein A. Artificial intelligence for home monitoring devices. Current Opinion in Ophthalmology. 2023;**34**:441-448

[21] Danese C et al. The impact of artificial intelligence on retinal disease management: Vision academy retinal expert consensus. Current Opinion in Ophthalmology. 2023;**34**:396-402

Chapter 3

Machine Learning Architectures and Their Applications in Optical Coherence Tomography

Ankit Butola

Abstract

Optical coherence tomography (OCT) is a powerful imaging technique that utilizes optical scattering to extract tomographic information of biological samples in their natural state. Over the past two decades, OCT has advanced both experimentally and computationally to improve its performance in terms of resolution, penetration depth, acquisition speed, and sensitivity. The interpretability of OCT particularly increased through its integration with artificial intelligence (AI). While fast and label-free nature of OCT becomes popular in optical imaging, AI assigned an artificial system to mimic human intelligence, such as classification, visualizations, and segmentation. In particular, the subfield of AI, i.e., machine learning (ML) is a data-driven approach, which is explicitly designed and optimized by fine-tuning the hyperparameters to reflect certain features through learning rule. In this chapter, we aim to provide a critical overview of OCT and machine learning model by presenting the scientific context, working principles, and current biomedical applications. The chapter will also cover types of convolutional neural networks (CNNs) that have been used in analyzing diverse OCT images.

Keywords: optical coherence tomography, optical microscopy, machine learning, deep neural network, ophthalmology, classification, segmentation

1. Introduction

Optical coherence tomography (OCT) is a non-contact and non-invasive optical technique to visualize the volumetric information of multilayered semitransparent objects [1, 2]. OCT is based on the principle of low-coherence interferometry (LCI) [1, 2]. There are different types of OCT techniques described in the literature that can provide volumetric information of the object, such as Time-Domain OCT (TD-OCT), Frequency Domain OCT (Spectral Domain OCT and Swept-Source OCT (SS-OCT)), and Full-Field OCT (FF-OCT) [1, 3]. In general, two types of scans must be performed in OCT to acquire the volumetric information of the specimen: the lateral-scan, which is performed by galvo scan, addresses laterally adjacent sample positions and the depth-scan to detect the depth information of the sample [4, 5]. In addition, the axial resolution of OCT is determined by the coherence length (l_c) of the light source rather than the depth of field of the objective lens.

OCT has found widespread use in ophthalmology, cardiology, dermatology, among other fields due to its ability to provide detailed cross-sectional images of tissue structures with micrometer resolution [5, 6]. The penetration depth of several millimeters in industrial sample and 1–2 mm in tissue makes it most suitable for the diverse biological applications [7, 8]; 1–2 mm of depth of penetration of OCT is primarily decided by the cellular and subcellular density. This penetration depth of 1–2 mm is helpful in many applications, for example, surgeon to anticipate tissue morphology beneath the surface and over large surface areas while conserving the tissue structure. In addition, it emerged as a gold standard technique for early diagnosis of retinal disease [3]. It provides cross-sectional images of the retina and optic nerve that enable early stage diagnosis and used to monitor conditions, such as macular degeneration, diabetic retinopathy, and glaucoma [9]. Over the last three decades, OCT has been developed both experimentally and computationally to improve its resolution, acquisition speed, depth of penetration, and therefore strengthen its applicability in various biological and biomedical applications [10, 11].

In recent years, the integration of artificial intelligence (AI) with OCT revolutionized its applicability in biophotonics [12–14]. AI has made remarkable progress in various domains that include image processing, natural language processing, autonomous systems, among others [15, 16]. The fast and label-free nature of OCT combined with the data analysis capabilities of machine learning brings forth systems that can mimic human intelligence, performing tasks, such as classification, virtual staining, identification of hidden features, and segmentation of objects [17, 18]. Machine learning involves the design and optimization of models through hyperparameter tuning that allow to extract specific features via learning rules [16, 19].

The application of machine learning to OCT has led to significant improvements in image interpretation, noise reduction, and feature extraction. Various machine learning techniques, such as supervised learning, unsupervised learning, and reinforcement learning, have been employed to enhance the performance of OCT systems [7]. For example, supervised learning models like support vector machines (SVMs) and random forests have been used to classify ocular diseases and breast cancer [20]. Unsupervised learning methods, such as K-means clustering and Principal Component Analysis (PCA), have been applied to segment images and identify patterns in large datasets [21].

Deep learning (DL), which is a subset of machine learning, has emerged as a powerful tool in the analysis of OCT images. Convolutional neural networks (CNNs) and recurrent neural networks (RNNs) are two prominent architectures that have shown significant promise in this area. CNNs with their ability to automatically learn hierarchical features from raw image data have been widely used for tasks, such as image classification, segmentation, and resolution enhancement [22, 23]. For instance, CNNs have been applied to identify pathological features in retinal OCT images, achieving high accuracy and robustness. RNNs, which are well suited for sequential data, have been utilized to analyze time-series OCT data, enabling dynamic tracking of changes in tissue morphology.

For example, AI-driven OCT systems can provide real-time diagnostic support to clinicians, aiding in the early detection and treatment of diseases. Furthermore, the ability to process and analyze large-scale OCT datasets with AI can lead to the discovery of novel biomarkers and therapeutic targets. The synergy between OCT and AI is also fostering advancements in personalized medicine, where imaging data can be used to tailor treatments to individual patients.

This chapter covers fundamental principles of OCT and machine learning models utilized for interpreting OCT images. It explores the foundational aspects of supervised and unsupervised learning models, along with advanced deep learning architectures, such as CNNs and RNNs. In addition, various applications of conventional and modern machine learning architectures are shown for the classifications and segmentation of OCT images. In addition to discussing the technical aspects of machine learning models, this chapter also addresses the practical considerations for implementing AI in OCT systems. The goal is to provide a comprehensive overview of the current state of AI in OCT and a roadmap for future research and development.

2. Principle of optical coherence tomography

OCT is based on the principle of low-coherence interferometry (LCI) [1, 2]. The experimental setup of LCI is shown in **Figure 1**. Light from a low-coherence (broadband) source is incident on the sample surface through the Michelson interferometer [24]. The light is split into reference and sample beams using 50:50 beam splitter. At each scan point, the back-scattered light intensity from multiple layers of the sample combines with the back-reflected light from the reference mirror to generate a 1D (one-dimensional) interference signal only when the optical path difference between two arms is less than the coherence length of the light source [1, 25]. The encoded depth information in the detected interference signal is reconstructed using Fourier transform analysis.

If $E_r = \frac{E_i}{\sqrt{2}} r_{ref} e^{i2kz_r}$ and $E_s = \frac{E_i}{\sqrt{2}} \sum_{n=1}^{N} r_{Sn} e^{i2kz_{sn}}$ represent the electric fields at the beam splitter after reflecting from reference and nth layer of the sample arm, respectively, the 1D interference signal at the detector can be written as

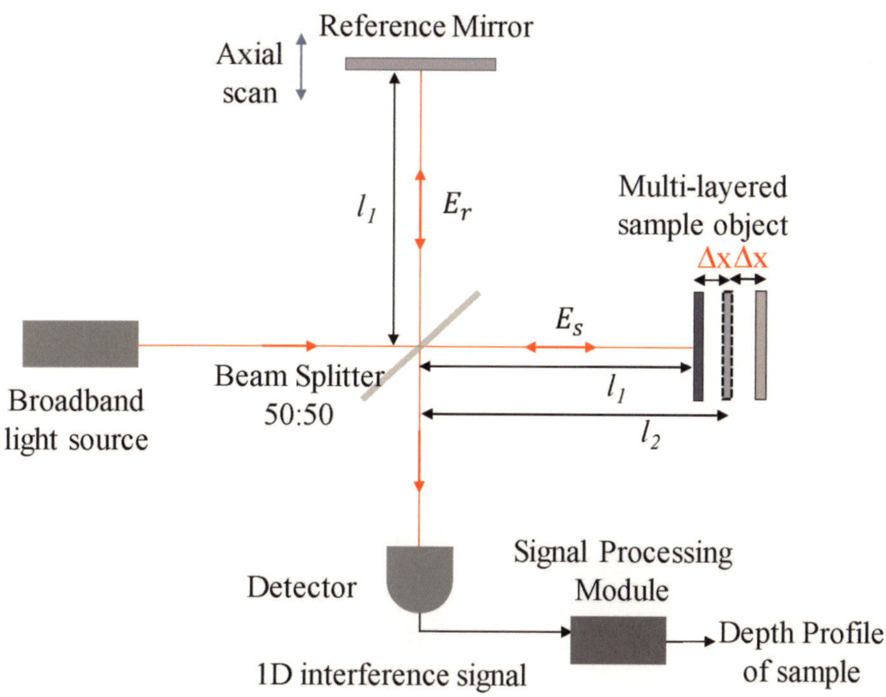

Figure 1.
Schematic diagram of low-coherence interferometry.

$$I(k,w) = \frac{\mu}{2}\left\langle \left| \frac{s(k,w)}{\sqrt{2}} r_{ref} e^{i(2kz_r - wt)} + \frac{s(k,w)}{\sqrt{2}} \sum_{n=1}^{N} r_{Sn} e^{i(2kz_{sn} - wt)} \right|^2 \right\rangle \tag{1}$$

where $s(k,w)$ represents the electric field amplitude and μ is the responsivity of the detector (Amperes/Watts). r_{ref} and r_{Sn} show the electric field reflectivity of the reference and nth layer of the sample arm, respectively. The above equation can be expanded as

$$\begin{aligned} I(k,w) = & \frac{\mu}{4}\left[S(k)\left(R_{ref} + R_{s1} + R_{s2} + \ldots + R_{sn}\right)\right] \\ & + \frac{\mu}{2}\left[S(k) \sum_{n=1}^{N} \sqrt{R_{ref}R_{sn}} \left(e^{i2k\left(z_{ref} - z_{sn}\right)} + e^{-i2k\left(z_{ref} - z_{sn}\right)}\right)\right] \\ & + \frac{\mu}{4}\left[S(k) \sum_{n \neq m = 1}^{N} \sqrt{R_{sn}R_{sn}} \left(e^{i2k(z_{sm} - z_{sn})} + e^{-i2k(z_{sm} - z_{sn})}\right)\right] \end{aligned} \tag{2}$$

The above equation can be rewritten as

$$\begin{aligned} I(k,w) = & \frac{\mu}{4}\left[S(k)\left(R_{ref} + R_{s1} + R_{s2} + \ldots + R_{sn}\right)\right] \\ & + \frac{\mu}{2}\left[S(k) \sum_{n=1}^{N} \sqrt{R_{ref}R_{sn}} \left(2\cos(2k\left(z_{ref} - z_{sn}\right))\right)\right] \\ & + \frac{\mu}{4}\left[S(k) \sum_{n \neq m = 1}^{N} \sqrt{R_{sn}R_{sn}} \left(2\cos(2k(z_{sm} - z_{sn}))\right)\right] \end{aligned} \tag{3}$$

Here, $S(k)$ represents Gaussian spectral profile i.e. square of the electric field amplitude encodes the spectral dependence of the light source. In addition, the degree of coherence for a light source with Gaussian spectral profile is given by

$$\gamma(\tau) = exp\left[-\left(\frac{\pi \Delta \nu \tau}{2\sqrt{ln\, 2}}\right)^2\right] . exp\,(-j2\pi \nu_0 \tau) \tag{4}$$

where $\Delta\nu$ is the width of the temporal frequency spectrum and ν_0 is the central frequency of the light source. The key point in OCT imaging system is the dominance of coherence function over axial point-spread function (at least for low numerical aperture lens); hence, the axial resolution of OCT system is defined by the coherence length of the light source [26].

An especial type of OCT is called SD-OCT, where the reflectivity of the sample can be calculated by taking the inverse Fourier transform of Eq. (2), mathematically

$$\begin{aligned} IFT[I(k,w)] = IFT & \left[\frac{\mu}{4}\left[S(k)\left(R_{ref} + R_{s1} + R_{s2} + \ldots R_{sn}\right)\right]\right. \\ & + \frac{\mu}{4}\left[S(k) \sum_{n=1}^{N} \sqrt{R_{ref}R_{sn}} \left(e^{i2k\left(z_{ref} - z_{sn}\right)} + e^{-i2k\left(z_{ref} - z_{sn}\right)}\right)\right] \\ & \left. + \frac{\mu}{4}\left[S(k) \sum_{n \neq m = 1}^{N} \sqrt{R_{sn}R_{sn}} \left(e^{i2k(z_{sm} - z_{sn})} + e^{-i2k(z_{sm} - z_{sn})}\right)\right]\right] \end{aligned} \tag{5}$$

Since cosine and delta functions are Fourier transform pair of each other, the above equation can be simplified as:

$$\begin{aligned} I(z) = {} & \frac{\mu}{8}\left[\gamma(z)\left(R_{ref} + R_{s1} + R_{s2} + \ldots R_{sn}\right)\right] \\ & + \frac{\mu}{4}\left[\gamma(z) \otimes \sum_{n=1}^{N} \sqrt{R_{ref}R_{sn}}\,\left(\delta\left(z \pm 2\left(z_{ref} - z_{sn}\right)\right)\right)\right] \\ & + \frac{\mu}{8}\left[\gamma(z) \otimes \sum_{n \neq m=1}^{N} \sqrt{R_{sn}R_{sn}}\,\left(\delta(z \pm 2(z_{sm} - z_{sn}))\right)\right] \end{aligned} \tag{6}$$

where $\left[\gamma(z)\left(R_{ref} + R_{s1} + R_{s2} + \ldots R_{sn}\right)\right]$ is the "DC term," $\frac{\mu}{8}\left[\gamma(z) \otimes \sum_{n=1}^{N} \sqrt{R_{ref}R_{sn}}\,\left(\delta\left(z \pm 2\left(z_{ref} - z_{sn}\right)\right)\right)\right]$ represents the "auto-correlation term" i.e. correlation between nth and mth layer of the sample. Additionally, $\frac{\mu}{4}\left[\gamma(z) \otimes \sum_{n=1}^{N} \sqrt{R_{ref}R_{sn}}\,\left(\delta\left(z \pm 2\left(z_{ref} - z_{sn}\right)\right)\right)\right]$ shows the "cross-correlation term" where desired sample field reflectivity i.e. $\sqrt{R_s(z_s)}$ is correlated with the reference field. Using the sifting property of the delta function i.e.

$$\gamma(z) \otimes \delta(z - z_0) = \gamma(z - z_0) \tag{7}$$

Eq. (11) referred to as "A-scan" can be written as

$$\begin{aligned} I(z) = {} & \frac{\mu}{8}\left[\gamma(z)\left(R_{ref} + R_{s1} + R_{s2} + \ldots R_{sn}\right)\right] \\ & + \frac{\mu}{4}\left[\sum_{n=1}^{N} \sqrt{R_{ref}R_{sn}}\left[\gamma\left[2\left(z_{ref} - z_{sn}\right)\right] + \gamma\left[-2\left(z_{ref} - z_{sn}\right)\right]\right]\right] \\ & + \frac{\mu}{8}\left[\sum_{n \neq m=1}^{N} \sqrt{R_{sn}R_{sn}}\left[\gamma[2(z_{sm} - z_{sn})] + \gamma[-2(z_{sm} - z_{sn})]\right]\right] \end{aligned} \tag{8}$$

SD-OCT has a dramatic sensitivity and speed advantage because depth-scan is not required. It also allows direct access to the spectrum, which enables numerical dispersion compensation and spectral shaping.

3. The necessity of machine learning for OCT image interpretation

Although OCT is a powerful label-free, non-invasive technique, the interpretation of OCT images poses several challenges. First, chemical specificity of OCT images is limited compared to the label-based imaging methods such as fluorescence microscopy. The primary bottleneck comes with mapping chemical composition with the OCT image of the object. Second, high-dimensional data produced by OCT scans can be overwhelming, making manual analysis time-consuming and prone to errors. Finally, subtle features indicative of early-stage diseases can be easily overlooked by the human eye. Therefore, traditional image analysis techniques often fall short of effectively distinguishing between fine structures and artifacts or noise, limiting the diagnostic utility of OCT.

Machine learning offers powerful solutions to these challenges. Modern deep learning models, such as convolutional neural networks (CNNs), are designed to automatically learn and extract hierarchical features from raw image data [27]. These models can be trained on large datasets of labeled OCT images to recognize patterns and structures associated with specific biological or pathological states. By doing so, machine learning algorithms can perform tasks, such as multilayer/object-specific segmentation, disease detection, and classification.

For example, machine learning models can analyze OCT images to segment retinal layers, detect fluid accumulation, and identify biomarkers for diseases like age-related macular degeneration, drusen, and diabetic retinopathy. These algorithms can also adapt to variations in image quality and patient-specific differences, providing robust and generalized solutions. Therefore, machine learning can bridge the technical gap by leveraging its ability to learn from data, automatically extract relevant features, and provide accurate and consistent analysis, thereby enhancing the diagnostic and research capabilities of OCT in biomedical applications.

4. Convolutional neural network

Convolutional neural networks (CNNs) consist of several types of layers, including convolutional layers, max-pooling layers, rectified linear unit (ReLU) layers, and fully connected layers followed by a soft-max layer for classification purposes [15]. **Figure 2** illustrates the architecture of CNNs. The learning process begins by applying a convolution operation to the input image using the filters in the first convolutional layer.

In general, convolution is an operation between two functions, f and k, which produces third function 's' that represents the modification of the shape of one function by the other. Mathematically, this is expressed as:

$$s(t) = \int f(x)k(t-x)\,dx \tag{9}$$

For a 2D (two-dimensional) image, f of size $M \times N$ and a 2d kernel k of size $m \times n$, the convolution operation is given by:

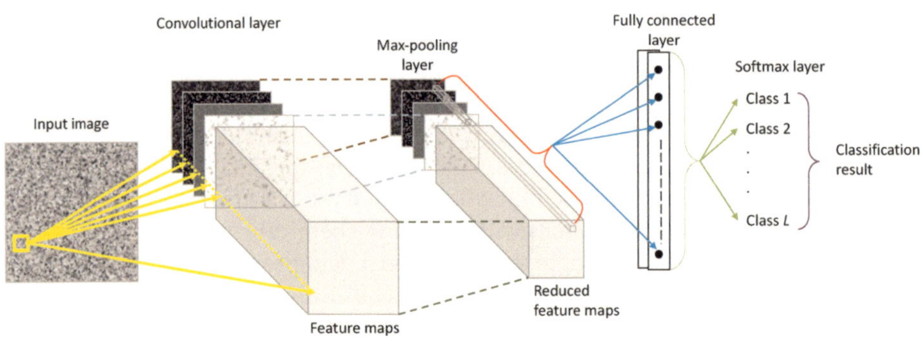

Figure 2.
Schematic diagram of convolutional neural network consisting of convolutional layer, max-pooling layer, fully connected layer, and soft-max layer.

$$s(i,j) = \sum_{a=0}^{m-1}\sum_{b=0}^{n-1} f(i+a, j+b) \bullet k(a,b) \tag{10}$$

This can be generalized for color images, where the convolution is performed across each channel.

$$s(i,j,c) = \sum_{a=0}^{m-1}\sum_{b=0}^{n-1}\sum_{d=0}^{D-1} f(i+a, j+b, d) k(a,b,c,d) \tag{11}$$

where D is the depth of the input image (number of channels) and c is the output channel.

To control the spatial dimensions of the output, padding and stride are used. Padding p involves usually adding zeros around the input image and stride s controls the step size of the convolution.

For a given input f of size $M \times N$ and a kernel k of size $m \times n$, with padding p and stride s, the output size (M', N') is calculated as:

$$M' = \left(\frac{M - m + 2p}{s}\right) + 1 \tag{12}$$

$$N' = \left(\frac{N - n + 2p}{s}\right) + 1 \tag{13}$$

Furthermore, ReLU activation function introduces non-linearity to the network, which is crucial for learning complex patterns. Mathematically, it can be defined as:

$$f(x) = \max(0, x) \tag{14}$$

Max-pooling operation followed the ReLU layer, which reduces the spatial dimensions while retaining the most critical information. For an input feature map f and a pooling window of size $m \times n$, the max-pooling operation is given by:

$$f_{i,j} = max\,\{f(i+a, j+b) | 0 \le a < m, 0 \le l < n\} \tag{15}$$

Furthermore, the fully connected layer aggregated the features extracted by previous layers to make the final prediction. It is represented as:

$$z = W \bullet x + b \tag{16}$$

where W is the weight matrix, x is the input vector, and b is the bias vector. Finally, the SoftMax function converts the raw scores from the fully connected layer into probabilities:

$$softmax(z_i) = \frac{e^{z_i}}{\sum_j e^{z_i}} \tag{17}$$

This ensures that the output probabilities sum to 1. The convolutional neural network combines multiple convolutional layers, each followed by ReLU and max-pooling layers, to learn spatial hierarchies of features. The fully connected layer then integrates these features to classify the input data accurately. Understanding these mathematical formulations can help to grasp how CNNs effectively process and interpret complex image data, such as those produced by OCT.

5. Machine learning approach for the analysis of OCT images

Table 1 provides the systematic review of different types of OCT techniques that have been used to acquire 3D images of different biological samples. These images are used by different machine learning methods for specific biological applications.

In the past two decades, various types of OCT techniques have been used for various biological applications where machine learning plays a pivotal role in data analysis and

OCT techniques	Biological sample	ML method	Key findings
SD-OCT	Retinal tissue [3, 9, 28, 29]	Convolutional neural networks (CNNs)	Classification of retinal diseases
		Support vector machine (SVM)	Detection of diabetic retinopathy
SS-OCT	Corneal tissue [20, 30, 31]	Support vector machine (SVM)	Detection of keratoconus
		Random forest	Classification of corneal diseases
Doppler OCT	Blood flow in retinal vessels [21, 32, 33]	Random forest	Analysis of blood flow dynamics
		K-means clustering	Segmentation of blood vessels
	Cardiovascular tissues [34]	CNNs	Detection of myocardial infarction
	Liver tissues [35]	CNNs	Detection of hepatic microvasculature
Polarization-Sensitive OCT	Skin tissue [23, 36]	Principal component analysis (PCA)	Assessment of burn depth
		K-means clustering	Differentiation of skin layers
Time-Domain OCT (TD-OCT)	Dental tissue [37]	k-Nearest Neighbors (k-NN)	Detection of dental caries
Full-Field OCT (FF-OCT)	Brain tissue [38, 39]	Linear discriminant analysis (LDA)	Imaging of neural structures
		SVM	Classification of brain tissue
OCT Angiography (OCTA)	Retinal vasculature [22, 40]	CNNs	Visualization of microvascular networks
			Automated segmentation of retinal layers
Multi-Modal OCT	Tumor tissue [41, 42]	Ensemble methods	Differentiation of tumor margin
		Random forest	Classification of tumor types

Table 1.
Detailed review of different types of OCT techniques and machine learning models that have been used to extract and analyze 3D images of diverse biological samples.

interpretation. For instance, Spectral-Domain OCT (SD-OCT) has been extensively applied in ophthalmology, particularly for imaging retinal tissues [3, 9, 28, 29]. Advance machine learning (ML) techniques, such as CNN and support vector machines (SVMs), assisted SD-OCT for automated classification of retinal diseases like diabetic retinopathy, drusen, etc. These algorithms analyze OCT images to detect multilayer structural changes, providing clinicians with accurate diagnostic information [29].

Another type of OCT technique i.e., Swept-Source OCT (SS-OCT) has been extensively used for retinal imaging due to its high-resolution and rapid acquisition capabilities [20, 30, 31]. CNNs significantly improved the classification of retinal diseases, such as diabetic retinopathy and age-related macular degeneration, by automatically identifying disease-specific patterns in OCT images. SS-OCT also offers deeper tissue penetration, making it suitable for imaging the cornea. Studies have used SVMs to detect keratoconus, a degenerative corneal disorder, with improved accuracy by analyzing the curvature and thickness of the corneal layers. Additionally, Random Forest algorithms have been applied to classify various corneal diseases, enhancing diagnostic precision.

On the other hand, researchers also used Doppler OCT to measure blood flow velocity and analyze retinal blood flow dynamics [21]. Different ML techniques, such as Random Forest algorithms, have facilitated the segmentation and analysis of blood vessels, providing insights into conditions like glaucoma and diabetic retinopathy. K-means clustering has also been employed for vessel segmentation, enhancing the visualization of retinal vasculature. Doppler OCT has also been applied to liver tissues for the assessment of fibrosis and detection of hepatic microvasculature, using Random Forest and CNN algorithms.

Polarization-Sensitive OCT (PS-OCT), which provides additional contrast based on tissue birefringence, has been used for assessing burn depth and differentiating skin layers [23, 36]. Principal Component Analysis (PCA) has been utilized to quantify changes in birefringence, aiding in the assessment of burn injuries. K-means clustering has helped in differentiating various skin layers, facilitating detailed structural analysis.

Time-Domain OCT (TD-OCT) has also been applied to dental imaging for the detection of dental caries [37]. Techniques like k-Nearest Neighbors (k-NN) have been employed to classify carious and non-carious regions, leveraging the detailed structural information provided by TD-OCT. Decision Trees have also been used to analyze dental tissues, aiding in the diagnosis and treatment planning.

For en face imaging, Full-Field OCT (FF-OCT) is explored to extract high-resolution imaging of neural structures in brain tissue [21]. Linear Discriminant Analysis (LDA) has facilitated the differentiation of various neural structures, aiding in neurological research. SVMs have also been applied to classify different types of brain tissues, providing valuable insights for neuroscientific studies.

Furthermore, detailed imaging of retinal microvascular networks is explored by using OCT Angiography (OCTA) [22, 40]. DL methods have been employed to automate the segmentation and visualization of these networks, enhancing the detection and monitoring of diseases, such as macular degeneration and diabetic retinopathy. Finally, Multi-Modal OCT combines various OCT techniques to provide comprehensive imaging of tumor tissues. Ensemble methods and Random Forest algorithms have been used to differentiate tumor margins and classify tumor types, improving the precision of oncological diagnoses.

The integration of OCT techniques with advanced machine learning methods has revolutionized its applicability for biological imaging. By leveraging the strengths of both technologies, researchers and clinicians can achieve more accurate diagnoses, better disease monitoring, and deeper insights into complex biological processes. The extensive range of applications highlighted in **Table 1** underscores the versatility and potential of combining OCT with machine learning in various domains of biological research and medical practice.

6. Practical prescription for machine learning in OCT images

A careful examination must be required to ensure accurate outcomes of using ML in OCT images. These challenges include technical, computation, and practical aspects of the integration of ML with OCT datasets.

For instance, OCT images often contain noise and artifacts due to the multiple components in the optical system, scanning, sample movement, and external vibrations. These artifacts can significantly affect the image quality and registration, as a consequence, can complicate the training process of ML models. Furthermore, establishing a reliable ground truth is critical for training and validation of ML models. Inconsistency in the ground truth labeling can lead to unreliable results and poor performance of the model. In addition, overfitting and underfitting are the common causes of training/testing failures. Such issues can be avoided by the appropriate

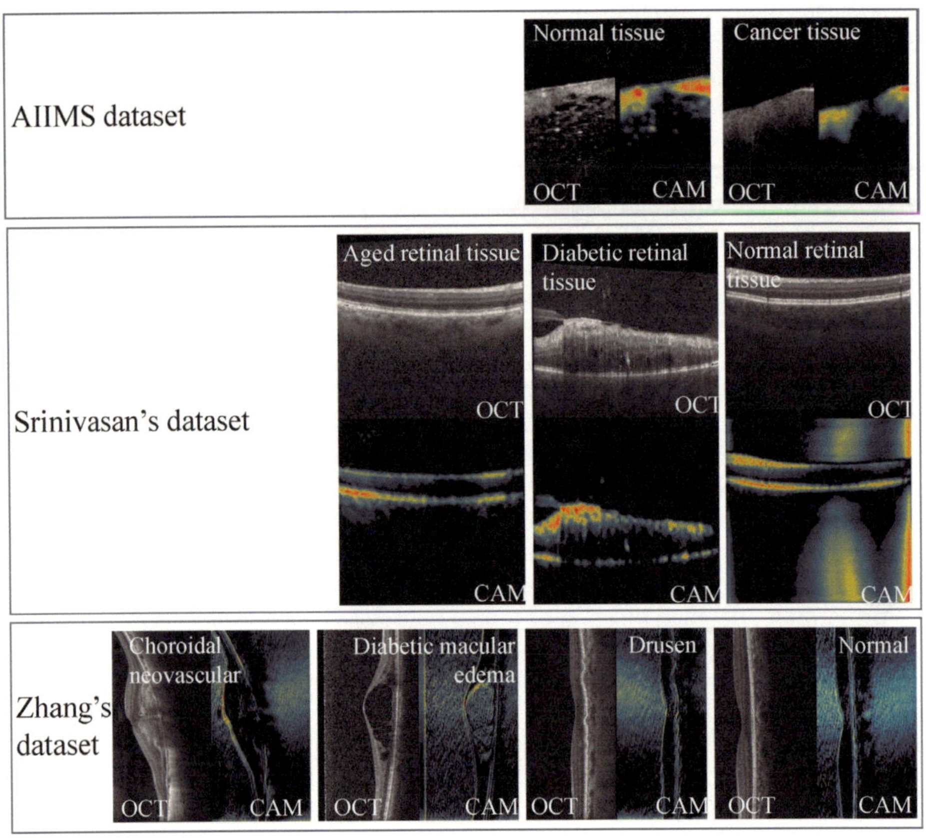

Figure 3.
OCT images (a_1–i_1) and class activation maps (CAMs) (a_2–i_2) to highlight the regions of an input image that are most relevant for predicting a specific class. OCT and CAMs images of normal/cancerous breast cancer tissue (All India Institute of Medical Sciences datasets) and ocular disease (Srinivasan and Zhang datasets) OCT images [9, 31, 44].

choice of ML models, and tuning the model's hyperparameters (such as the number of layers and learning rate).

Furthermore, visualization in deep learning is important to highlight the regions of an input image that are most relevant for predicting a specific class. Class activation maps (CAMs) help interpret and understand the decision-making process of CNNs by indicating which parts of the image contribute most to the network's final classification decision [43]. CAMs (see **Figure 3**) represent the firing strength of various regions that help in the conclusion regarding the class label [45]. For objects with well-defined boundaries in both the training and test datasets, researchers have employed activation maps to explore and interpret the behavior of CNN models. By visualizing the areas of an image that contribute most to the network's classification, CAMs help bridge the gap between complex neural network operations and interpretability.

7. Conclusion

Optical Coherence Tomography (OCT) combined with machine learning offers a powerful tool for the automated classification of biological samples into diagnostically relevant classes. OCT is a promising, label-free imaging technique that provides volumetric information, offering advantages over conventional label-free methods. In the future, fully automated classification using OCT and machine learning can serve as a valuable intermediate tool for experts across multiple medical applications, including ophthalmology and to distinguish between normal and abnormal tissues.

Furthermore, deep learning-based methods for classification, segmentation, virtual staining, and resolution enhancement hold broad applications in biomedical imaging. These data-driven approaches can improve the robustness, reduce computational artifacts, and enhance selectivity and sensitivity in optical imaging. However, it is crucial to be aware of the limitations of AI in biomedical imaging to fully understand the potential benefits of data-driven learning. Therefore, machine learning models must undergo rigorous validation to meet regulatory standards for clinical use. Ensuring that these models are reliable, safe, and effective across diverse clinical environments is essential for achieving regulatory approval. By overcoming practical challenges and integrating machine learning with OCT can enhance diagnostic accuracy, improve patient outcomes, and drive advancements in the field of biomedical imaging.

Acknowledgements

The author would like to acknowledge the European Research Council Starting Grant (ID 804233).

Author details

Ankit Butola
Department of Physics and Technology, UiT The Arctic University of Norway, Tromsø, Norway

*Address all correspondence to: ankit.butola@uit.no; ankitbutola321@gmail.com

References

[1] Drexler W, Fujimoto JG. Optical Coherence Tomography: Technology and Applications. Berlin, Heidelberg: Springer; 2008

[2] Huang D, Swanson EA, Lin CP, Schuman JS, Stinson WG, Chang W, et al. Optical coherence tomography. Science. 1991;**254**:1178-1181

[3] Lee CS, Baughman DM, Lee AY. Deep learning is effective for classifying normal versus age-related macular degeneration OCT images. Ophthalmology Retina. 2017;**1**: 322-327

[4] Boppart SA. Optical coherence tomography. In: Optical Imaging and Microscopy: Techniques and Advanced Systems. Berlin, Heidelberg: Springer; 2003. pp. 309-337

[5] Welzel J. Optical coherence tomography in dermatology: A review. Skin Research and Technology. 2001;7:1-9

[6] De Carlo TE, Romano A, Waheed NK, Duker JS. A review of optical coherence tomography angiography (OCTA). International Journal of Retina and Vitreous. 2015;**1**:1-15

[7] Joshi D, Butola A, Kanade SR, Prasad DK, Mithra SA, Singh N, et al. Label-free non-invasive classification of rice seeds using optical coherence tomography assisted with deep neural network. Optics & Laser Technology. 2021;**137**:106861

[8] Mehta DS, Butola A, Singh V. Quantitative Phase Microscopy and Tomography: Techniques Using Partially Spatially Coherent Monochromatic Light. Bristol, United Kingdom: IOP Publishing; 2022

[9] Kermany DS, Goldbaum M, Cai W, Valentim CC, Liang H, Baxter SL, et al. Identifying medical diagnoses and treatable diseases by image-based deep learning. Cell. 2018;**172**:1122-1131. e1129

[10] Fujimoto JG. Optical coherence tomography for ultrahigh resolution in vivo imaging. Nature Biotechnology. 2003;**21**:1361-1367

[11] Butola A, Coucheron DA, Szafranska K, Ahmad A, Mao H, Tinguely J-C, et al. Multimodal on-chip nanoscopy and quantitative phase imaging reveals the nanoscale morphology of liver sinusoidal endothelial cells. Proceedings of the National Academy of Sciences. 2021;**118**:e2115323118

[12] Maloca PM, Lee AY, de Carvalho ER, Okada M, Fasler K, Leung I, et al. Validation of automated artificial intelligence segmentation of optical coherence tomography images. PLoS One. 2019;**14**:e0220063

[13] Lee CS, Tyring AJ, Wu Y, Xiao S, Rokem AS, DeRuyter NP, et al. Generating retinal flow maps from structural optical coherence tomography with artificial intelligence. Scientific Reports. 2019;**9**:5694

[14] Dubey K, Singla N, Butola A, Lathe A, Quaiser D, Srivastava A, et al. Ensemble classifier for improve diagnosis of the breast cancer using optical coherence tomography and machine learning. Laser Physics Letters. 2019;**16**:025602

[15] Bengio Y, Goodfellow I, Courville A. Deep Learning. Cambridge, MA, USA: MIT press; 2017

[16] LeCun Y, Bengio Y, Hinton G. Deep learning. Nature. 2015;**521**:436-444

[17] Butola A, Popova D, Prasad DK, Ahmad A, Habib A, Tinguely JC, et al. High spatially sensitive quantitative phase imaging assisted with deep neural network for classification of human spermatozoa under stressed condition. Scientific Reports. 2020;**10**:13118

[18] Butola A, Kanade SR, Bhatt S, Dubey VK, Kumar A, Ahmad A, et al. High space-bandwidth in quantitative phase imaging using partially spatially coherent digital holographic microscopy and a deep neural network. Optics Express. 2020;**28**: 36229-36244

[19] Zuo C, Qian J, Feng S, Yin W, Li Y, Fan P, et al. Deep learning in optical metrology: A review. Light: Science & Applications. 2022;**11**:1-54

[20] Butola A, Ahmad A, Dubey V, Srivastava V, Qaiser D, Srivastava A, et al. Volumetric analysis of breast cancer tissues using machine learning and swept-source optical coherence tomography. Applied Optics. 2019;**58**: A135-A141

[21] Mariampillai A, Standish BA, Moriyama EH, Khurana M, Munce NR, Leung MK, et al. Speckle variance detection of microvasculature using swept-source optical coherence tomography. Optics Letters. 2008;**33**: 1530-1532

[22] Kashani AH, Lee SY, Moshfeghi A, Durbin MK, Puliafito CA. Optical coherence tomography angiography of retinal venous occlusion. Retina. 2015;**35**: 2323-2331

[23] Marvdashti T, Duan L, Aasi SZ, Tang JY, Bowden AKE. Classification of basal cell carcinoma in human skin using machine learning and quantitative features captured by polarization sensitive optical coherence tomography. Biomedical Optics Express. 2016;**7**: 3721-3735

[24] Usmani K, Ahmad A, Joshi R, Dubey V, Butola A, Mehta DS. Relationship between the source size at the diffuser plane and the longitudinal spatial coherence function of the optical coherence microscopy system. JOSA A. 2019;**36**:D41-D46

[25] Butola A, Joshi T, Ahmad A, Dubey V, Senthilkumaran P, Mehta DS. 3D topography and tomography of multilayered freeform optical surfaces using large-range measurement swept-source low-coherence interferometry. Laser Physics. 2018;**28**:116101

[26] Qin Y, Butola A, Agarwal K. 3D refractive index reconstruction from phaseless coherent optical microscopy data using multiple scattering-based inverse solvers—A study. Inverse Problems. 2023;**40**:015003

[27] Jo Y, Cho H, Lee SY, Choi G, Kim G, Min H-S, et al. Quantitative phase imaging and artificial intelligence: A review. IEEE Journal of Selected Topics in Quantum Electronics. 2018;**25**:1-14

[28] Archana R, Rajalakshmi T, Vijay Sai P. Non-invasive technique to detect diabetic retinopathy based on electrooculography signal using machine learning classifiers. Proceedings of the Institution of Mechanical Engineers, Part H: Journal of Engineering in Medicine. 2022;**236**:882-895

[29] Abramoff MD, Fort PE, Han IC, Jayasundera KT, Sohn EH, Gardner TW. Approach for a clinically useful comprehensive classification of vascular and neural aspects of diabetic retinal disease. Investigative Ophthalmology & Visual Science. 2018;**59**:519-527

[30] Tan O, Li G, Lu AT-H, Varma R, Huang D, A. I. f. G. S. Group. Mapping of macular substructures with optical coherence tomography for glaucoma diagnosis. Ophthalmology. 2008;**115**: 949-956

[31] Butola A, Prasad DK, Ahmad A, Dubey V, Qaiser D, Srivastava A, et al. Deep learning architecture "LightOCT" for diagnostic decision support using optical coherence tomography images of biological samples. Biomedical Optics Express. 2020;**11**:5017-5031

[32] Mariampillai A, Leung MK, Jarvi M, Standish BA, Lee K, Wilson BC, et al. Optimized speckle variance OCT imaging of microvasculature. Optics Letters. 2010;**35**:1257-1259

[33] Leitgeb RA, Werkmeister RM, Blatter C, Schmetterer L. Doppler optical coherence tomography. Progress in Retinal and Eye Research. 2014;**41**:26-43

[34] Tsai M-T, Chen Y, Lee C-Y, Huang B-H, Trung NH, Lee Y-J, et al. Noninvasive structural and microvascular anatomy of oral mucosae using handheld optical coherence tomography. Biomedical Optics Express. 2017;**8**:5001-5012

[35] Mason C, Markusen J, Town M, Dunnill P, Wang R. Doppler optical coherence tomography for measuring flow in engineered tissue. Biosensors and Bioelectronics. 2004;**20**:414-423

[36] Iftimia N, Ferguson RD, Mujat M, Patel AH, Zhang EZ, Fox W, et al. Combined reflectance confocal microscopy/optical coherence tomography imaging for skin burn assessment. Biomedical Optics Express. 2013;**4**:680-695

[37] Katkar RA, Tadinada SA, Amaechi BT, Fried D. Optical coherence tomography. Dental Clinics. 2018;**62**: 421-434

[38] Möller J, Bartsch A, Lenz M, Tischoff I, Krug R, Welp H, et al. Applying machine learning to optical coherence tomography images for automated tissue classification in brain metastases. International Journal of Computer Assisted Radiology and Surgery. 2021;**16**:1517-1526

[39] Maldiney T, Greigert H, Martin L, Benoit E, Creuzot-Garcher C, Gabrielle P-H, et al. Full-field optical coherence tomography for the diagnosis of giant cell arteritis. PLoS One. 2020;**15**: e0234165

[40] Le D, Son T, Yao X. Machine learning in optical coherence tomography angiography. Experimental Biology and Medicine. 2021;**246**: 2170-2183

[41] Tucker-Schwartz JM, Beavers KR, Sit WW, Shah AT, Duvall CL, Skala MC. In vivo imaging of nanoparticle delivery and tumor microvasculature with multimodal optical coherence tomography. Biomedical Optics Express. 2014;**5**:1731-1743

[42] Yashin K, Karabut M, Fedoseeva V, Khalansky A, Matveev L, Elagin V, et al. Multimodal optical coherence tomography in visualization of brain tissue structure at glioblastoma (experimental study). Современные технологии в медицине. 2016;**8**:73-80

[43] Ma X, Ji Z, Niu S, Leng T, Rubin DL, Chen Q. MS-CAM: Multi-scale class activation maps for weakly-supervised segmentation of geographic atrophy lesions in SD-OCT images. IEEE Journal of Biomedical and Health Informatics. 2020;**24**:3443-3455

[44] Srinivasan PP, Kim LA, Mettu PS, Cousins SW, Comer GM, Izatt JA, et al.

Fully automated detection of diabetic macular edema and dry age-related macular degeneration from optical coherence tomography images. Biomedical Optics Express. 2014;**5**: 3568-3577

[45] Sunija A, Kar S, Gayathri S, Gopi VP, Palanisamy P. Octnet: A lightweight cnn for retinal disease classification from optical coherence tomography images. Computer Methods and Programs in Biomedicine. 2021;**200**:105877

Section 2

OCT and Anterior Segment Diseases

Chapter 4

Application of Optical Coherence Tomography in Corneal Ectasia Diseases

Jinhai Huang, Yiran Wang, Kexin Li and Xinning Yang

Abstract

This chapter explores the application of anterior segment optical coherence tomography (OCT) in the diagnosis and treatment of corneal ectasia diseases, with a particular focus on keratoconus, post-refractive corneal ectasia, and pellucid marginal degeneration (PMD). OCT provides high-resolution imaging of corneal sublayers, assisting in early detection and tracking of disease progression. For corneal ectasia diseases, OCT assists in identifying characteristic changes in corneal thickness and morphology, guiding treatment strategies such as contact lens fitting, intrastromal corneal ring segments (ICRS) implantation, corneal crosslinking (CXL), and corneal transplantation. OCT's precision and reliability make it a valuable tool in managing these challenging corneal conditions, facilitating improved patient outcomes.

Keywords: keratoconus, optical coherence tomography, corneal ectasia, pellucid marginal degeneration, anterior segment

1. Introduction

Corneal ectasia diseases include keratoconus, post-refractive surgery corneal ectasia, and pellucid marginal degeneration (PMD), often accompanied by corneal thickness and morphology changes.

Topography is an important means of evaluating corneal ectasia diseases, including instruments based on Placido and Scheimpflug principles. However, the imaging results are somewhat affected by patients with poor ocular surface conditions, such as corneal opacity or scarring. The reproducibility of peripheral corneal imaging is not as good as that of central corneal. Furthermore, it does not provide corneal sublayer imaging.

Anterior segment optical coherence tomography (OCT) tends to use long wavelengths and fast axial scanning speeds to offer high-resolution cross-sectional images of various corneal layers, including the epithelium, Bowman's layer, stroma, and endothelium. It can be further subdivided into time-domain OCT and Fourier-domain OCT. High-resolution images from OCT aid clinicians in assessing corneal thickness, morphology, and structure, facilitating the diagnosis of corneal ectasia diseases with changes in cornea features. In addition, regular OCT examinations

IntechOpen

enable clinicians to observe changes in corneal structure, evaluate disease severity, and monitor progression, allowing for timely adjustments to treatment strategies. Furthermore, OCT can be utilized to assess surgical suitability and postoperative outcomes. In treating certain progressive corneal diseases, such as corneal transplantation, OCT helps clinicians determine surgical approaches, assess graft suitability, and monitor postoperative recovery.

Based on clinical case reports, this chapter will explain the application of OCT in corneal ectasia diseases from keratoconus, post-refractive corneal dilation, and PMD.

2. Keratoconus

Keratoconus is a progressive corneal disease typically in adolescents or young adults. The main characteristic of this condition is the progressive thinning and bulging of the cornea, which forms a cone-shaped protrusion, impairs vision, and causes visual distortions. In patients with severe keratoconus, signs such as Vogt's striae, Fleischer's ring, and Munson's sign can be seen under the slit-lamp.

2.1 Diagnosis

The increase in anterior surface curvature, posterior surface elevation, and abnormal corneal or corneal epithelium thickness distribution are typical characteristics of keratoconus. Among these, the importance of thickness measurement in diagnosing keratoconus is increasingly recognized [1]. As the severity of the keratoconus increases, the corneal topography becomes obviously abnormal. But forme fruste keratoconus (FFKC), sometimes referred to as preclinical keratoconus, is challenging to diagnose by a single corneal topography parameter, because the anterior surface morphology has not changed significantly (**Figure 1** Right eye). Yang et al. [2] noted that keratoconus could be identified by distinctive patterns seen on OCT pachymetric and epithelial thickness maps, revealing focal thinning occurring at the same or adjacent locations, even in the early stages. Li et al. [3] determined five pachymetric parameters using OCT, which showed high sensitivity and specificity in diagnosing

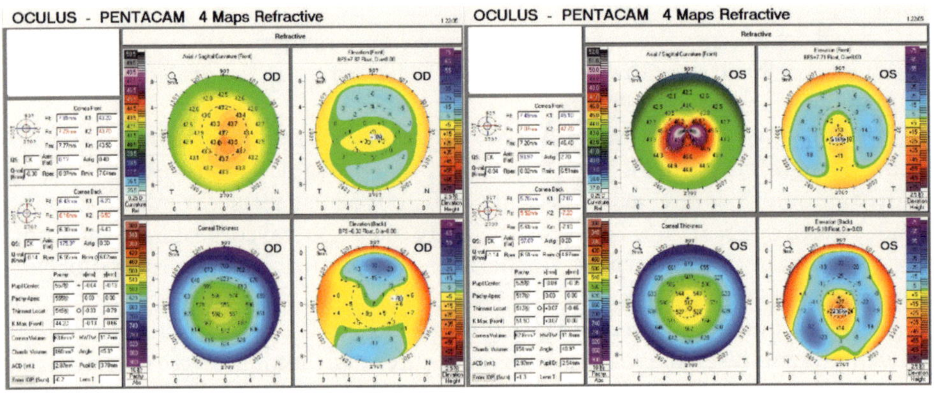

Figure 1.
Topography measured by Pentacam (Oculus, Wetzler, Germany). The anterior axial curvature and posterior corneal elevation of the left eye significantly increased. However, there are no obvious signs in the right eye. The maximum curvature (Kmax) reaching 51.9 diopter (D) and the elevation of the posterior surface 36 um for left eye; the corresponding parameters for the right eye are 44.2 D and 7 μm.

keratoconus. OCT imaging analysis of corneal sublayers aids in the early diagnosis of keratoconus. The corneal epithelium at the cone's apex undergoes thinning in the early stages to compensate for irregularities in the anterior surface caused by thinning and steepening of the stromal layer. OCT can detect changes in the epithelium at the cone's apex, presenting a "doughnut-like" thinning, [4, 5] overall reduction in epithelial thickness, and an increase in the difference between the minimum and maximum epithelial thickness. Epithelial remodeling occurs not only in patients with keratoconus but also after refractive surgery and wearing contact lenses [6, 7]. OCT can also differentiate between early keratoconus and corneal warpage induced by contact lens wear, as the positions of maximum corneal curvature correspond to the minimum and maximum epithelial thickness locations, respectively. Changes in corneal thickness can be used to monitor the progression of keratoconus. The evaluation of changes in epithelial thickness in the subcentral zone of the cornea using OCT is more sensitive for assessing disease progression. Two cases with different stages of keratoconus are presented (**Figures 1–5**).

Case 1. A 22-year-old male with binocular keratoconus. According to Topographic Keratoconus Classification: OD Keratoconus stage FFKC, OS Keratoconus stage 1.

Case 2. A 23-year-old binocular keratoconus male patient. According to Topographic Keratoconus Classification: OD Keratoconus stage 3–4, OS Keratoconus stage 2.

Additionally, histological changes, such as wing cells with irregularly shaped nuclei, elongated epithelial cells, and the disruption of Bowman's layer, were caused by keratoconus [8]. OCT can visualize morphological changes in the anterior elastic layer, presenting a "moth-like" appearance, thinning, and increased light scattering [9, 10]. Considering corneal structural changes occurring in keratoconus, Sandali et al. [11] developed a five-stage classification of keratoconus using OCT, which has been confirmed to have high repeatability.

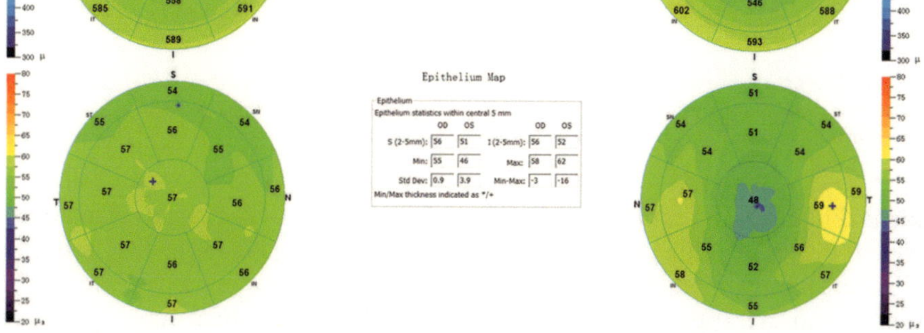

Figure 2.
Corneal Thickness Map measured by RTVue OCT (Optovue, Fremont, USA). Compared with the right eye, the left eye's overall corneal and epithelial thickness is thinner. The thinnest corneal thickness of the right eye and the left eye is 541 µm and 509 µm. The central epithelium thickness of the left eye was significantly thinner, corresponding to the position of the corneal cone. The epithelium of the right eye appears to be partially thin and irregular.

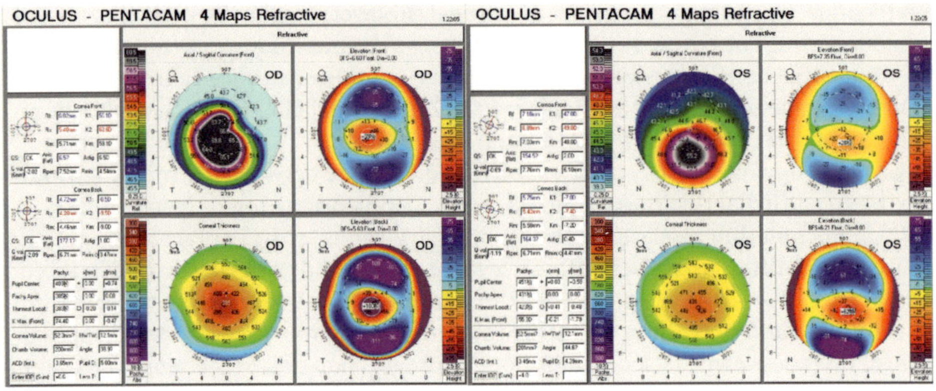

Figure 3.
Topography measured by Pentacam. The curvature of front surface and the height of the posterior surface increased for both eyes. The grade of the right eye was more severe, with the Kmax reaching 74.4 D and the elevation of the posterior surface 100 μm, while the Kmax of the left eye reached 55.3 D and the elevation of the posterior surface was 62 μm.

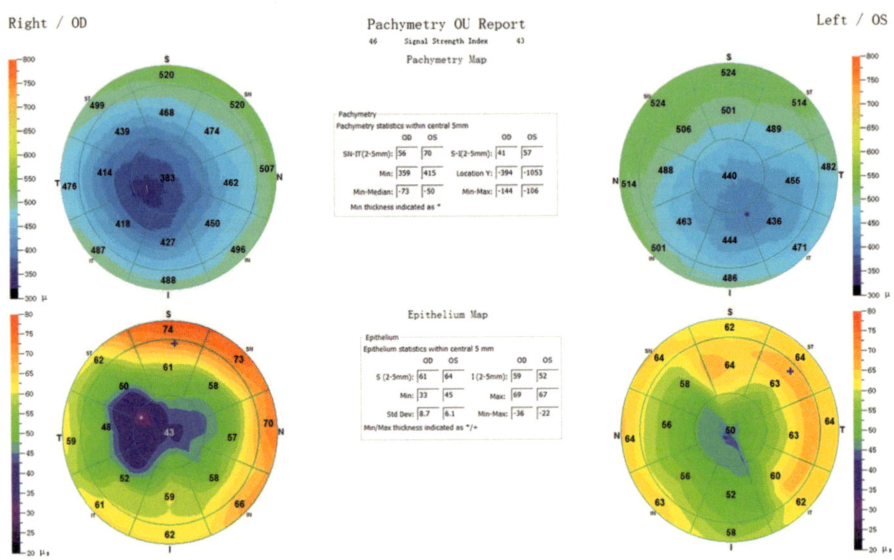

Figure 4.
Corneal Thickness Map measured by RTVue OCT. The thinnest corneal thickness and epithelial thickness of the right eye were 359 μm and 33 μm, respectively, while those of the left eye were 415 μm and 43 μm. The thinning cornea corresponds to increased curvature. More severe eye with thinner corneal and epithelial thickness.

Corneal hydrops, an acute complication of keratoconus, is characterized by significant bullous edema of the cornea resulting from breaks in the Descemet's membrane, leading to an influx of aqueous into the stroma and epithelium. Diagnostic and therapeutic guidance is provided through corneal imaging techniques such as anterior segment OCT, Scheimpflug tomography, and ultrasound biomicroscopy [12]. OCT, in particular, offers the advantage of noncontact imaging for precise localization of intrastromal aqueous influx. Therapeutic interventions have been developed to alleviate symptoms and accelerate healing. These include

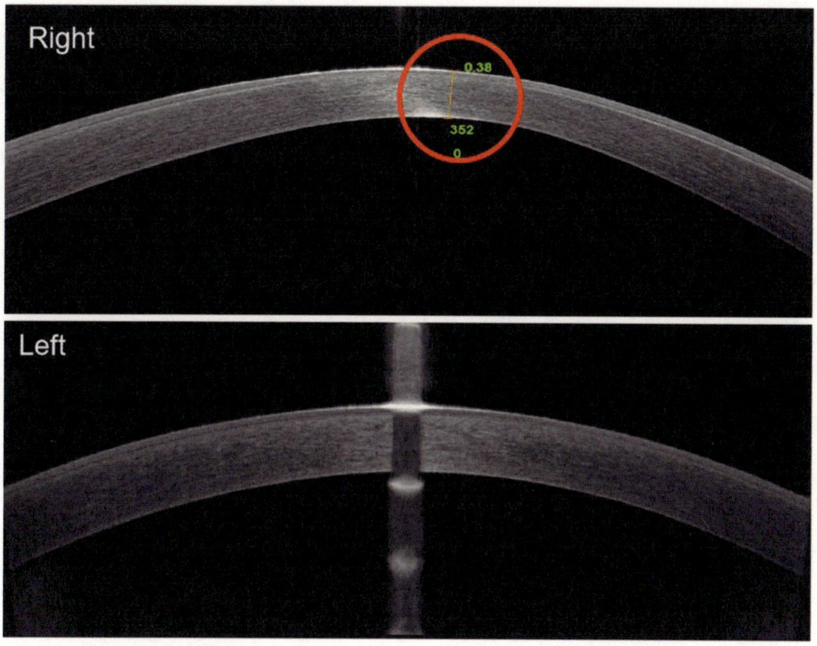

Figure 5.
Cross-sectional images show a significant thinning of the cornea thickness in the right eye. The thinning area is the position of the red circle in the figure, and the thickness is 352 μm.

both medical and surgical approaches as well as conservative methods. Intracameral gas injection is utilized to create a gas tamponade and compression sutures, such as pre-Descemet's membrane sutures [13]. Conservative methods involve using hypertonic saline eye drops/ointments or antiglaucoma agents. Hypertonic saline aids in drawing fluid from the cornea, while antiglaucoma agents reduce hydrodynamic pressure on the cornea's posterior surface. OCT could evaluate the appearance of acute corneal edema (**Figure 6**). The typical pattern is rupture of the Descemet's membrane swelling and thickening of the basal layer large fissure formed by infiltration of aqueous humor. The severity and detachment depth of the Descemet's membrane determine the recovery time of corneal edema. OCT can also show corneal scars, indicating healing status. The following anatomical features associated with the risk of corneal edema in keratoconus: increased epithelial thickness, stromal thinning, anterior hyperreflectives at the Bowman's layer level, and the absence of stromal scarring, could be identified by OCT [14]. OCT can also guide the treatment by monitoring the repair of Descemet's membrane after anterior chamber gas injection.

Case 3. A 25-year-old male patient with left keratoconus, sudden acute corneal edema.

It is necessary to appropriately grade patients to prevent clinical mistakes, as the accuracy of OCT in detecting epithelial thickness diminishes with disease severity. Ning et al. [15] set the cut-off values of mild, moderate, and severe keratoconus to 4.9 μm, 5.2 μm, and 7.4 μm for the different grades of the thinnest epithelial thickness. When the measurement difference is less than these thresholds, it is considered that the severity of the disease causes the difference within the permissible range. Otherwise, it is not clinically acceptable.

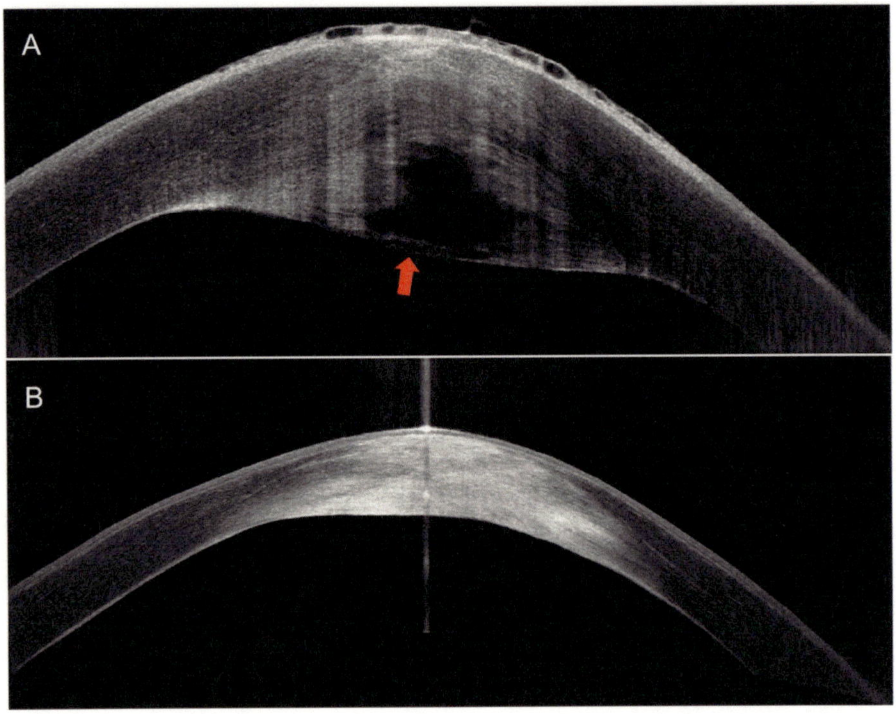

Figure 6.
A. Initial follow-up. The corneal thickness increased, the Descemet's membrane was broken (red arrow), and the interstromal fluid was accumulated. B. Six months later. The picture shows that the interlaminar fluid vanished and was replaced with dense white shadows caused by corneal scarring.

2.2 Treatment

OCT plays a vital role in the treatment monitoring of patients with keratoconus.

Frame glasses and soft contact lenses are difficult to provide good visual quality due to the irregularity of the front surface of keratoconus patients. Rigid gas permeable (RGP) and scleral lens (SL) are the most suitable ways to improve vision. OCT can measure the thickness of epithelium, stroma, and tear lens, which provides quantitative means for RGP matching [16]. A previous study showed that ideal central and edge tear film thicknesses were 35.1 ± 7.3 μm and 102.5 ± 12.1 μm for post-RGP patients, respectively [17]. OCT measurement is beneficial for RGP fitting and disease management. Parameters such as scleral curvature, scleral sagittal height or elevation, and corneal and scleral angle measured by OCT guide the selection of SL [18]. Approximately 20–30% of scleral lens wearers experience midday fogging in the post-lens tear layer. This condition involves the accumulation of debris or particulate matter, such as conjunctival lipid or mucin, which can reduce contrast sensitivity and visual acuity [19]. OCT is an evaluable method to instruct when to remove, rinse, refill, and reinsert the SL to maintain ideal vision. Since the thickness of the SL affects the oxygen exchange between the cornea and the air, OCT can be used to accurately measure the distribution of the thickness of the SL, to truly evaluate the overall permeability. The thickness of the tear lens, the material, and the time of wearing SL can all lead to corneal edema, but the corneal edema will quickly subside after the removal of SL. OCT can evaluate the time course and nature of corneal edema when wearing SL, which is helpful to explore the cause [20]. Furthermore, Controlling SL decentration is particularly important for customized front surface wavefront-guided correction of keratoconus. OCT imaging can quantify lens dispersion during SL wear by calculating the distance change between the normal to the anterior corneal apex and the normal to the apex of the anterior lens surface [21].

Intrastromal corneal ring segments (ICRS) implantation implants the ring into the corneal stroma to stabilize the cornea, improve the irregular corneal, and reduce the curvature, eventually improving visual quality for mild to moderate keratoconus [22]. Treating keratoconus with stromal ring is a reversible and adjustable surgical method. However, if the ICRS is placed too shallowly, it can compress the anterior stroma and may cause perforation of the anterior elastic layer, among other complications. Placing too deep can lead to complications such as perforation of the posterior elastic layer and acute corneal edema [23]. Therefore, preoperative assessment of corneal stromal thickness and intraoperative evaluation of the depth of tunnel creation are crucial. OCT can guide the placement of ICRS to ensure the safety and accuracy of the surgery. In addition, postoperatively, OCT can be used to detect whether the ICRS has shifted to ensure the visual quality of the patient after surgery. Analysis of epithelial remodeling after ICRS implantation by OCT helps to determine whether ICRS implantation regularizes the cornea and helps to analyze asymmetric stromal effects [24].

To halt the progression of keratoconus, CXL is the only way. It uses photosensitizers and light reactions to crosslink corneal tissue, thereby improving biomechanics. The most prominent feature in OCT after CXL surgery is the appearance of a boundary line within the stromal layer. The stromal boundary line is typically clearly visible at one month postoperatively, but may disappear at three months, sometimes replaced by faint irregular high-reflective lines within the deep stroma (**Figure 7**) [25]. It is generally believed to represent the boundary between crosslinked and uncrosslinked corneal stroma, and its depth is closely related to the therapeutic effect, allowing for comparison of the effectiveness of different crosslinking protocols. Thorsrud et al. proposed that OCT is more accurate than Scheimpflug and has a more extensive range than *in vivo* confocal microscopy (IVCM) in measuring demarcation line depth [26]. OCT after CXL surgery can also show reshaping of the corneal epithelium, manifested primarily as a more regular distribution of overall thickness, indicating surgical efficacy and explaining postoperative changes in corneal curvature and thickness [27].

Case 4. A 23-year-old male with corneal crosslinking.

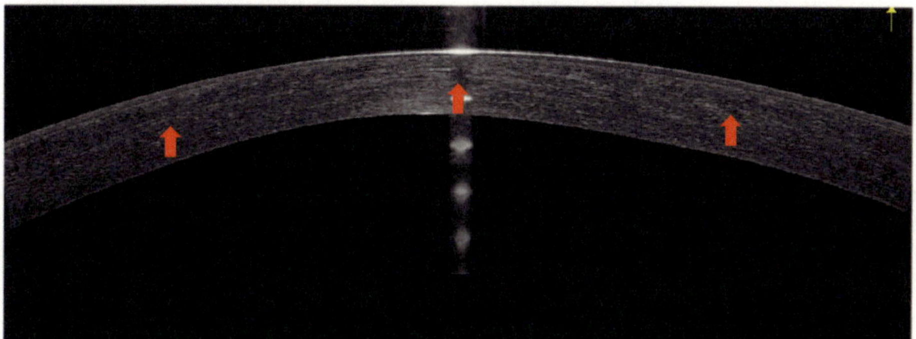

Figure 7.
OCT image demonstrates a white high-reflective line (red arrows), indicating the boundary between crosslinked and uncrosslinked areas.

For patients with corneal scarring and risk of corneal edema, keratoplasty is the only way to restore vision. Deep anterior lamellar keratoplasty (DALK) retains the Descemet's membrane and endothelial cell layer, replacing the stromal layer with the donor to reduce the risk of rejection. Penetrating keratoplasty (PKP) replaces the entire diseased corneal layer with donor tissue. However, the probability of rejection is relatively high, and progressive loss of donor endothelial cells may occur in the late stage [28]. Accurate imaging of OCT before surgery can guide the selection of surgical procedures: if there is a full-layer corneal scar, PKP should be selected. If a scar exists in the posterior cornea, large-bubble method should not be used to assist DALK, because it will affect the formation of large bubbles. In addition, OCT can also be used to evaluate the thickness, surface regularity, and the presence and location of corneal opacity for donor cornea to determine whether the donor is suitable for transplantation. During the operation, OCT can guide the manually separated or large-bubble assisted DALK drill ring to reach the deepest position to completely remove the stroma layer of the recipient for better visual effect. After the operation, OCT can be used to evaluate the effect of corneal transplantation by corneal thickness, opacity, and optical density distribution. OCT can also display poor graft-host interface adherence and identify double anterior chambers resulting from late spontaneous Descemet's membrane detachment.

3. Corneal ectasia after refractive surgery

Corneal refractive surgery, may lead to corneal ectasia, which manifests as a keratoconus-like condition characterized by progressive corneal distortion and compromised optical quality. Corneal ectasia is a rare but serious postoperative complication reported to occur in 0.02% to 0.6% of patients. It can occur as early as one week till years after surgery, 50% of cases within the first year, and up to 80% of cases within two years [29]. The precise pathogenesis of post-LASIK and photorefractive keratectomy (PRK) ectasia remains unclear, likely consequent to a combination of the factors. In some cases, the cornea may have had an underlying predisposition to keratoconus that was either undiagnosed preoperatively or presented as forme fruste keratoconus. Alternatively, tissue removal during LASIK or PRK may thin the cornea sufficiently, destabilizing its structural integrity and leading to subsequent ectasia. Remarkable risk factors for ectasia include high preoperative myopia, thin residual stromal bed, extent of tissue alteration, and particularly forme fruste keratoconus evident on preoperative topography [30].

Similar to keratoconus, the formation of the cone is associated with exhibit collagen fibril loss or slippage and alterations in the extracellular matrix within the stroma, contributing to biomechanical instability and subsequent changes in corneal anatomy and topography [31]. Post-LASIK ectasia typically manifests these changes predominantly in the residual stromal bed. To prevent refractive dilatation, it is essential to ensure the thickness of postoperative residual stroma through preoperative OCT measurement. In addition, due to a history of refractive surgery, a characteristic thickness change can be seen on OCT thickness maps: extensive corneal thickness thinning and cone area thinner (**Figures 8** and **9**).

Case 5. A 27-year-old female with corneal ectasia in her right eye, who had previously had corneal refractive surgery.

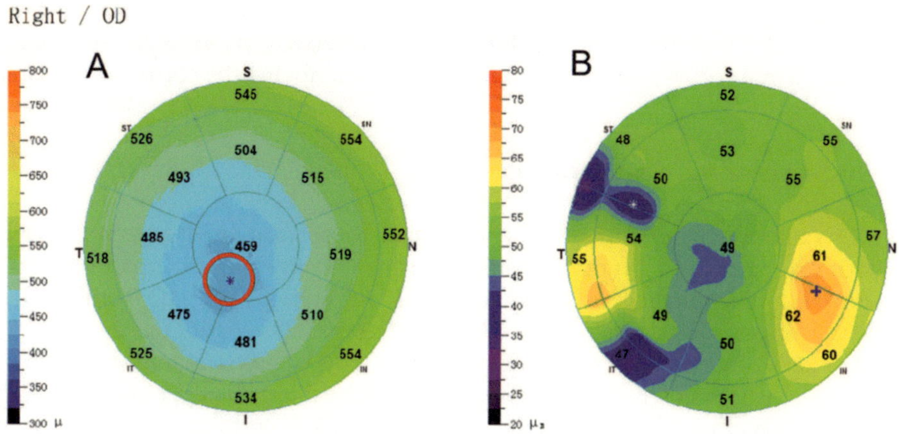

Figure 8.
A. Corneal thickness map. The decrease in corneal thickness is shown in blue, which is the characteristic manifestation after refractive surgery. Furthermore, a thinner area circled in red is the cone area. B. Corneal epithelial thickness map. The patient's epithelium was highly irregular, possibly due to epithelial remodeling after corneal dilation.

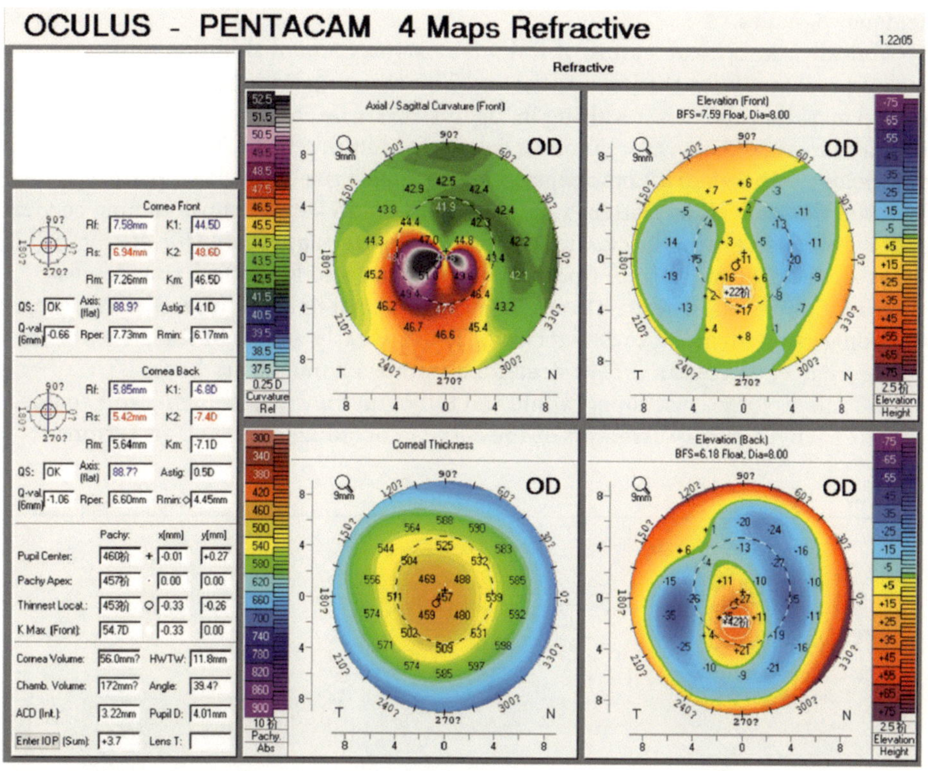

Figure 9.
The topography showed an increase in central anterior curvature and posterior corneal elevation. Kmax 54.7 D, Back elevation 42 μm.

There has been no definitive treatment to halt the progression of ectasia; however, CXL, a method commonly employed for keratoconus management, is believed to confer benefits in managing ectasia by reinforcing and stabilizing the corneal structure.

4. Pellucid marginal degeneration

PMD is a rare, non-inflammatory, and progressive corneal disease characterized by ectatic cornea thinning, typically found inferiorly. Its prevalence remains uncertain due to frequent misdiagnosis as keratoconus. The etiology of PMD is still unclear, and there is ongoing debate regarding whether it represents a distinct disease or a variant of keratoconus. In contrast to keratoconus, PMD tends to manifest later in life and progresses more slowly, with fewer associated visual impairments and a lower risk of corneal hydrops. The histopathology of PMD is similar to that of keratoconus, such as normal corneal epithelium and Descemet's membrane, significant thinning of the stromal layer and interruption of Bowman's layer, etc., but there are also differences. The difference in ultrastructural features, such as the architecture of collagen fibrils, proteoglycans, and keratocytes between PMD and keratoconus, have been identified, indicating potential distinct pathophysiological mechanisms. At the same time, PMD is typically considered bilateral, while unilateral cases have been reported. Gender preference is not clearly established, although some studies suggest a higher incidence in males.

Clinically, the critical feature of PMD is a narrow band of thinning typically located 1 to 2 mm from the inferior limbus. This thinning leads to a flattening of the vertical meridian above it, resulting in "against-the-rule" astigmatism. Additionally, an area of increased curvature is often below the thinning band. This characteristic morphology creates a distinct topographic map called the "crab claw" pattern. However, the "crab claw" pattern can also be present in keratoconus, making corneal topographic indices and the classical "crab claw" pattern unreliable for distinguishing PMD from keratoconus. In keratoconus, Vogt's striae and Fleischer's ring deposition can be observed, whereas these changes are absent in PMD. Nevertheless, these symptoms can be difficult to detect clinically in the early or subclinical stages of the disease. Hence, there is an urgent need for accurate diagnostic methods.

OCT allows for precise topographic and tomographic measurements and enables accurate pachymetric assessments of the cornea, including epithelial and stromal

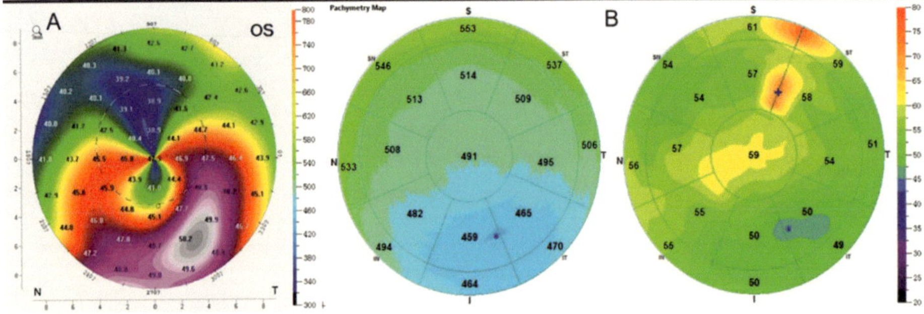

Figure 10.
A. The anterior surface curvature of this patient shows a classic "crab-claw" change. B. Corneal and epithelial thickness maps showed thinning of the inferior cornea.

thickness mapping, with high resolution and reliability. Mohr et al. [32] showed that the sublayer thickness of the infratemporal paracentral and inferior cornea measured by OCT helps to distinguish PMD from keratoconus. However, no evident corneal thinning was detected using Scheimpflug images [33]. The possible reason is that OCT has an advantage over traditional Scheimpflug imaging, owing to its superior axial and transversal resolution. It is worth mentioning that wide-field OCT measurements should be used to avoid misdiagnosis due to the inability to cover peripheral changes (**Figure 10**).

Case 6. A 32-year-old male with pellucid marginal degeneration (PMD).

PMD treatment is similar to keratoconus, including contact lenses, corneal crosslinking, stromal ring implantation, corneal transplantation, etc. The role of OCT in these treatment options has been described in detail in the previous article. Overall, OCT has played an important auxiliary role in diagnosing and treating PMD.

5. Conclusions

In summary, the application of OCT in corneal ectasia diseases aids in early diagnosis, disease monitoring, and evaluation of treatment efficacy, ultimately improving patient outcomes and quality of life.

Acknowledgements

This work was supported by the Project of National Natural Science Foundation of China (Grant No. 82271048); Science and Technology Commission of Shanghai Municipality (Grant No. 22S11900200, 23XD1420500); EYE & ENT Hospital of Fudan University High-level Talents Program (Grant No. 2021318); Program for Professor of Special Appointment (Eastern Scholar, TP2022046) at Shanghai Institutions of Higher Learning.

Conflict of interest

The authors declare no conflict of interest.

Nomenclature

OCT	optical coherence tomography
PMD	pellucid marginal degeneration
ICRS	intrastromal corneal ring segments
CXL	corneal crosslinking
DALK	deep anterior lamellar keratoplasty
IVCM	*in vivo* confocal microscopy
PKP	penetrating keratoplasty
PRK	photorefractive keratectomy
FFKC	forme fruste keratoconus

Author details

Jinhai Huang[1,2,3,4*], Yiran Wang[1,2,3,4], Kexin Li[1,2,3,4] and Xinning Yang[1,2,3,4]

1 Eye Institute and Department of Ophthalmology, Eye and ENT Hospital, Fudan University, Shanghai, China

2 NHC Key Laboratory of Myopia and Related Eye Diseases, Shanghai, China

3 Key Laboratory of Myopia and Related Eye Diseases, Chinese Academy of Medical Sciences, Shanghai, China

4 Shanghai Research Center of Ophthalmology and Optometry, Shanghai, China

*Address all correspondence to: vip999vip@163.com

References

[1] José APG, Donald T, Christopher JR, et al. Global consensus on keratoconus and ectatic diseases. Cornea. 2015;**34**(4):359-369. DOI: 10.1097/ico.0000000000000408

[2] Yang Y, Pavlatos E, Chamberlain W, Huang D, Li Y. Keratoconus detection using OCT corneal and epithelial thickness map parameters and patterns. Journal of Cataract and Refractive Surgery. 2021;**47**(6):759-766. DOI: 10.1097/j.jcrs.0000000000000498

[3] Li Y, Meisler D, Tang M, et al. Keratoconus diagnosis with optical coherence tomography pachymetry mapping. Ophthalmology. 2008;**115**(12):2159-2166. DOI: 10.1016/j.ophtha.2008.08.004

[4] Reinstein D, Gobbe M, Archer T, Silverman R, Coleman D. Epithelial, stromal, and total corneal thickness in keratoconus: Three-dimensional display with Artemis very-high frequency digital ultrasound. Journal of Refractive Surgery. 2010;**26**(4):259-271. DOI: 10.3928/1081597x-20100218-01

[5] Reinstein D, Archer T, Gobbe M. Rate of change of curvature of the corneal stromal surface drives epithelial compensatory changes and remodeling. Journal of Refractive Surgery. 2014;**30**(12):799-802. DOI: 10.3928/1081597x-20141113-02

[6] Huang D, Tang M, Shekhar R. Mathematical model of corneal surface smoothing after laser refractive surgery. American Journal of Ophthalmology. 2003;**135**(3):267-278. DOI: 10.1016/s0002-9394(02)01942-6

[7] Reinstein D, Gobbe M, Archer T, Couch D, Bloom B. Epithelial, stromal, and corneal pachymetry changes during orthokeratology. Optometry and Vision Science. 2009;**86**(8):E1006-E1014. DOI: 10.1097/OPX.0b013e3181b18219

[8] Sykakis E, Carley F, Irion L, Denton J, Hillarby M. An in depth analysis of histopathological characteristics found in keratoconus. Pathology. 2012;**44**(3):234-239. DOI: 10.1097/PAT.0b013e3283511b42

[9] Pircher N, Beer F, Holzer S, et al. Large field of view corneal epithelium and Bowman's layer thickness maps in Keratoconic and healthy eyes. American Journal of Ophthalmology. 2020;**209**:168-177. DOI: 10.1016/j.ajo.2019.05.025

[10] Yadav R, Kottaiyan R, Ahmad K, Yoon G. Epithelium and Bowman's layer thickness and light scatter in keratoconic cornea evaluated using ultrahigh resolution optical coherence tomography. Journal of Biomedical Optics. 2012;**17**(11):116010. DOI: 10.1117/1.Jbo.17.11.116010

[11] Sandali O, El Sanharawi M, Temstet C, et al. Fourier-domain optical coherence tomography imaging in keratoconus: A corneal structural classification. Ophthalmology. 2013;**120**(12):2403-2412. DOI: 10.1016/j.ophtha.2013.05.027

[12] Sharma N, Mannan R, Jhanji V, et al. Ultrasound biomicroscopy-guided assessment of acute corneal hydrops. Ophthalmology. 2011;**118**(11):2166-2171. DOI: 10.1016/j.ophtha.2011.03.040

[13] Sharma N, Maharana P, Jhanji V, Vajpayee R. Management of acute corneal hydrops in ectatic corneal disorders. Current Opinion in Ophthalmology.

2012;**23**(4):317-323. DOI: 10.1097/ICU.0b013e328354a2a8

[14] Fuentes E, Sandali O, El Sanharawi M, et al. Anatomic predictive factors of acute corneal hydrops in Keratoconus: An optical coherence tomography study. Ophthalmology. 2015;**122**(8):1653-1659. DOI: 10.1016/j.ophtha.2015.04.031

[15] Ning R, Wang Y, Xu Z, et al. Assessing progression limits in different grades of keratoconus from a novel perspective: Precision of measurements of the corneal epithelium. Eye and Vision. 2024;**11**(1):1. DOI: 10.1186/s40662-023-00368-9

[16] Valdes G, Romaguera M, Serramito M, Cerviño A, Gonzalo CG. OCT applications in contact lens fitting. Contact Lens & Anterior Eye. 2022;**45**(4):101540. DOI: 10.1016/j.clae.2021.101540

[17] Elbendary A, Abou SW. Evaluation of rigid gas permeable lens fitting in keratoconic patients with optical coherence tomography. Graefe's Archive for Clinical and Experimental Ophthalmology. 2013;**251**(6):1565-1570. DOI: 10.1007/s00417-013-2271-1

[18] Vincent S, Alonso-Caneiro D, Collins M. Optical coherence tomography and scleral contact lenses: Clinical and research applications. Clinical & Experimental Optometry. 2019;**102**(3):224-241. DOI: 10.1111/cxo.12814

[19] Carracedo G, Serramito-Blanco M, Martin-Gil A, Wang Z, Rodriguez-Pomar C, Pintor J. Post-lens tear turbidity and visual quality after scleral lens wear. Clinical & Experimental Optometry. 2017;**100**(6):577-582. DOI: 10.1111/cxo.12512

[20] Vincent S, Alonso-Caneiro D, Collins M. The time course and nature of corneal oedema during sealed miniscleral contact lens wear. Contact Lens & Anterior Eye. 2019;**42**(1):49-54. DOI: 10.1016/j.clae.2018.03.001

[21] Vincent S, Alonso-Caneiro D, Collins M. The temporal dynamics of miniscleral contact lenses: Central corneal clearance and centration. Contact Lens & Anterior Eye. 2018;**41**(2):162-168. DOI: 10.1016/j.clae.2017.07.002

[22] Modi N, Haneen J-H. Depth of intrastromal corneal ring segments by OCT. European Journal of Ophthalmology. 2012;**23**(2):171-176. DOI: 10.5301/ejo.5000212

[23] Barbara R, Barbara A, Naftali M. Depth evaluation of intended vs actual intacs intrastromal ring segments using optical coherence tomography. Eye (London, England). 2015;**30**(1):102-110. DOI: 10.1038/eye.2015.202

[24] Abdelmajid B, Sofiene K, Clementine D, et al. Asymmetric Intrastromal corneal ring segments with Progressive Base width and thickness for Keratoconus: Evaluation of efficacy and analysis of epithelial Remodeling. Journal of Clinical Medicine. 2023;**12**(4):1673. DOI: 10.3390/jcm12041673

[25] Hafezi F, Kling S, Gilardoni F, et al. Individualized corneal cross-linking with riboflavin and UV-A in ultrathin corneas: The Sub400 protocol. American Journal of Ophthalmology. 2021;**224**:133-142. DOI: 10.1016/j.ajo.2020.12.011

[26] Thorsrud A, Sandvik G, Hagem A, Drolsum L. Measuring the depth of crosslinking demarcation line in vivo: Comparison of methods and devices. Journal of Cataract and Refractive Surgery. 2017;**43**(2):255-262. DOI: 10.1016/j.jcrs.2017.01.003

[27] Haberman I, Lang P, Broncano A, Kim S, Hafezi F, Randleman J. Epithelial remodeling after corneal crosslinking using higher fluence and accelerated treatment time. Journal of Cataract and Refractive Surgery. 2018;**44**(3):306-312. DOI: 10.1016/j.jcrs.2017.12.021

[28] Christin H, Mayank AN. Systematic review comparing penetrating keratoplasty and deep anterior lamellar keratoplasty for management of keratoconus. Contact Lens & Anterior Eye. 2016;**40**(1):3-14. DOI: 10.1016/j.clae.2016.10.001

[29] Giri P, Azar D. Risk profiles of ectasia after keratorefractive surgery. Current Opinion in Ophthalmology. 2017;**28**(4):337-342. DOI: 10.1097/icu.0000000000000383

[30] Hersh P, Stulting R, Muller D, Durrie D, Rajpal R. U.S. Multicenter clinical trial of corneal collagen crosslinking for treatment of corneal ectasia after refractive surgery. Ophthalmology. 2017;**124**(10):1475-1484. DOI: 10.1016/j.ophtha.2017.05.036

[31] Meek K, Tuft S, Huang Y, et al. Changes in collagen orientation and distribution in keratoconus corneas. Investigative Ophthalmology & Visual Science. 2005;**46**(6):1948-1956. DOI: 10.1167/iovs.04-1253

[32] Mohr N, Shajari M, Krause D, et al. Pellucid marginal degeneration versus keratoconus: Distinction with wide-field SD-OCT corneal sublayer pachymetry. The British Journal of Ophthalmology. 2021;**105**(12):1638-1644. DOI: 10.1136/bjophthalmol-2020-316496

[33] Niklas P, Jan L, Stephan H, Andreas G, Gerald S. Corneal crosslinking for pellucid marginal degeneration. Journal of Cataract and Refractive Surgery. 2019;**45**(8):1163-1167. DOI: 10.1016/j.jcrs.2019.03.018

Chapter 5

OCT Imaging for Measuring Structural Changes in the Cornea for Evaluating Tonometers

Han Saem Cho, Sae Chae Jeoung and Yun Sik Yang

Abstract

Intraocular pressure (IOP), which is a hydrodynamic pressure inside the anterior chamber of the eye, is a fundamental measurement to evaluate an eye condition. If the anterior chamber is described as a closed system surrounded by a soft cornea, the structural characteristics of the cornea, including corneal radius of curvature (CRC) and central corneal thickness (CCT), should be governed by the IOP changes. In this chapter, we have proposed a theoretical framework in analytical form to describe the circumferential motion of the cornea in terms of the Young's modulus and the Poisson's ratio. The proposed model has successfully been applied to describe corneal structural changes observed by optical coherence tomography (OCT) images. This chapter will discuss the application of OCT technology to investigate deformations of central corneal structures with high resolution at high speed.

Keywords: cornea, intraocular pressure (IOP), optical coherence tomography (OCT), central corneal thickness (CCT), corneal radius of curvature (CRC)

1. Introduction

The eye is a spherical structure filled with liquid and gel-like substances. Aqueous humor, the liquid within the eye, circulates internally. If this circulation is disrupted, it results in increased internal pressure in the eye, leading to glaucoma, which can damage the optic nerve [1–4]. Early diagnosis of this type of glaucoma is crucial because once the optic nerve is damaged, it cannot be restored. The primary method to diagnose glaucoma involves measuring intraocular pressure (IOP), which is the internal pressure of the eye [1, 2]. Devices used for this measurement are called tonometers, with the Goldmann tonometer and non-contact tonometer being commonly used in clinical settings. Accurate measurement of IOP is vital for early-stage glaucoma diagnosis. Thus, evaluating the accuracy of tonometers is crucial. Since it is challenging to measure IOP directly, it is done indirectly through the cornea. The cornea, a flexible tissue, structurally deforms when IOP increases, which can affect the IOP measurement. To measure IOP accurately, it is necessary to analyze these structural changes in the cornea. Optical coherence tomography (OCT) is the most optimized technology for this purpose. OCT is an imaging technology that uses light interference signals, capable of detecting signals backscattered from the sample and generating high-resolution tomographic images in axial direction. This technology allows for imaging subtle structural changes in the cornea caused by changes in IOP. In this chapter, we provide an overview of the anatomy of the eye and the flow of aqueous humor, which is strongly related to the IOP (Sections 2.1–2.2). We also discuss measurement methods of IOP (Sections 2.3–2.4). Additionally, we review currently available methods, including OCT, to investigate corneal structure quantitatively (Sections 3.1–3.2). Furthermore, we highlight the details of how to quantitatively measure and evaluate the structural deformation of the cornea changes caused by IOP alteration using OCT technology (Sections 4.1–4.2). We will further propose the methods for measuring and evaluating tonometers using this technology (Section 4.3).

2. Basic knowledge of ophthalmology

2.1 The eye

The human eyeball (shown in **Figure 1**) is a spherical structure filled with liquid and gel. Its antero-posterior diameter is approximately 24 mm, with a horizontal axis longer than the vertical axis [3, 5]. The eyeball comprises three main parts: the outer membrane, the middle membrane, and the inner membrane [3]. The outer membrane includes the transparent cornea, which receives light from the outside, and the sclera, a tough, opaque white tissue that maintains the shape of the eye. The middle membrane consists of the iris, ciliary body, and choroid. The iris is a circular membrane around the pupil that contracts and relaxes to regulate the amount of light entering the eye. The ciliary body connects the choroid to the iris's outer edge and is triangular in cross-section, comprising the ciliary epithelium, ciliary stroma, and ciliary muscle. It surrounds the lens and aids in controlling its shape by contracting and relaxing. Additionally, the anterior surface of the ciliary body produces aqueous humor, while its posterior surface interfaces with the gel-like vitreous body. The choroid is a thin membrane rich in blood vessels located between the sclera and the retina, supplying oxygen and nutrients to the eye. The innermost membrane is the retina, where the optic nerve distributes and serves as nerve tissue crucial for light reception. Light detected by the photoreceptors in the retina is transmitted as signals through the optic nerve to the brain. The optic nerve

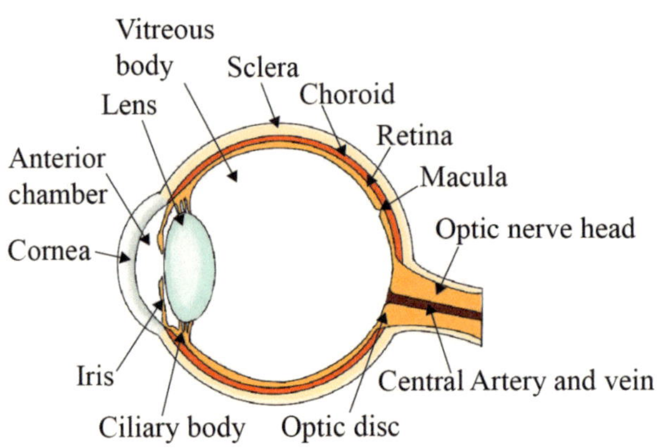

Figure 1.
Structure of the eyeball.

head, where these nerves converge and connect to the brain, forms a blind spot incapable of detecting light due to the absence of optic nerve fibers.

The eye is broadly divided into two parts based on the lens: the anterior segment and the posterior segment [3, 5]. The anterior segment includes the cornea, iris, anterior chamber, ciliary body, and lens. The space between the cornea and iris, filled with aqueous humor, is known as the anterior chamber. On the other hand, the posterior segment includes the vitreous body, retina, choroid, sclera, and optic nerve located behind the lens. This segment is primarily examined to diagnose abnormalities related to the optic nerve. The posterior segment is mainly associated with vision and is examined when diagnosing vision-related abnormalities. On the other hand, because the anterior segment contains areas where aqueous humor circulates and is produced and drained, it is observed when diagnosing abnormalities in aqueous humor circulation and intraocular pressure.

2.2 Anterior segment of the eye

As mentioned earlier, the anterior segment of the eye refers to the part in front of the vitreous body and includes the cornea, iris, anterior chamber, ciliary body, and lens. The anterior chamber, located between the iris and the cornea, is filled with aqueous humor produced by the ciliary body shown in **Figure 2**. The average volume of the anterior chamber is approximately 0.25–0.3 mL [3, 6, 7]. Additionally, aqueous humor drains through the trabecular meshwork. This production and drainage of aqueous humor facilitate its circulation.

The cornea depicted in **Figure 3** is transparent and has a higher curvature compared to other parts of the eye, allowing it to transmit light to the retina inside the eye. It is convex but slightly oval in shape. The size of the cornea varies considerably among individuals, but on average, its diameter is approximately 10.6 mm vertically and 11.7 mm horizontally [3, 5]. The posterior part of the cornea is concave and circular, with a diameter of about 11.7 mm [3]. The central portion of the cornea is thinnest, measuring approximately 0.4–0.7 mm, while the peripheral part is thicker. The radius of curvature of the anterior surface of the cornea is approximately 7.5–8.5 mm, and the radius of curvature of the posterior surface is about 6.5–7.5 mm. Structurally, the cornea is composed of five layers: epithelium, Bowman's layer, stroma, Descemet's membrane, and endothelium. The cornea is avascular and lacks lymphatic drainage. It

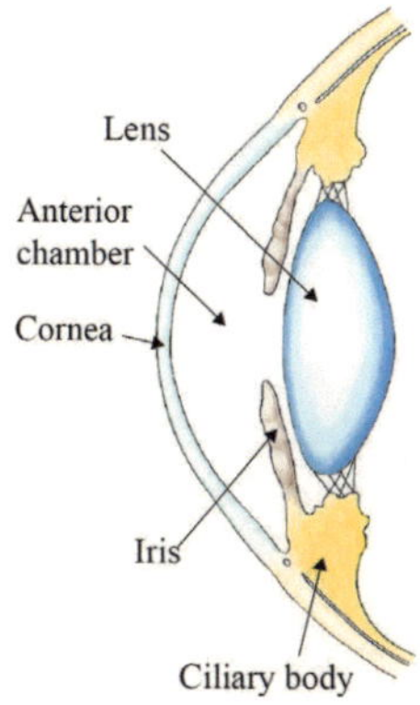

Figure 2.
Structure of the anterior segment of the eye.

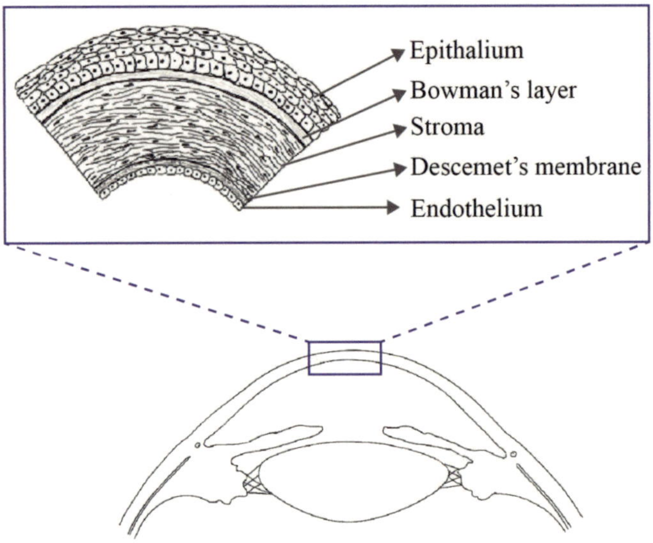

Figure 3.
Structure of the cornea.

receives nourishment from the anterior ciliary arteries of the conjunctiva and sclera, as well as from the aqueous humor.

The ciliary body shown in **Figure 4(a)** is a tissue that connects the choroid and iris. It forms a complete ring shape and has a triangular cross-section. The ciliary processes of the ciliary body are characterized by numerous folds or ridges and are responsible for producing aqueous humor [3, 5]. Additionally, the ciliary zonules, which are part of the ciliary body, attach to the lens and play a role in suspending and positioning it. Moreover, the ciliary muscle is involved in controlling the shape of the lens and functions to adjust focus for objects at varying distances.

The limbus shown in **Figure 4(b)** is the transitional zone between the cornea and sclera of the eye. It forms a narrow ring surrounding the cornea. Within the limbus are the trabecular meshwork and Schlemm's canal, which are involved in draining aqueous

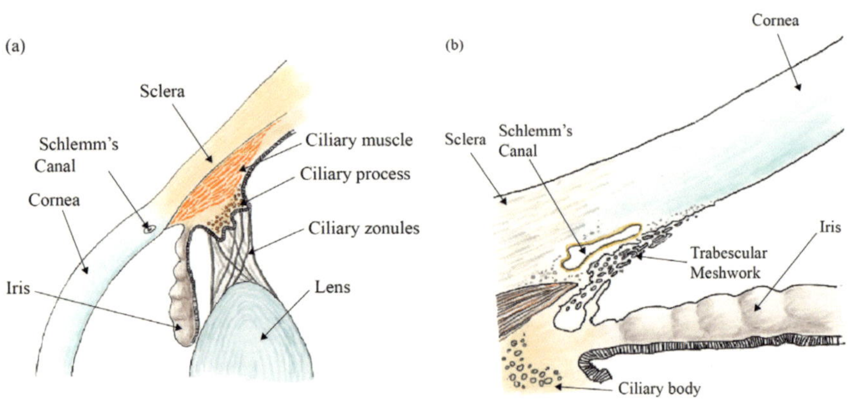

Figure 4.
Structure of (a) the ciliary body and (b) the limbus.

humor. The trabecular meshwork is a spongy tissue composed of thin, column-shaped structures that create a network of channels through which aqueous humor flows [3, 5, 6]. This tissue acts like a sieve, facilitating the movement of aqueous humor from the anterior chamber to Schlemm's canal. It is a circular channel located circumferentially around the cornea near the iris. It functions as the primary drainage pathway for aqueous humor that has passed through the trabecular meshwork [3, 6, 8].

As mentioned earlier, aqueous humor is produced by the ciliary body (see **Figure 5**). It flows between the suspensory ligaments of the lens and enters the anterior chamber through the pupil. Approximately 90% of the aqueous humor outflow occurs through the trabecular meshwork, Schlemm's canal, and the aqueous veins [3, 6, 8]. The remaining 10% exits through the anterior surface of the ciliary body [3]. Some aqueous humor may be absorbed into the vortex veins through the scleral fenestra. A small amount can enter the blood vessels of the iris or diffuse through the vitreous and reach the blood vessels of the retina and optic nerve. Diffusion through the cornea is also a possible route of outflow [3, 6].

2.3 Intraocular pressure

Intraocular pressure (IOP) refers to the pressure of the fluid inside the eye. Maintaining stable IOP is crucial for the health and function of the eye. The normal range of IOP is generally considered to be between 10 and 21 mmHg [1, 2, 7, 9]. Elevated IOP can lead to deformation of the retina and optic nerve head, which are susceptible to external pressure, increasing the risk of developing glaucoma—a condition that damages the optic nerve [1, 4, 6]. There are various causes of increased IOP [3, 6, 8, 10]. Firstly, impaired drainage of aqueous humor can occur. The trabecular meshwork and Schlemm's canal are the primary pathways for aqueous humor drainage in the anterior chamber of the eye. If these pathways become blocked or function improperly,

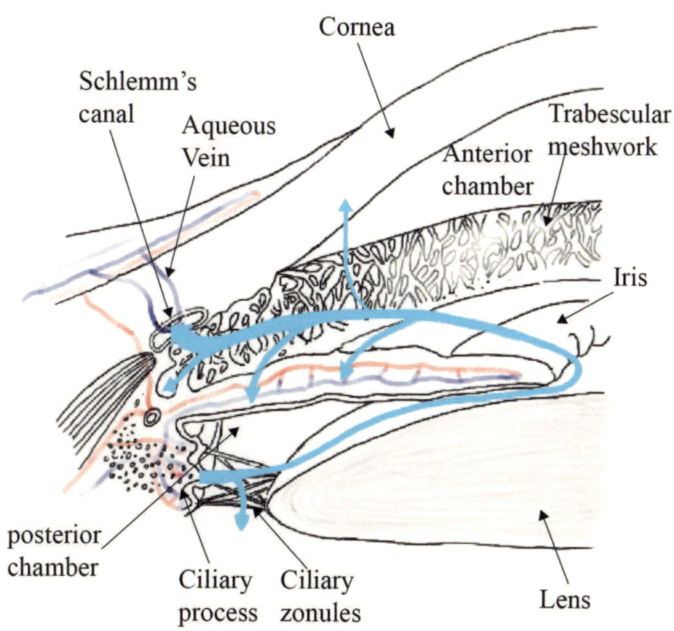

Figure 5.
Circulation of aqueous humor in the anterior chamber of the eye.

IOP can rise. Secondly, overproduction of aqueous humor can lead to elevated IOP. Aqueous humor is produced in the ciliary body, and conditions like neovascular glaucoma or uveitis can cause excessive production. Inflammatory eye diseases such as uveitis or iridocyclitis can also increase IOP by disrupting the normal drainage of aqueous humor. Additionally, genetic factors and systemic diseases, including hypertension or diabetes, can affect IOP [11, 12]. Monitoring and managing IOP is crucial for preventing vision loss and managing glaucoma. Since measuring IOP is a fundamental diagnostic method for many eye conditions, numerous methods have been developed to quantitatively measure IOP. The most well-known and still considered the gold-standard method is Goldmann applanation tonometry [13, 14]. Non-contact tonometry is another widely used method for measuring IOP during health check-ups. Additionally, rebound tonometry is an easy-to-use method suitable for measuring IOP in difficult-to-measure situations. Recently, a disposable lens-type portable tonometer has been developed, allowing users to self-measure IOP in daily life.

2.4 Types of tonometers currently used clinically

2.4.1 Goldmann tonometer

The Goldmann tonometer (GAT), of which conceptual force balance is depicted in **Figure 6**, is a method developed by Hans Goldmann and Theo Schmidt in 1957 to measure the force required to flatten a specific area of the cornea and convert it into IOP [1, 13, 14]. This technique is based on the Imbert-Fick principle [15], described by the equation:

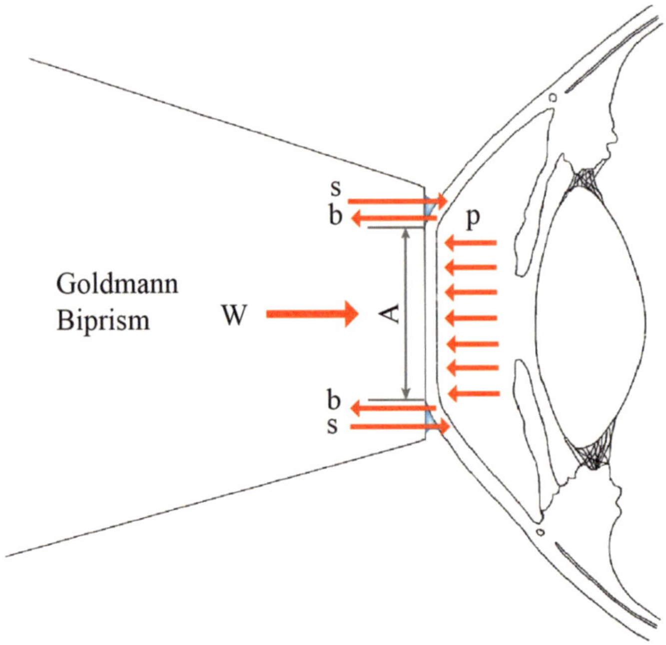

Figure 6.
Forces for Goldmann applanation tonometry. While flattening the corneal surface, the sum of the forces (W) caused by the biprism and surface tension (s) due to the tear films between the corneal surface and the biprism is balanced with those due to the intraocular pressure (p) and corneal rigidity (b).

DOI: http://dx.doi.org/10.5772/intechopen.1007803

$$W = pA \tag{1}$$

where W is the applanation force, p is the pressure of a body of fluid encapsulated within a sphere, and A is the area of applanation. This principle assumes that the surface containing the fluid is infinitely thin, perfectly elastic, and flexible. However, in reality, not all surfaces behave this way. When applying this principle to flatten the cornea, the specific characteristics of the cornea must be considered. Goldmann adjusted the equation to incorporate these factors:

$$W + s = PA + b \tag{2}$$

where W is the tonometer force, s is the surface tension of corneal tear film, P is the intraocular pressure, A is the area of applanation, and b represents the corneal rigidity to bending.

In Eq. (2), the area A was calculated to be 7.35 mm^2, considering the balance between corneal rigidity and tear film surface tension forces, which formed the basis for designing the GAT [1]. The GAT setup includes a slit lamp, microscope, and biprism. Fluorescent dye is applied to the cornea under examination, and blue light from the slit lamp is directed onto it. The biprism is used to flatten the corneal surface. During this process, the desired applanation area is verified by observing the fluorescent tear meniscus through the microscope. When viewed through the biprism, the meniscus appears as two divided semicircular rings. The correct amount of pressure is applied when the inner edges of these two semicircles just touch, as shown in **Figure 7(c)**.

2.4.2 Non-contact tonometer

This is a method of flattening the cornea using a non-contact tonometer (NCT) with an air puff, developed in the 1970s [1]. As shown in **Figure 8**, the air puffs are delivered rapidly to enable much quicker measurements compared to GAT. It is non-contact and simple to use, making it widely employed in primary health check-ups. The NCT consists primarily of an air-puff generator, infrared light emitter, and detector. Without any external stimulation, the convex cornea surface scatters the lights from the emitter in all directions. Meanwhile, if the air puffs flatten the cornea, the corneal surface acts like a flat mirror, reflecting light that can be detected. This reflection allows measurement of IOP based on the time it takes for the corneal surface to flatten after the air pulse is sprayed. Modern devices use pressure transducers to directly measure the air pulse pressure needed to achieve corneal flattening. While NCT offers faster measurements compared to GAT, it is less accurate and precise in IOP measurement due to its instantaneous and dynamic nature. Recently, several devices have been developed that not only measure IOP but also assess corneal characteristics. One such device is the ocular response analyzer (ORA), which measures the dynamic properties of the cornea using air pulses and evaluates corneal hysteresis and resistance factor to assess the viscoelastic and biomechanical properties of the cornea [1, 16]. Another device is the CORVIS ST tonometer, which records corneal deformation caused by air pulses using a high-speed camera to evaluate the biomechanical properties of the cornea [1, 17].

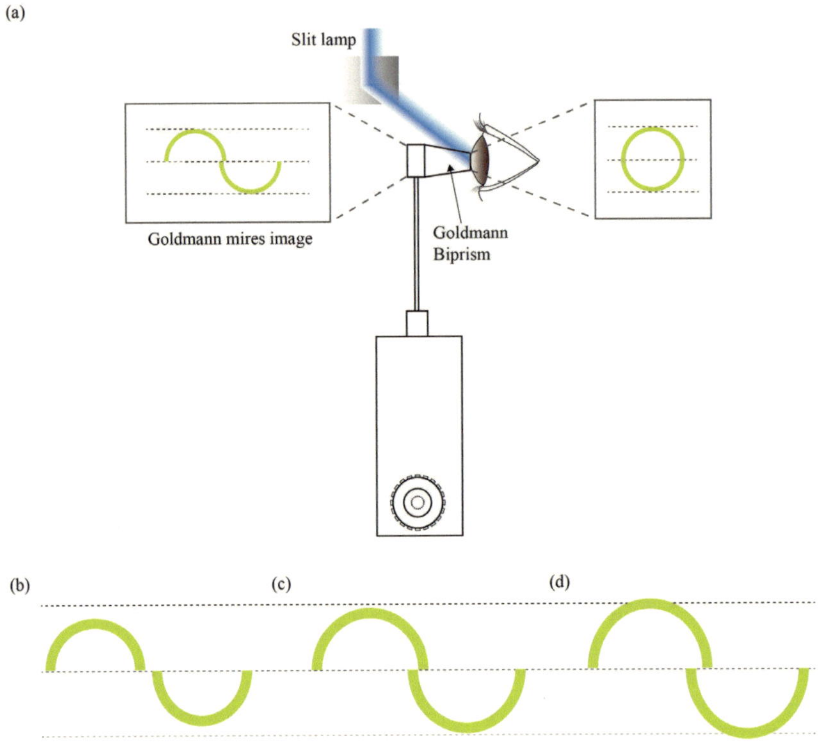

Figure 7.
(a) The operating principle of the Goldmann applanation tonometer (GAT) and the images of fluorescein-stained meniscus when the flattening force is (b) low, (c) proper, and (d) high compared to the intraocular pressure (IOP).

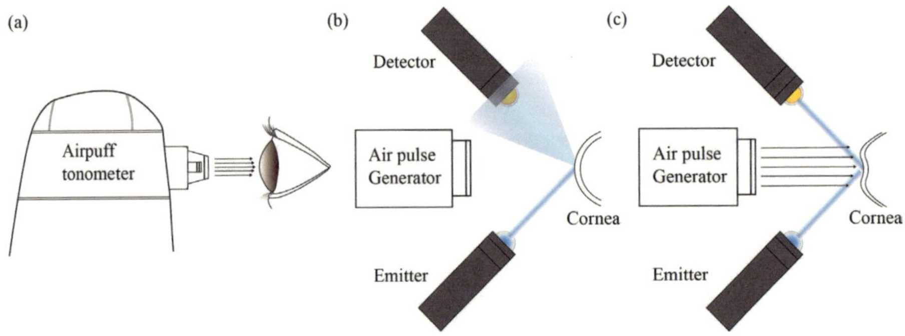

Figure 8.
(a) The operating principle of the non-contact tonometer (NCT). The light intensity detected has varied before (b) and after (c) issuing an air puff due to the changes in the curvature of the corneal surface.

2.4.3 Other types of tonometers

It has been reported that the highest values of IOP mainly contribute to the progression of glaucoma. Therefore, it is essential to continuously monitor IOP to verify and control the risk factor of the progression [18, 19]. Meanwhile, the GAT as a gold-standard medical instrument for IOP measurement as well as the NCT are subject to time and space constraints because patients should visit a hospital. This makes it difficult for patients to continuously monitor their IOP. To overcome these limitations, much effort has been made to develop other non-invasive ways to routinely measure the IOP. The use of home tonometry like a rebound-type tonometer is widely used. And also, the contact-lens type method has been introduced as a promising candidate for wearable IOP sensors.

2.4.3.1 Rebound tonometers

As shown in **Figure 9(a)**, a rebound tonometer consisting of a solenoid propelling coil, a sensing coil, and a thin probe [1, 20]. A brief electrical current into the solenoid causes the magnetized probe to shortly extend toward the cornea. Upon contact with the cornea, the probe rebounds, and this impact is detected by the sensing coil through electromagnetic induction. The duration of the impact is measured and converted into IOP. This method was introduced and commercialized as the hand-held tonometer like the 'Tono-Pen' and 'iCare' products [1, 21]. Unlike the GAT or NCT, the rebound tonometer does not require the patient to be seated during measurement. This makes it suitable for measuring the IOP in the supine position of the disabled patients and young children who cannot sit still. The correlation between IOP measurements using the tonometer and the Goldmann tonometer was reported to be acceptable [22]. Most portable tonometers available at home require that the patient or guardian take manual measurements. And also, the IOP measured by the patients using the rebound tonometers may differ by 5 mmHg compared with the IOP measured by a physician using the tonometers [23, 24]. Although the rebound-type tonometry can provide promising performance for measuring the IOP in supine position, there are still some issues, including lower accuracy and sensitivity compared to other methods, which limits its suitability for precise intraocular pressure measurements.

2.4.3.2 Contact-lens type tonometry

The rebound tonometry can be applied to routinely measure the IOP. However, the tonometry is not able to provide real-time continuous measurements of the IOP. To overcome these limitations, extensive efforts have been made to develop contact-lens

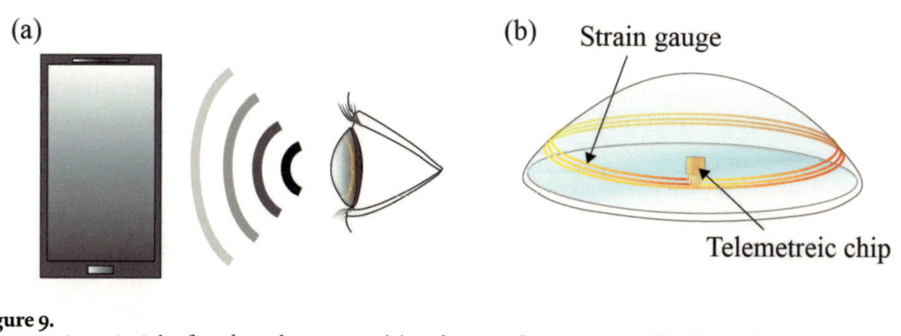

Figure 9.
The operating principle of a rebound tonometer (a) and contact-lens tonometer (b). The probe can strike the surface of the cornea due to the injection of a brief current into the solenoidal coil. The rebound tonometers detected the changes in the variation of the induction accompanied by an abrupt change in the motion of the probe, which is dependent on the IOP. For contact-lens tonometry, the strain sensors, which are embedded in soft contact lenses, can detect the changes in the limbal strain alterations accompanied by IOP changes.

sensors, which provide continuous real-time monitoring of the IOP. As shown in **Figure 9(b)**, the sensors can detect the changes in a strain due to an expansion of the corneal limbus accompanied by the IOP increment [25]. 'Triggerfish' is the commercialized contact-lens sensors for IOP changes after FDA approval [26]. This device with a wireless antenna and a ring-shaped strain gauge embedded into a soft hydrophilic silicone contact lens is rigid, bulky, partially blocking vision area, or insufficiently sensitive to monitoring the deformation of only 0.03% in tensile strain per mmHg of human subjects. More sophisticated designs of the devices were introduced to improve the performance of the contact-lens sensors [27]. More recently, T. Y. Kim reported a wireless theranostic smart contact lens that can monitor continuous real-time IOP measures and even take appropriate drug treatment in response to the IOP increment [28]. Meanwhile, the knowledge about the structural changes accompanied with IOP changes of human subjects is very limited to fully describe the detailed dependence of the strain and the IOP for the patients, whose eyes have different structural and mechanical characteristics. The deformation of the limbus strain of the human subjects less than 0.03% led us to suppose that the deeper understandings on the dependence of mechanical and structural changes in the human cornea on the IOP are crucial to improving the performance of the contact-lens sensors to monitor the IOP.

3. Technologies for measuring structural changes in the cornea

When the pressure within the eye, filled with liquid and gel, fluctuates, the three layers surrounding the eye also undergo changes. Among these layers, the cornea is the most flexible and exposed to external conditions. Consequently, variations in IOP affect the cornea the most. Accurate measurement of these changes in the cornea can help detect fluctuations in IOP, and understanding the mechanical properties of the cornea enables estimation of true IOP. Therefore, monitoring and imaging structural changes in the cornea are crucial for precise measurement of intraocular pressure and diagnosis of glaucoma.

3.1 Previous instruments for measuring structural changes in the cornea

Methods for quantitatively measuring structural changes in the cornea include assessing changes in corneal thickness or measuring corneal curvature. The earliest method used to measure corneal thickness was optical pachymetry, which operates on the principle of specular reflection. However, this method lacks precision and faces limitations such as variability due to corneal curvature or clarity. In the 1960s, ultrasound technology introduced ultrasonic pachymetry, a method using ultrasound waves to measure corneal thickness that provided more stable measurements compared to optical methods [29]. Despite its stability, ultrasound pachymetry requires direct contact with the cornea and the use of a gel medium to prevent air-tissue reflections. To address these limitations, non-contact optical methods for measuring corneal thickness have been developed [30–33]. These methods utilize slit scanning and Scheimpflug imaging technology, offering higher resolution and greater convenience compared to ultrasound-based approaches. In the nineteenth century, the development of the keratometer marked a significant advancement in measuring corneal curvature in clinical settings [34]. Introduced by Emile Javal and Hjalmar Schiotz, this device focused on the corneal vertex, enabling curvature measurements approximately 3 mm from the center [35]. Subsequently, Antonio Placido introduced the Placido disc, which measures corneal curvature by analyzing the distortion of concentric black and white rings projected onto the cornea [30, 31]. In 1896, Allvar Gullstrand developed the photokeratoscope, which qualitatively assessed corneal curvature based on images captured with a Placido disc [36, 37]. Advancements in digital technology led to the videokeratoscope in the 1980s, which quantifies ring images as color maps [31]. By the 1990s, advancements in slit scanning technology enabled equipment to analyze the posterior corneal surface, expanding capabilities beyond simple topography to monolayer assessments of the cornea [31, 38]. In the 2000s, Scheimpflug imaging technology further improved accuracy in measuring the posterior corneal surface, enhancing aerial photography-based techniques [30, 31].

3.2 OCT imaging for measuring structural changes in the cornea

OCT is a technology that utilizes light interference signals to produce tomographic images of the object [39, 40]. It excels in detecting even the faintest light signals emitted from the sample, owing to its heterodyne gain characteristic, where signal intensity is determined by the interaction between the light from the sample and the light from a reference mirror. While traditional confocal microscopy typically achieves sensitivity levels between −50 and 70 dB, OCT achieves sensitivity ranging from approximately −90–110 dB [41]. Moreover, OCT can rapidly capture a single tomographic image in the axial direction, making it widely adopted as a bioimaging technique. With a resolution of about ten micrometers, OCT is suitable for imaging tissue structures rather than individual cells [42]. Consequently, its most impactful applications in the human body have been in ophthalmology [43–53]. Since its introduction as a novel imaging modality in ophthalmology, OCT has been extensively studied for imaging the posterior segment of the eye [43, 45–48, 52]. However, recognizing the diagnostic utility of OCT in the anterior segment of the eye, ongoing development of OCT imaging systems for anterior segment observation has progressed [44, 49–51]. These systems are valuable for monitoring corneal pathology development as well as for imaging and measuring the anterior chamber angle and structural changes in the iris. The configuration of an OCT system for anterior segment of an eye imaging is depicted in **Figure 10**. OCT systems for the anterior segment of the eye currently in active use are a second-generation configuration, primarily categorized into Fourier domain OCT (FD-OCT) and swept-source OCT (SS-OCT).

The FD-OCT comprises a broadband light source and an interferometer, as illustrated in **Figure 10(a)**. The sample arm, responsible for imaging the sample, includes a scanning unit such as galvano mirrors and an objective lens, enabling two-dimensional and three-dimensional imaging. The reference arm is designed with an optical path similar to the sample arm, ending with a reference mirror where light backscattered from the sample and reflected from the mirror interfere. The interference signal is detected and acquired using a spectrometer, capturing spectralized interference signals. In contrast, SS-OCT utilizes a wavelength-swept light source, and its detection part involves a single detector instead of a spectrometer. SS-OCT (**Figure 10(b)**) is being increasingly introduced in ophthalmic OCT and offers the advantage of high-speed imaging compared to FD-OCT systems using CCDs. Recent research and development in SS-OCT enable imaging at speeds in the MHz range, which is approximately 10–100 times faster than conventional systems [54, 55]. This high-speed capability allows for precise measurement of structural changes in the cornea. In comparison, Scheimpflug imaging, which measures corneal radius of curvature (CRC) or central corneal thickness (CCT), lags behind OCT in imaging

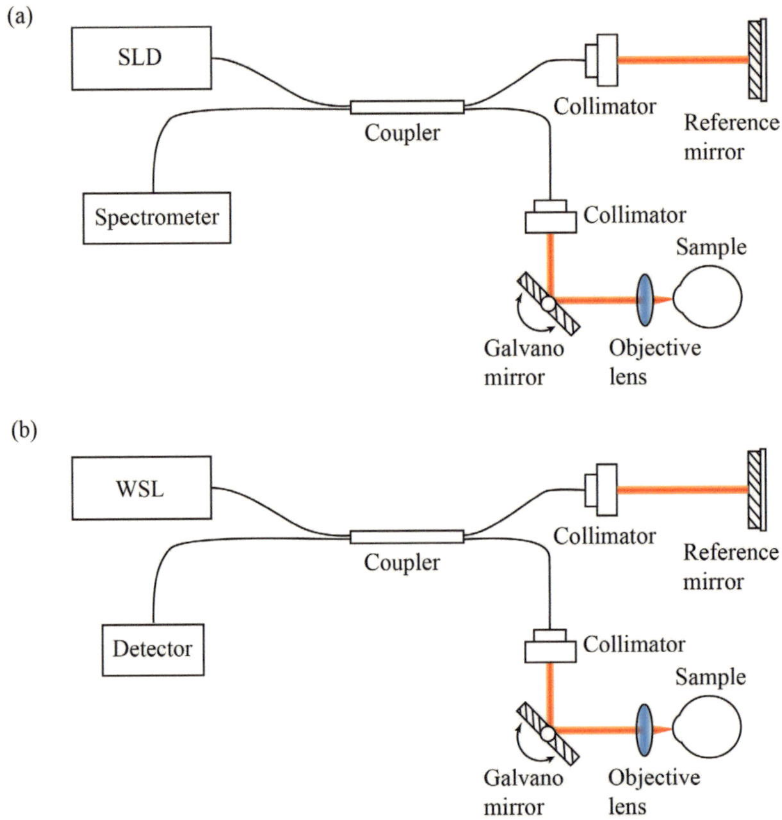

Figure 10.
The configuration of (a) Fourier domain optical coherence tomography (FD-OCT) and (b) swept-source optical coherence tomography (SS-OCT) for anterior segment of the eye imaging (SLD: super-luminescent diode laser, WSL: wavelength swept laser).

speed and is thus less suitable for dynamic measurements [56]. Conversely, the OCT imaging systems currently in commercial use excel in dynamic measurement, capable of acquiring 2D images at over 100 frames per second. Algorithms based on OCT images of the corneal area enable simultaneous measurement of CCT and CRC using manual or automatic methods.

4. Utilization of OCT imaging for tonometry evaluation

4.1 OCT imaging with eye phantoms for mimicking cornea deformation

IOP is a fundamental and crucial parameter in diagnosing eye diseases. Therefore, it is critical to assess whether the tonometer accurately measures IOP values. The evaluation procedures for tonometers are outlined in the ISO 8612 standard document. The essence of this procedure involves comparing the tonometer under evaluation with the GAT by measuring the eyes of living humans. This evaluation process necessitates extensive clinical trials and involves measuring a wide range of live human eyes. However, a challenge with this approach is that because the subjects are living individuals, the measurement conditions cannot be precisely controlled, which compromises the accuracy of the measurements. Moreover, variations in individual eye conditions inevitably affect IOP measurement values, making accurate measurement and comparison challenging. Therefore, to achieve precise comparative measurements, it is crucial to control the conditions of the measurement subjects. Furthermore, conducting clinical trials involving 120 eyes incurs significant costs, which poses a substantial challenge when developing new tonometers. To address these challenges, this study developed eye phantoms that mimic the human cornea to evaluate tonometers, aiming to enable comparisons with a standard tonometer without the need for large-scale clinical trials.

To develop eye phantoms that accurately simulate the human cornea for evaluating tonometers, it is essential that the external appearance resemble the cornea and that it effectively replicates structural changes in response to IOP variations. Previously, eye phantoms were used for evaluation of tonometers. The eye phantoms mimic human corneas using materials with mechanical properties, CCT, and CRC similar to those of the human cornea. The cornea of these phantoms are made from a soft, flexible material similar to the actual human cornea. However, for ease of fabrication, the non-corneal area is constructed from a rigid material unlike human eyes. Additionally, the corneas of these phantoms are fixed to the rigid parts. These phantoms are referred to as the cornea eye phantom (CEP). Unlike human eyes, where the cornea and sclera are continuously connected, in CEP, only the flexible corneal part deforms with changes in IOP. Although the sclera is tougher than the cornea, it is not too hard like metal or hard plastic. We anticipated that developing an eye phantom where all parts of the eye are continuous and not fixed would more closely resemble the human eye. Creating such an eye phantom requires a continuous spherical shape filled internally with liquid to mimic the aqueous humor and gel-like vitreous body. Technically, this was achieved using molding techniques based on polymer materials like polydimethylsiloxane (PDMS) and applying Archimedes' buoyancy principle. These new phantoms are known as a full eye phantom (FEP). The characteristics of CEP and FEP can be summarized as depicted in **Figure 11**.

Two types of eye phantoms were created to mimic the physical characteristics of the human cornea and observe how structural changes vary with changes in IOP.

These eye phantoms were designed with CCT values of 350, 450, and 550 μm and a CRC of 8.5 mm. Recognizing that CCT would significantly influence corneal

	Full eye phantom (FEP)	Cornea eye phantom (CEP)
Structure	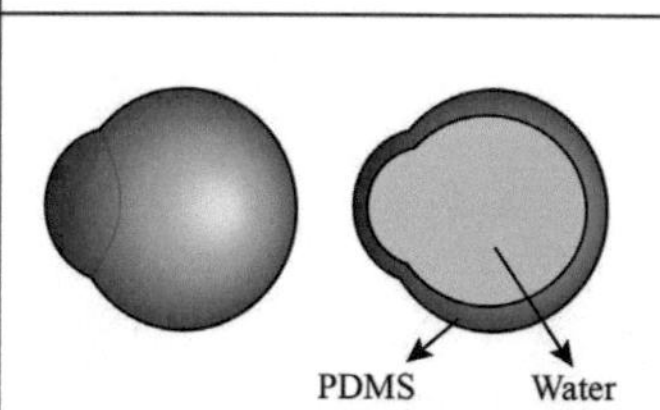 	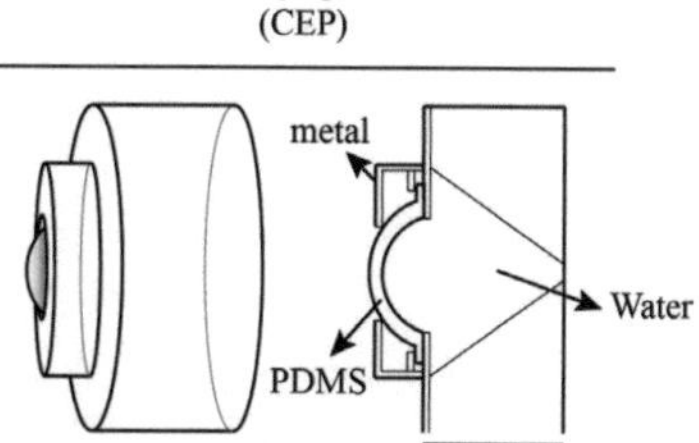
Young's modulus	380 kPa	380 kPa (only cornea)
CCT	370, 470, 570 μm	
CRC	8.5 mm	

Figure 11.
Comparison of full eye phantom (FEP) and cornea eye phantom (CEP): Structure, Young's modulus, central corneal thickness (CCT), and corneal radius of curvature (CRC).

structural deformation, three different CCT values were chosen to encompass the typical range found in humans. To replicate the mechanical properties of the human cornea, PDMS (Sylgard 184) was used. The mechanical properties were adjusted by varying the mixing ratio of the silicone elastomer and curing agent in the PDMS formulation. Tensile test specimens were fabricated according to the ASTM D 412 standard, and mechanical testing was conducted to identify a mixing ratio that could achieve mechanical properties similar to those of the human cornea. The Young's modulus of the PDMS produced was measured at 380 kPa, demonstrating mechanical properties comparable to those of the human cornea. Meanwhile, to observe how structural changes occur in the two types of eye phantoms due to variations in IOP, the pressure control and measurement device in the form of a syringe pump was employed. This device was connected to the eye phantom to adjust IOP, while OCT images of the cornea of the phantoms were obtained.

The pressure was adjusted in increments of 1 mmHg within the range of 0 to 45 mmHg using a pressure control device, and OCT images were acquired (see **Figure 12**). The images were acquired using an FD-OCT imaging system, driven by a light source with a central wavelength of 1300 nm and a bandwidth of approximately 100 nm, operating at a transverse scan speed of about 18 frames per second with an imaging range of approximately 10 mm and an imaging depth of approximately 2.528 mm. The axial resolution of this system was measured to be approximately 4.9 μm in air. From the acquired OCT images, CCT and CRC data were obtained using an automated segmentation algorithm implemented in Python. CCT was determined by detecting the anterior and posterior surfaces of the cornea using an edge detection algorithm and automatically measuring the

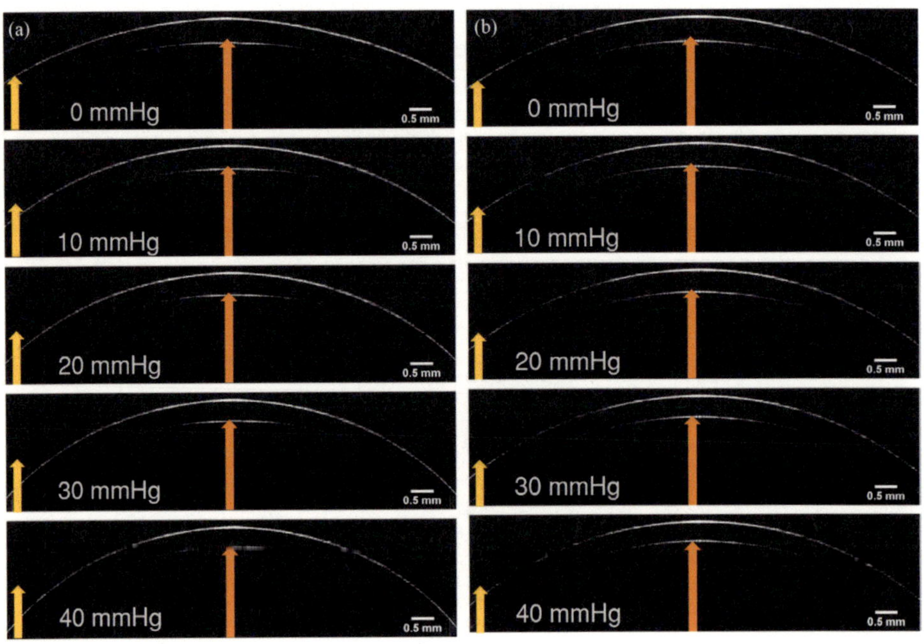

Figure 12.
OCT images of (a) cornea eye phantom (CEP) and (b) full eye phantom (FEP) as intraocular pressure (IOP) changes (0, 10, 20, 30, and 40 mmHg). Arrows of the same color displayed in a row of images have the same size to easily recognize changes in surface. (Scale bar: 0.5 mm). Reproduced with permission from [57].

distance between these surfaces. CRC was calculated by fitting the corneal surface to a circular function to determine its curvature.

The acquired OCT images and the changes in CCT and CRC according to the variations in IOP are illustrated in **Figure 13**. As IOP increases, the CCT of both types of eye phantoms tends to decrease linearly. Moreover, it is evident that each type exhibits a similar slope depending on CCT. In contrast, CRC demonstrates different trends between the two eye phantoms. The CEP shows a significant decrease in CRC as IOP increases. Conversely, the FEP tends to decrease slightly or remain stable as internal pressure increases. The distinct CRC behaviors of these two types of eye phantoms are illustrated in **Figure 14**.

In the CEP, the cornea material is soft and flexible, while the non-corneal part is rigid, and the cornea is fixed to this rigid part. Thus, when IOP increases, only the cornea undergoes significant deformation, as depicted in **Figure 14(a)**. Consequently, the CRC of the CEP gradually decreases, reflecting the substantial deformation possible in the cornea, which is the only part capable of deformation. Conversely, the FEP is constructed entirely from soft and flexible materials, with all parts interconnected and not fixed. Therefore, all parts can deform in response to changes in IOP, resulting in less pronounced deformation of the cornea compared to CEP (see **Figure 14(b)**). However, in cases where the cornea is very thin, it can deform more easily relative to other parts, leading to a deformation pattern similar to that of CEP (see **Figure 14(c)**). FEP, with an average CCT similar to that of normal human corneas (540–550 μm), shows minimal change or a slight decrease in CRC as IOP increases. Based on clinical studies, human corneas are known to exhibit changes similar to those observed in FEP in response to variations in IOP [58]. Consequently,

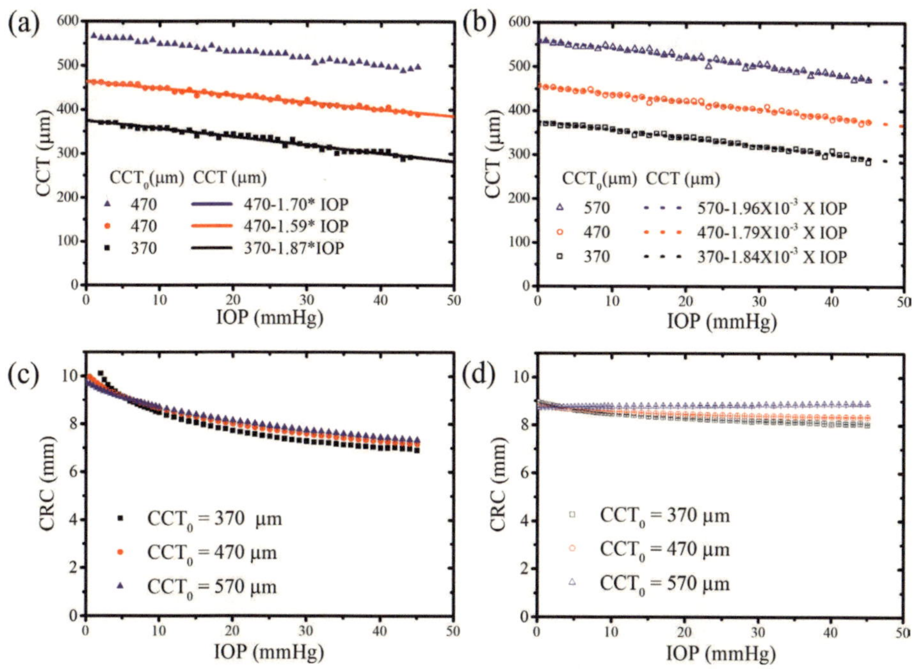

Figure 13.
The changes of central corneal thickness (CCT) and corneal radius of curvature (CRC) in the cornea eye phantom (CEP) ((a), (c)) and full eye phantom (FEP) ((b), (d)) as intraocular pressure (IOP) varies (CCTo: the measured central corneal thickness when internal pressure is 0). Reproduced with permission from [57].

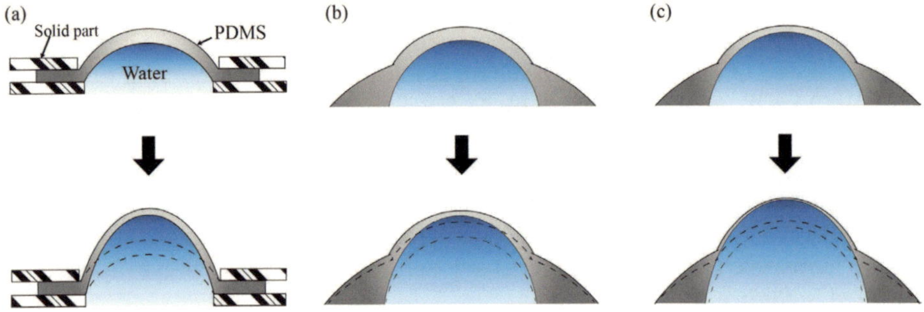

Figure 14.
The different structural change of the cornea between cornea eye phantom (CEP) (a) and full eye phantom (FEP) ((b) and (c)). (c) shows a case with a relatively thin central corneal thickness (CCT) compared to (b). Reproduced with permission from [57].

FEP appears to more accurately simulate the structural changes of the human eye compared to CEP. Two types of eye phantoms were assessed using an NCT, and the results are depicted in **Figure 15**. Both types exhibit an increase in measured values as IOP increases. However, it is evident that the slope of increase for the CEP is approximately 1.5 times greater on average compared to the FEP. This disparity arises because the CEP experiences a significant decrease in CRC as IOP increases, requiring greater force from the NCT to flatten the cornea with an air puff. In contrast, the actual human cornea does not exhibit significant changes in CCT based on variations in IOP. Therefore, the FEP may be more suitable than CEP for evaluating hydrodynamic-based tonometers.

4.2 In vivo OCT imaging for measuring structural changes in the cornea

To verify whether changes in CCT and CRC corresponded to the results obtained from measuring eye phantoms, changes in IOP were induced in actual human eyes, and OCT images were acquired. **Figure 16(a)** illustrates CRC before and 4 hours after treatment to restore normal IOP. Dashed lines connect data points measured from the same patient. CRC appears to slightly increase or remain constant as IOP rises. **Figure 16(b)** demonstrates the relationship between the CRC and the CCT based on

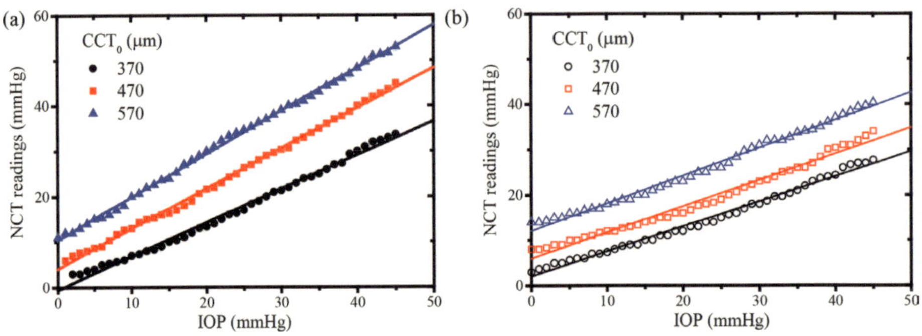

Figure 15.
The result data of non-contact tonometry (NCT) for (a) cornea eye phantom (CEP) and (b) full eye phantom (FEP). The slope of increase for the CEP is approximately 1.5 times greater on average compared to the FEP (CCTo: the measured central corneal thickness when internal pressure is 0). Reproduced with permission from [57].

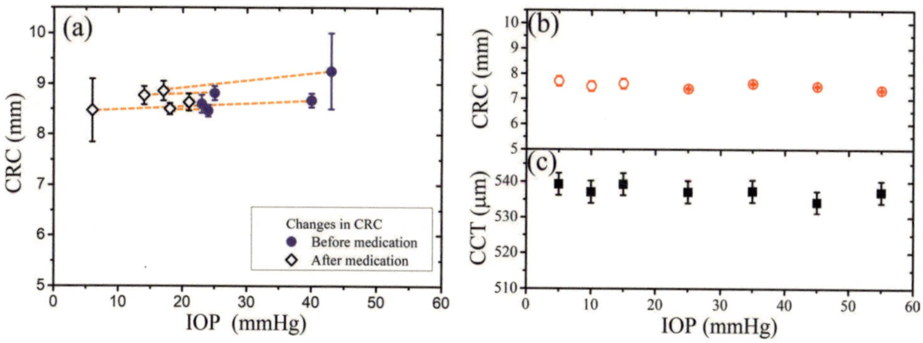

Figure 16.
(a) The cornea deformation of human subjects as intraocular pressure (IOP) changes. The averaged corneal radius of curvature (CRC) of the human eye before (closed blue circle) and after (open black diamond) medication. The data pairs connected by dashed lines are measured from the same patients. The dependence of (b) CRC and (c) central corneal thickness (CCT) on IOP observed from the cannulated human subjects. Reproduced with permission from [57].

IOP in cannulated human subjects. The values of the CRC and the CCT values were determined from OCT images taken within 1 minute after the change in IOP, whereas the results in **Figure 16(a)** were observed in human subjects more than 4 hours after the change in IOP. Regardless of the experimental conditions, the in vivo experimental results closely resemble the structural deformation observed in the FEP, as CRC shows a tendency to increase or remain stable with changes in IOP.

4.3 Evaluation of IOP with OCT imaging

Assuming the eye phantom behaves like a very thin spherical shell, the force balance equation can be formulated as follows (see **Figure 17**) [59]:

$$IOP \times \pi \times CRC^2 = \sigma_C \times 2\pi \times CRC \times CCT \quad (3)$$

Here, IOP represents intraocular pressure, CRC denotes corneal radius of curvature, and CCT stands for central corneal thickness. From the above equation, IOP can be expressed as:

$$IOP = \frac{2 \times \sigma_c \times CCT}{CRC} \quad (4)$$

where σ_C is circumferential stress.

Additionally, assuming the volume of the finite element at the cornea vertex remains constant, when deformation is minimal, the circumferential strain (ε_c) relative to CCT can be expressed as:

$$\varepsilon_c = \left(\frac{CCT_0}{CCT}\right)^{1/2} - 1 \quad (5)$$

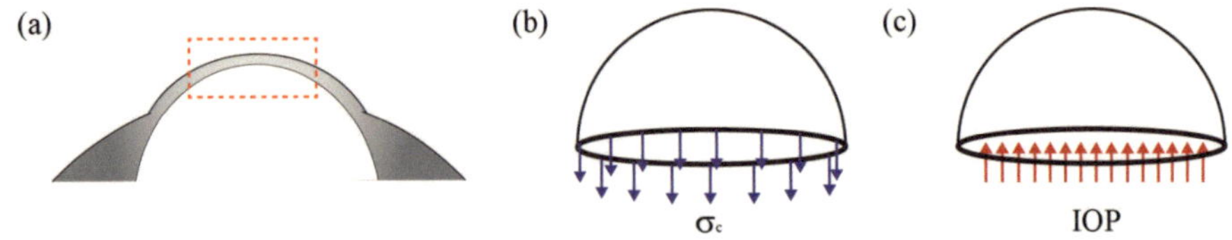

Figure 17.
(a) Cross-sectional diagram of the cornea part of the eyeball phantom and the free body diagram of the cornea. It consists of two forces: (b) circumferential stress (σ_c) and (c) intraocular pressure (IOP). Reproduced with permission from [57].

Here, ε_c denotes circumferential strain, and CCT_0 represents CCT when IOP is 0 mmHg.

Moreover, according to Hooke's law, the relationship between Young's modulus (E) and Poisson's ratio (ν) can be expressed as:

$$\frac{E}{(1-\nu)} = \frac{\sigma_c}{\varepsilon_c} \tag{6}$$

If information regarding Poisson's ratio and Young's modulus of the cornea is known σ_C can be derived using the above equation. Consequently, IOP can be calculated using CRC, CCT, and σ_C obtained from OCT images. In essence, OCT images allow for the estimation of IOP. By comparing the IOP calculated from OCT images with the IOP calculated through tonometry, it becomes possible to determine the measurement accuracy of tonometers. Given the various variables involved and the economic expense of evaluating using living human eyes, the use of FEP, which accurately simulates the human eye, enables precise comparative measurement evaluations. Meanwhile, a method to measure and evaluate IOP through speckle changes on OCT corneal images due to changes in IOP was also recently proposed [60, 61]. This research method was evaluated for effectiveness in porcine corneas and shows another way to measure IOP noninvasively by measuring speckles of biomechanical changes within the cornea on OCT images.

4.4 Future research prospects

It is reasonable to suppose that the changes in IOP alter the dimensional characteristics of the eyeball, including the CCT and the CRC, if the eyeball is considered a pressurized bulb with thin and soft tissue. Fully understandings of the deformation mechanisms resulted from IOP changes will provide a new opportunity to monitor IOP. A smart contact lens like Triggerfish, which was commercialized with Food and Drug Administration approval in 2016, has already been reported to continuously monitor the IOP based on the assumption that the strain of the cornea is dependent on the IOP [27, 28]. Without complete knowledge of the structural deformations in a living human subject caused by IOP changes, however, it is not easy to determine the exact correlation function between the strain of the cornea and the IOP. Previous works to assess the capabilities of smart contact lenses for monitoring the IOP have utilized living rabbit eyes as an animal model and CEP as an artificial eyeball. The results from these performance tests cannot be directly applied to human subjects since the dimensional and mechanical characteristics of the models differ from those of human eyes. A detailed understanding of the structural deformations resulting from IOP changes is crucial to overcoming these limitations by developing more sophisticated model eyes that mimic human subjects. It is expected that the proposed method, including the OCT technology to quantitatively evaluate deformation characteristics, can be applied to performance tests of commercialized tonometers.

Acknowledgements

This work was supported in part by the Korea Research Institute of Standards and Science (No. 24011099 and 24071003). The authors thank J. W. Kim for his assistance with the calibration of the pressure controller.

Conflict of interest

The authors declare no conflict of interest.

Author details

Han Saem Cho[1], Sae Chae Jeoung[1*] and Yun Sik Yang[2]

1 Division of Biomedical Metrology, Korea Research Institute of Standards and Science (KRISS), Yuseong-gu, Daejeon, Republic of Korea

2 Department of Ophthalmology, Wonkwang University School of Medicine, Iksan, Republic of Korea

*Address all correspondence to: scjeoung@kriss.re.kr

References

[1] Kotecha A, Lim KS, Hirn C, Garway-Heath D. 10—Tonometry and intraocular pressure fluctuation. In: Shaarawy TM, Sherwood MB, Hitchings RA, Crowston JG, editors. Glaucoma. 2nd ed. Philadelphia: W.B. Saunders; 2015. pp. 98-108. DOI: 10.1016/B978-0-7020-5193-7.00010-8

[2] Harper R, Henson DB. Chapter 8—Diagnosis of the glaucomas 2: Intraocular pressure. In: Edgar DF, Rudnicka AR, editors. Glaucoma Identification and Co-Management. Edinburgh: Butterworth-Heinemann; 2007. pp. 107-118. DOI: 10.1016/B978-0-7506-3782-4.50011-9

[3] Snell RS, Lemp MA. The Eyeball. Clinical Anatomy of the Eye. New Jersey: John Wiley and Sons, Ltd; 2013. pp. 132-213. DOI: 10.1002/9781118690987.ch6

[4] Grieshaber MC, Pienaar A, Olivier J, Stegmann R. Clinical evaluation of the aqueous outflow system in primary open-angle glaucoma for canaloplasty. Investigative Ophthalmology and Visual Science. 2010;**51**:1498-1504. DOI: 10.1167/iovs.09-4327

[5] Forrester JV, Dick AD, McMenamin PG, Roberts F, Pearlman E. Chapter 1—Anatomy of the eye and orbit. In: Forrester JV, Dick AD, McMenamin PG, Roberts F, Pearlman E, editors. The Eye. 4th ed. Philadelphia: W.B. Saunders; 2016. pp. 1-102.e2. DOI: 10.1016/B978-0-7020-5554-6.00001-0

[6] Toris CB. 6—Aqueous humor dynamics and intraocular pressure elevation. In: Shaarawy TM, Sherwood MB, Hitchings RA, Crowston JG, editors. Glaucoma. 2nd ed. Philadelphia: W.B. Saunders; 2015. pp. 47-56. DOI: 10.1016/B978-0-7020-5193-7.00006-6

[7] Maus TL, Brubaker RF. Measurement of aqueous humor flow by fluorophotometry in the presence of a dilated pupil. Investigative Ophthalmology and Visual Science. 1999;**40**(2):542-546

[8] Goel M, Picciani RG, Lee RK, Bhattacharya SK. Aqueous humor dynamics: A review. The Open Ophthalmology Journal. 2010;**4**:52-59. DOI: 10.2174/1874364101004010052

[9] Liu H, Fan S, Gulati V, Camras LJ, Zhan G, Ghate D, et al. Aqueous humor dynamics during the day and night in healthy mature volunteers. Archives of Ophthalmology. 2011;**129**:269-275. DOI: 10.1001/archophthalmol.2011.4

[10] Brubaker RF. Flow of aqueous humor in humans [the friedenwald lecture]. Investigative Ophthalmology and Visual Science. 1991;**32**:3145-3166

[11] Yasukawa T, Hanyuda A, Yamagishi K, Yuki K, Uchino M, Ozawa Y, et al. Relationship between blood pressure and intraocular pressure in the JPHC-NEXT eye study. Scientific Reports. 2022;**12**:17493. DOI: 10.1038/s41598-022-22301-1

[12] Zhao D, Cho J, Kim MH, Friedman DS, Guallar E. Diabetes, fasting glucose, and the risk of glaucoma: A meta-analysis. Ophthalmology. 2015;**122**:72-78. DOI: 10.1016/j.ophtha.2014.07.051

[13] Papritz F, Goldmann H, Schmidt T. Apparatus for measuring the intraocular or tonometric pressure of an eye. U.S. Patent No. 3,070,997. United States; 1980

[14] Moses RA. The Goldmann applanation tonometer*. American Journal of Ophthalmology. 1958;**46**:865-869. DOI: 10.1016/0002-9394(58)90998-X

[15] Gloster J, Perkins ES. The validity of the imbert-fick law as applied to applanation tonometry. Experimental Eye Research. 1963;**2**:274-283. DOI: 10.1016/S0014-4835(63)80048-2

[16] Kaushik S, Pandav SS. Ocular response analyzer. Journal of Current Glaucoma Practice. 2012;**6**:17-19. DOI: 10.5005/jp-journals-10008-1103

[17] Hong J, Xu J, Wei A, Deng SX, Cui X, Yu X, et al. A new tonometer—The Corvis ST tonometer: Clinical comparison with noncontact and Goldmann applanation tonometers. Investigative Ophthalmology & Visual Science. 2013;**54**:659-665. DOI: 10.1167/iovs.12-10984

[18] CGV DM, Juthani VJ, Liebmann JM, Teng CC, Tello C, Susanna R Jr, et al. Risk factors for visual field progression in treated glaucoma. Archives of Ophthalmology. 2011;**129**:562-568. DOI: 10.1001/archophthalmol.2011.72

[19] Renard E, Palombi K, Gronfier C, Pepin J-L, Noel C, Chiquet C, et al. Twenty-four hour (nyctohemeral) rhythm of intraocular pressure and ocular perfusion pressure in normal-tension glaucoma. Investigative Ophthalmology and Visual Science. 2010;**51**:882-889. DOI: 10.1167/iovs.09-3668

[20] Kontiola A. A new electromechanical method for measuring intraocular pressure. Documenta Ophthalmologica. 1997;**93**:265-276. DOI: 10.1007/BF02569066

[21] Nakakura S. Icare® rebound tonometers: Review of their characteristics and ease of use. Clinical Ophthalmology. 2018;**12**:1245-1253

[22] Kao SF, Lichter PR, Bergstrom TJ, Rowe S, Musch DC. Clinical comparison of the oculab tono-pen to the Goldmann applanation tonometer. Ophthalmology. 1987;**94**:1541-1544. DOI: 10.1016/S0161-6420(87)33249-X

[23] Muir KW. Home tonometry—Can we? Should we? JAMA Ophthalmology. 2017;**135**:1036. DOI: 10.1001/jamaophthalmol.2017.3194

[24] Pronin S, Brown L, Megaw R, Tatham AJ. Measurement of intraocular pressure by patients with glaucoma. JAMA Ophthalmology. 2017;**135**:1030-1036. DOI: 10.1001/jamaophthalmol.2017.3151

[25] Flatau A, Solano F, Idrees S, Jefferys JL, Volpe P, Damion C, et al. Measured changes in limbal strain during simulated sleep in face down position using an instrumented contact lens in healthy adults and adults with glaucoma. JAMA Ophthalmology. 2016;**134**:375-382. DOI: 10.1001/jamaophthalmol.2015.5667

[26] Dunbar GE, Shen BY, Aref AA. The sensimed triggerfish contact lens sensor: Efficacy, safety, and patient perspectives. Clinical Ophthalmology. 2017;**11**:875-882. DOI: 10.2147/OPTH.S109708

[27] Kim J, Park J, Park Y-G, Cha E, Ku M, An HS, et al. A soft and transparent contact lens for the wireless quantitative monitoring of intraocular pressure. Nature Biomedical Engineering. 2021;**5**:772-782. DOI: 10.1038/s41551-021-00719-8

[28] Kim TY, Mok JW, Hong SH, Jeong SH, Choi H, Shin S, et al. Wireless theranostic smart contact lens for monitoring and control of intraocular

pressure in glaucoma. Nature Communications. 2022;**13**:6801. DOI: 10.1038/s41467-022-34597-8

[29] Salz JJ, Azen SP, Berstein J, Caroline P, Villasenor RA, Schanzlin DJ. Evaluation and comparison of sources of variability in the measurement of corneal thickness with ultrasonic and optical pachymeters. Ophthalmic Surgery. 1983;**14**:750-754

[30] Martin R. Cornea and anterior eye assessment with placido-disc keratoscopy, slit scanning evaluation topography and scheimpflug imaging tomography. Indian Journal of Ophthalmology. 2018;**66**:360-366

[31] Fan R, Chan TC, Prakash G, Jhanji V. Applications of corneal topography and tomography: A review. Clinical and Experimental Ophthalmology. 2018;**46**:133-146. DOI: 10.1111/ceo.13136

[32] Randleman JB, Akhtar J, Lynn MJ, Ambrósio R Jr, Dupps WJ Jr, Krueger RR, et al. Comparison of objective and subjective refractive surgery screening parameters between regular and high-resolution Scheimpflug imaging devices. Journal of Cataract and Refractive Surgery. 2014;**41**:286-294. DOI: 10.1016/j.jcrs.2014.06.026

[33] Kanellopoulos AJ. Scheimpflug vs scanning-slit corneal tomography: Comparison of corneal and anterior chamber tomography indices for repeatability and agreement in healthy eyes. Clinical Ophthalmology. 2020;**14**:2583-2592. DOI: 10.2147/OPTH.S251998

[34] Gutmark R, Guyton DL. Origins of the keratometer and its evolving role in ophthalmology. Survey of Ophthalmology. 2010;**55**:481-497. DOI: 10.1016/j.survophthal.2010.03.001

[35] Keeler CR, Helland M, Albert DM. Hjalmar Schiøtz, the great Norwegian innovator and his ophthalmoscope. Acta Ophthalmologica. 2014;**92**:588-592. DOI: 10.1111/aos.12274

[36] El HSG. A new photokeratoscopic technique. Optical Engineering. 1976;**15**:154308. DOI: 10.1117/12.7971981

[37] Sen M, Honavar SG. Allvar gullstrand: Prize and prejudice. Indian Journal of Ophthalmology. 2021;**69**:1366-1367. DOI: 10.4103/ijo.IJO_1076_21

[38] Seitz B, Behrens A, Langenbucher A. Corneal topography. Current Opinion in Ophthalmology. 1997;**8**:8-24

[39] Fujimoto JG, Brezinski ME, Tearney GJ, Boppart SA, Bouma B, Hee MR, et al. Optical biopsy and imaging using optical coherence tomography. Nature Medicine. 1995;**1**:970-972. DOI: 10.1038/nm0995-970

[40] Huang D, Swanson EA, Lin CP, Schuman JS, Stinson WG, Chang W, et al. Optical coherence tomography. Science. 1979;**1991**(254):1178-1181. DOI: 10.1126/science.1957169

[41] Choma MA, Sarunic MV, Yang C, Izatt JA. Sensitivity advantage of swept source and Fourier domain optical coherence tomography. Optics Express. 2003;**11**:2183-2189. DOI: 10.1364/OE.11.002183

[42] Bouma B. Handbook of Optical Coherence Tomography. Abington, UK: Taylor and Francis; 2001

[43] Hee MR, Izatt JA, Swanson EA, Huang D, Schuman JS, Lin CP, et al. Optical coherence tomography of the human retina. Archives of Ophthalmology. 1995;**113**:325-332. DOI: 10.1001/archopht.1995.01100030081025

[44] Bechmann M, Thiel MJ, Neubauer AS, Ullrich S, Ludwig K, Kenyon KR, et al. Central corneal thickness measurement with a retinal optical coherence tomography device versus standard ultrasonic pachymetry. Cornea. 2001;**20**:50-54

[45] Hee MR, Puliafito CA, Duker JS, Reichel E, Coker JG, Wilkins JR, et al. Topography of diabetic macular edema with optical coherence tomography. Ophthalmology. 1998;**105**:360-370. DOI: 10.1016/S0161-6420(98)93601-6

[46] Rutledge BK, Puliafito CA, Duker JS, Hee MR, Cox MS. Optical coherence tomography of macular lesions associated with optic nerve head pits. Ophthalmology. 1996;**103**:1047-1053. DOI: 10.1016/S0161-6420(96)30568-X

[47] Toth CA, Birngruber R, Boppart SA, Hee MR, Fujimoto JG, Dicarlo CD, et al. Argon laser retinal lesions evaluated In vivo by optical coherence tomography. American Journal of Ophthalmology. 1997;**123**:188-198. DOI: 10.1016/S0002-9394(14)71035-9

[48] Wilkins JR, Puliafito CA, Hee MR, Duker JS, Reichel E, Coker JG, et al. Characterization of epiretinal membranes using optical coherence tomography. Ophthalmology. 1996;**103**:2142-2151. DOI: 10.1016/S0161-6420(96)30377-1

[49] Izatt JA, Hee MR, Swanson EA, Lin CP, Huang D, Schuman JS, et al. Micrometer-scale resolution imaging of the anterior eye In vivo with optical coherence tomography. Archives of Ophthalmology. 1994;**112**:1584-1589. DOI: 10.1001/archopht.1994.01090240090031

[50] Goldsmith JA, Li Y, Chalita MR, Westphal V, Patil CA, Rollins AM, et al. Anterior chamber width measurement by high-speed optical coherence tomography. Ophthalmology. 2005;**112**:238-244. DOI: 10.1016/j.ophtha.2004.09.019

[51] Maldonado MJ, Ruiz-Oblitas L, Munuera JM, Aliseda D, García-Layana A, Moreno-Montañés J. Optical coherence tomography evaluation of the corneal cap and stromal bed features after laser in situ keratomileusis for high myopia and astigmatism. Ophthalmology. 2000;**107**:81-87; discussion 88. DOI: 10.1016/s0161-6420(99)00022-6

[52] Schuman JS, Hee MR, Puliafito CA, Wong C, Pedut-Kloizman T, Lin CP, et al. Quantification of nerve fiber layer thickness in normal and glaucomatous eyes using optical coherence tomography. Archives of Ophthalmology. 1995;**113**:586-596. DOI: 10.1001/archopht.1995.01100050054031

[53] Konstantopoulos A, Hossain P, Anderson DF. Recent advances in ophthalmic anterior segment imaging: A new era for ophthalmic diagnosis? The British Journal of Ophthalmology. 2007;**91**:551-557. DOI: 10.1136/bjo.2006.103408

[54] Klein T, Wieser W, Reznicek L, Neubauer A, Kampik A, Huber R. Multi-MHz retinal OCT. Biomedical Optics Express. 2013;**4**:1890-1908. DOI: 10.1364/BOE.4.001890

[55] Klein T, Wieser W, Eigenwillig CM, Biedermann BR, Huber R. Megahertz OCT for ultrawide-field retinal imaging with a 1050nm Fourier domain mode-locked laser. Optics Express. 2011;**19**:3044-3062. DOI: 10.1364/OE.19.003044

[56] Kanellopoulos AJ, Asimellis G. Comparison of high-resolution

Scheimpflug and high-frequency ultrasound biomicroscopy to anterior-segment OCT corneal thickness measurements. Clinical Ophthalmology. 2013;7:2239-2247. DOI: 10.2147/OPTH.S53718

[57] Cho HS, Jeoung SC, Yang YS. Development of eye phantom for mimicking the deformation of the human cornea accompanied by intraocular pressure alterations. Scientific Reports. 2022;**12**:20670. DOI: 10.1038/s41598-022-24948-2

[58] Hjortdal JO, Jensen PK. In vitro measurement of corneal strain, thickness, and curvature using digital image processing. Acta Ophthalmologica Scandinavica. 1995;**73**:5-11. DOI: 10.1111/j.1600-0420.1995.tb00004.x

[59] Hibbeler RC. Mechanics of Materials. New Jersey: Pearson Education; 2011

[60] Niemczyk M, Danielewska ME, Kostyszak MA, Lewandowski D, Iskander DR. The effect of intraocular pressure elevation and related ocular biometry changes on corneal OCT speckle distribution in porcine eyes. PLoS One. 2021;**16**:e0249213. DOI: 10.1371/journal.pone.0249213

[61] Niemczyk M, Iskander DR. Measuring intraocular pressure with OCT: The first approach. Biomedical Optics Express. 2023;**14**:4531-4541. DOI: 10.1364/BOE.500546

Chapter 6

SS-OCT Enhances the Diagnosis and Treatment of Anterior Segment Diseases

Feiyan Chai and Xiaogang Wang

Abstract

Swept-source optical coherence tomography (SS-OCT) is a non-contact imaging technology that has emerged as a novel tool for visualizing the anterior segment of the eye. This technology is characterized by its rapid scanning speed, high resolution, and excellent penetration capabilities. As a result, swept-source OCT is now widely utilized in the diagnosis, treatment, and follow-up of various anterior segment diseases, such as iridoschisis, posterior lenticonus, intraocular lens dislocation, and capsular block syndrome. Given the limitations of conventional measurement instruments regarding measurement methods and precision, the use of non-contact swept-source OCT offers quantitative data that enhances the assessment of disease severity and progression.

Keywords: swept-source OCT, iridoschisis, posterior lenticonus, intraocular lens dislocation, capsular block syndrome

1. Introduction

Swept-source optical coherence tomography (SS-OCT) utilizes coherent light to generate high-resolution images of anterior segment structures. This technology offers excellent penetration capabilities for corneal tissues and allows for the measurement of various biological parameters, including those of the cornea, anterior chamber, angle, iris, and lens. Unlike previous imaging technologies, such as ultrasound biomicroscopy (UBM) and Scheimpflug imaging, SS-OCT employs a non-invasive, non-contact approach, thereby minimizing the discomfort often associated with contact examinations (**Table 1**).

With ongoing technological advancements, SS-OCT provides rapid scanning speeds and wide scanning ranges, establishing it as a commonly used tool for the clinical examination of anterior segment structures. This technology assists clinicians in formulating precise surgical plans for the anterior segment and effectively monitoring disease progression. This chapter aims to provide an overview of the applications of SS-OCT in the diagnosis and follow-up of some specific anterior segment diseases and conditions. It is important to specify that all OCT images presented in this section have been obtained using the ANTERION SS-OCT device (Heidelberg, Germany) at Shanxi Eye Hospital.

	SS-OCT	UBM	Pentacam
Imaging principle	Low-coherence interferometry	High-frequency ultrasound	Scheimpflug rotating camera
Axial resolution	3–20 μm	>50 μm	—
Examination method	Seated, non-contact	Supine, contact	Seated, non-contact
Penetration capability	Obstructed by the iris	Can penetrate the iris	Obstructed by the iris
Scanning depth	12–16 mm	3.5–5 mm	6–8 mm

Table 1.
Comparison of common anterior segment imaging systems.

2. Examples of SS-OCT applications in anterior segment diseases and special conditions

2.1 Corneal perforation

Overview: Corneal perforation is a common emergency in ophthalmology that, if not treated promptly, can lead to serious complications. It can result from several corneal diseases, including infectious keratitis, neurotrophic keratitis, trauma, inflammatory conditions, and persistent epithelial defects. Therefore, actively managing the underlying condition is clinically significant in preventing corneal perforation.

Case presentation: A 13-year-old male presented with redness, pain, and vision loss in his left eye that had persisted for 1 day. A slit-lamp examination revealed significant conjunctival congestion and a perforation in the inferior temporal cornea, with iris tissue incarcerated in the perforation site (**Figure 1A**).

OCT imaging and comments: The SS-OCT horizontal scan image of the perforation displayed uneven corneal thickness, highlighting a significant thickening of the

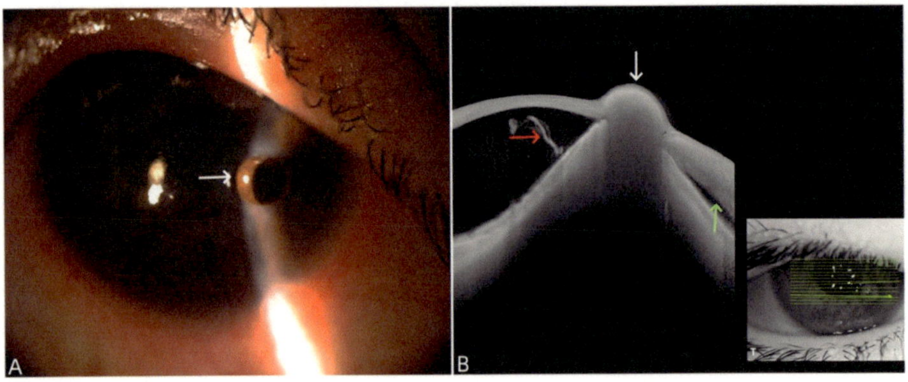

Figure 1.
(A) Slit-lamp and SS-OCT images of the corneal perforation. (B) The OCT image demonstrates the iris tissue protruding in a "figure-eight" shape and being incarcerated in the perforation (B, white arrow), with fluffy exudates observed on the surface of the iris (B, red arrow). The anterior chamber depth varied on either side of the incarceration site, with the nasal side gradually becoming shallower from the center toward the temporal side, while the temporal side appeared slit-like (B, green arrow).

temporal cornea compared to the nasal side. The OCT imaging confirmed corneal perforation and iris tissue prolapse (**Figure 1B**).

2.2 Post-cataract surgery corneal edema

Overview: The primary treatment for cataracts is phacoemulsification combined with artificial lens implantation. The use of ultrasound energy during the procedure can result in varying degrees of corneal damage, with corneal edema being the most common complication. This condition primarily affects the corneal stroma and can subsequently impact early postoperative vision recovery [1, 2].

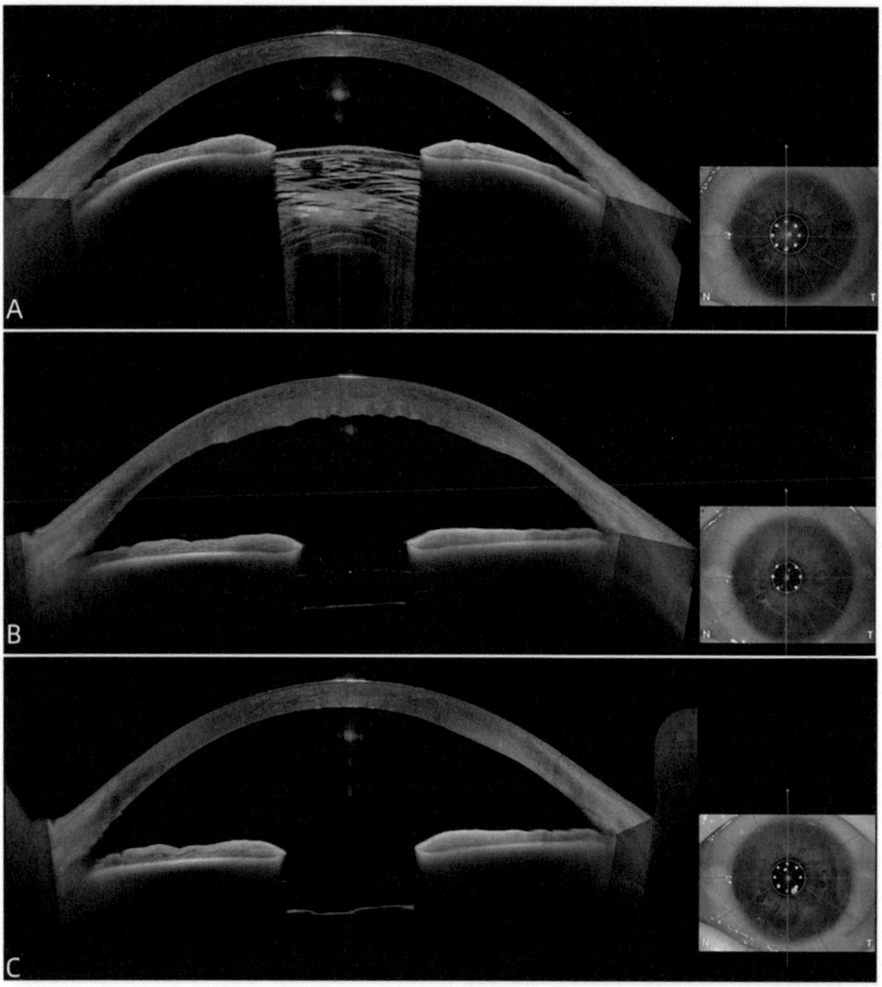

Figure 2.
OCT images of a patient with age-related cataract complicated by postoperative corneal edema. (A) The SS-OCT examination indicated that the preoperative left eye had a smooth corneal surface, with a central corneal thickness of 544 μm and enhanced reflective signals from the anterior cortical lens. One day postoperatively, the central corneal stroma was swollen and thickened, reaching a thickness of 915 μm. (B) The Descemet's membrane and endothelial layer appeared irregularly wavy. (C) By 1 week postoperatively, corneal thickness gradually approached normal, measuring 605 μm, although the central corneal endothelial surface remained uneven.

Case presentation: A 78-year-old male presented with blurred vision in his left eye, which had persisted for over 3 years. Upon slit-lamp examination, a cloudy lens in the left eye was observed, which was diagnosed as an age-related cataract. The patient underwent phacoemulsification combined with artificial lens implantation.

OCT imaging and comments: Preoperative OCT images displayed a normal cornea, with the anterior cortex of the lens exhibiting layered high-reflectance signals. The lens nucleus and posterior cortex appeared as low-reflectance signals, obscured by the anterior high-reflectance signals (**Figure 2A**). Due to significant lens opacity, a larger amount of ultrasound energy was utilized during cataract surgery, resulting in corneal tissue damage and subsequent postoperative corneal edema. One day postoperatively, OCT revealed thickening of the corneal stroma, with the corneal endothelial surface appearing irregularly wavy (**Figure 2B**). One week after surgery, the condition stabilized; although mild edema was still present in the central corneal stroma, corneal thickness approached normal levels (**Figure 2C**).

2.3 Iridoschisis

Overview: Iridoschisis is a rare disorder characterized by the separation of the anterior stromal layer of the iris from the posterior stroma and muscle layers. Examination typically reveals floating fibrillar material in the anterior chamber [3, 4]. The term "iridoschisis" was first proposed by Lowenstein and Foster in 1945, who described a deep, parallel split between the anterior and posterior stromal layers of the iris [5]. The condition usually begins unilaterally but often progresses to affect both eyes [6]. Mansour reported that iridoschisis occurs most frequently in the inferior quadrant (37%, 37/100), followed by the inferonasal quadrant (18%, 18/100), the superior quadrant (9%, 9/100), and the inferotemporal quadrant (7%, 7/100). Additionally, 29% (29/100) of patients present with diffuse iridoschisis [7].

Case presentation: A 74-year-old female patient reported blurred vision in her right eye for over 2 years. A slit-lamp examination revealed iridoschisis in the inferotemporal area of both eyes, accompanied by lens opacities and pigment deposits on the anterior lens capsule. She was diagnosed with bilateral senile cataracts and iridoschisis. The examination showed a "shredded appearance" for the iris of the right eye and loose iris tissue in the left eye (**Figure 3A, B**). Phacoemulsification and intraocular lens implantation were performed to treat the cataract in the right eye.

OCT imaging and comments: OCT scans of the iridoschisis area in the right eye demonstrated diffuse iris atrophy, stromal disorganization, and splitting in the affected region, with the anterior layer appearing shredded and floating in the anterior chamber. In severe cases, this floating iris material may adhere to the corneal endothelium (**Figure 3C**). The left eye exhibited milder changes, consistent with the early stage of the disease (**Figure 3C, D**).

2.4 Anterior uveitis

Overview: Anterior uveitis is the most common type of uveitis, accounting for approximately 50% of all cases [8]. Depending on its duration, it can be classified as

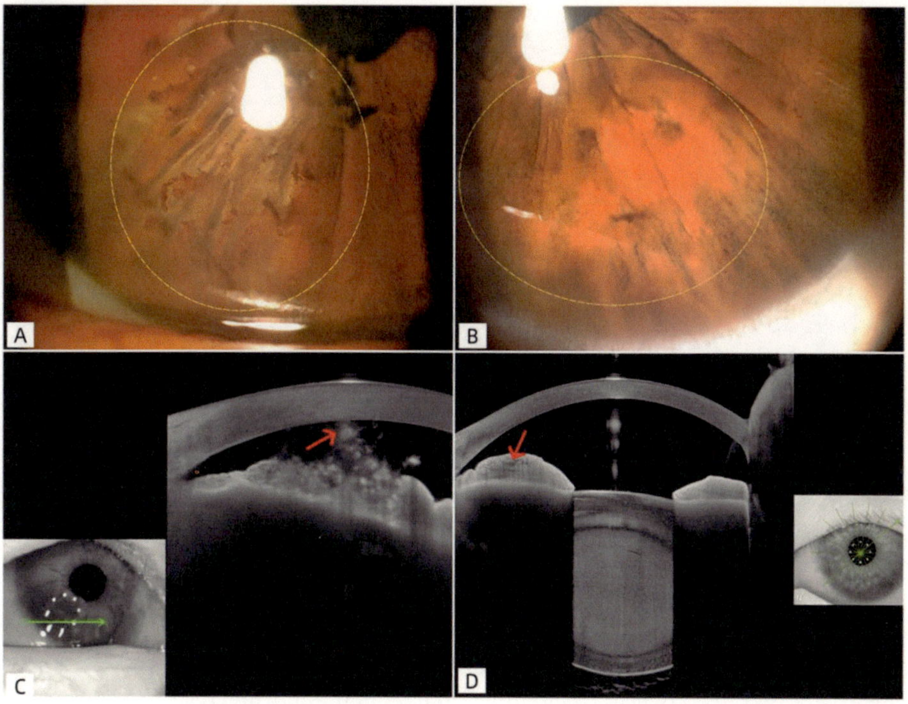

Figure 3.
Slit-lamp and SS-OCT images of a patient with iridoschisis. (A, B) The slit-lamp images show loose iris tissue in both eyes, with significant iris atrophy in the right eye (highlighted by yellow-dashed lines). (C) OCT scans of the iridoschisis area in the right eye reveal stromal disorganization and shredded, floating iris tissue, some of which adhere to the corneal endothelium (red arrow). (D) In the left eye, OCT shows cystic spaces within the stroma, appearing as areas of low reflectivity (red arrow).

acute, chronic, or recurrent. Patients typically present with symptoms such as eye redness, pain, and vision loss, and usually require anti-inflammatory and symptomatic treatments.

2.4.1 Case presentation

Case 1: A 37-year-old female presented with a 1-week history of redness, pain, and vision loss in her left eye. A slit-lamp examination revealed ciliary injection, intense aqueous flare (+++), and posterior synechiae in the left eye. The clinical diagnosis was acute anterior uveitis in the left eye.

OCT imaging and comments: OCT imaging showed generally normal corneal thickness and shape, with significant inflammation in the anterior chamber and iris tissue (**Figure 4**).

Case 2: A 78-year-old female reported blurred vision in her right eye for over 2 years. The slit-lamp examination revealed an extremely shallow anterior chamber, posterior synechiae, and lens opacities. The clinical diagnosis was cataract, which was treated with phacoemulsification and IOL implantation. Anterior uveitis was noted after cataract surgery.

OCT imaging and comments: This patient presented with a significantly shallow anterior chamber preoperatively, limiting the surgical space in the surgical procedure.

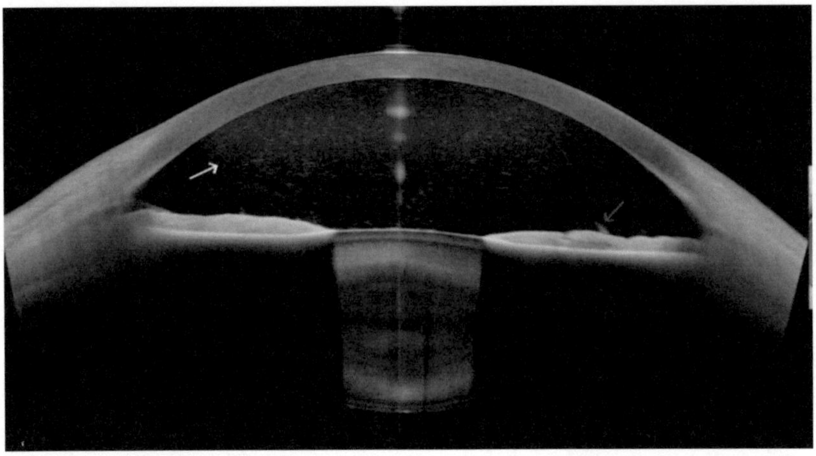

Figure 4.
SS-OCT image of Case 1 with anterior uveitis. The OCT image displays dense high-reflectivity spots in the anterior chamber (white arrow), most prominent in the central area, along with dot-like exudates on the iris surface (red arrow).

The use of ultrasound during the phacoemulsification caused damage to the corneal tissue, resulting in postoperative corneal edema and uveitis. Postoperative OCT images demonstrated corneal thickening, an irregular endothelial surface, and a reticular exudative membrane in the anterior chamber (**Figure 5**).

2.5 Posterior lenticonus

Overview: Posterior lenticonus is a rare congenital anomaly characterized by a conical or hemispherical protrusion of the posterior visual axis region of the lens into the vitreous cavity [9, 10]. This condition is often associated with localized thinning or even defects in the posterior lens capsule. In advanced stages, spontaneous rupture

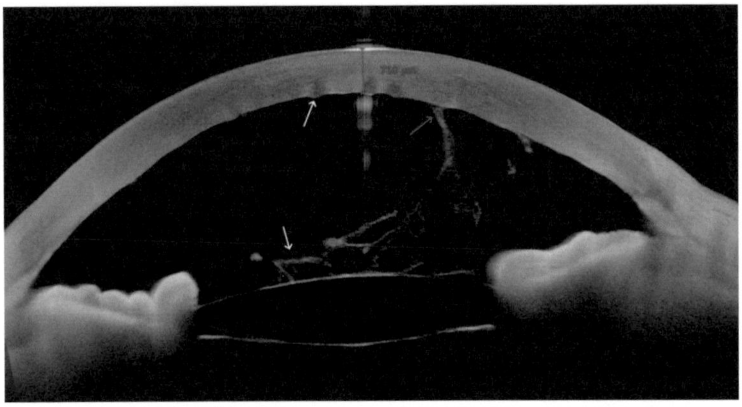

Figure 5.
SS-OCT image of Case 2 with pseudophakic eye and anterior uveitis. The OCT image reveals corneal edema and thickening, with a central corneal thickness of approximately 710 μm and an uneven endothelial surface (white arrow). A reticular exudative membrane with high reflectivity is visible on the IOL surface (yellow arrow), with portions of the membrane adhering to the corneal endothelium (red arrow).

of the posterior lens capsule may occur. The timing of treatment varies depending on the severity of the condition.

Case presentation: An 8-year-old female presented with blurred vision in her right eye since early childhood. A slit-lamp examination revealed a conical localized posterior bulge near the central part of the posterior lens capsule, accompanied by subcapsular cortical opacities (**Figure 6A**). Retro-illumination showed a localized dark area (**Figure 6B**). The clinical diagnosis was right eye posterior lenticonus with congenital cataract, which was treated with phacoemulsification and IOL implantation. During surgery, the surgeon did the posterior capsule capsulorhexis. Postoperatively,

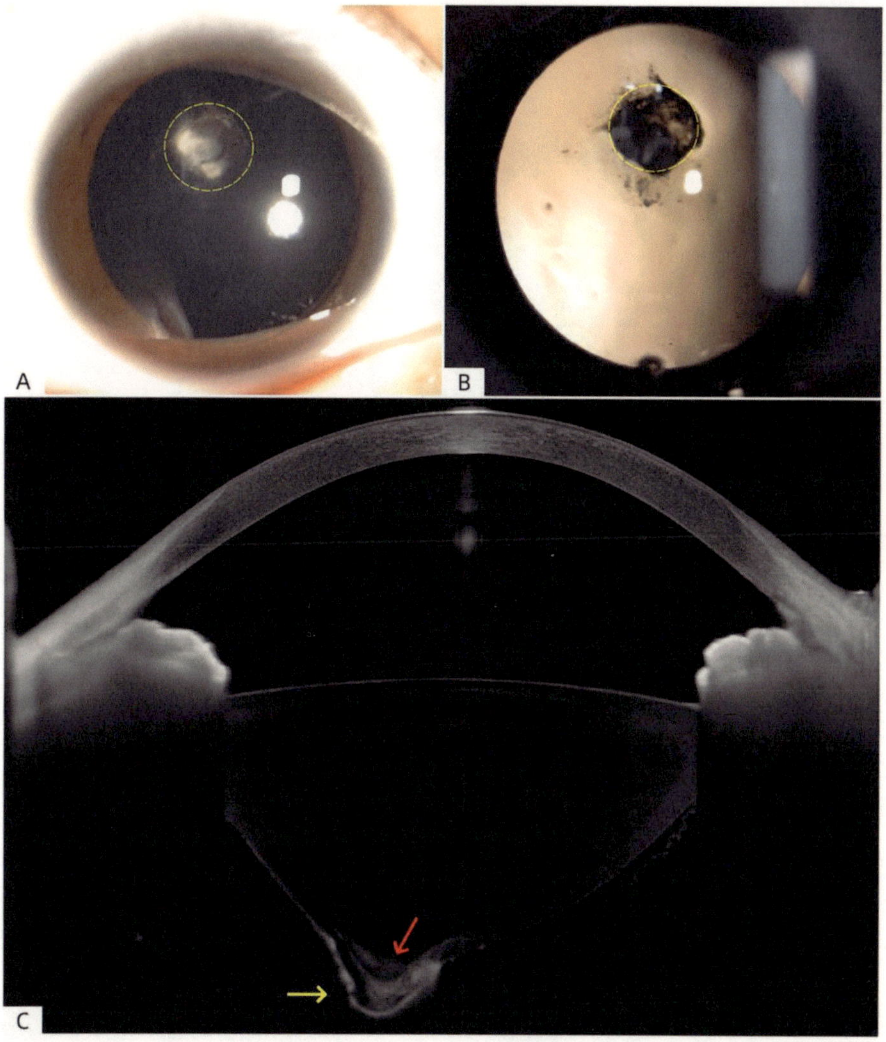

Figure 6.
Preoperative slit-lamp and SS-OCT images of posterior lenticonus. (A) The slit-lamp examination revealed a conical localized posterior bulge of the posterior capsule, with subcapsular cortical opacification appearing grayish-white (yellow-dashed line). (B) Retro-illumination showed a corresponding dark area in the lens at that location (yellow-dashed line). (C) SS-OCT scans demonstrated significant posterior bulging of the posterior capsule toward the vitreous cavity around the visual axis region, with a marked increase in local curvature (yellow arrow). The corresponding subcapsular cortex exhibited a high-reflectivity signal (red arrow).

slit-lamp examination with side illumination confirmed that the central posterior cone had been completely removed (**Figure 7A**), and retro-illumination revealed a nearly circular defect in the center of the posterior lens capsule (**Figure 7B**).

OCT imaging and comments: SS-OCT images of posterior lenticonus indicated localized posterior bulging of the posterior capsule, with high-reflectivity signals corresponding to the lens cortex in that area (**Figure 6C**). After surgery, the intraocular lens was well-positioned, the posterior cone had disappeared, and the posterior capsule capsulorhexis was clearly visible (**Figure 7C**).

2.6 Posterior polar cataract

Overview: Posterior polar cataract represents a distinct subtype of congenital cataracts, which can be further categorized into non-progressive and progressive

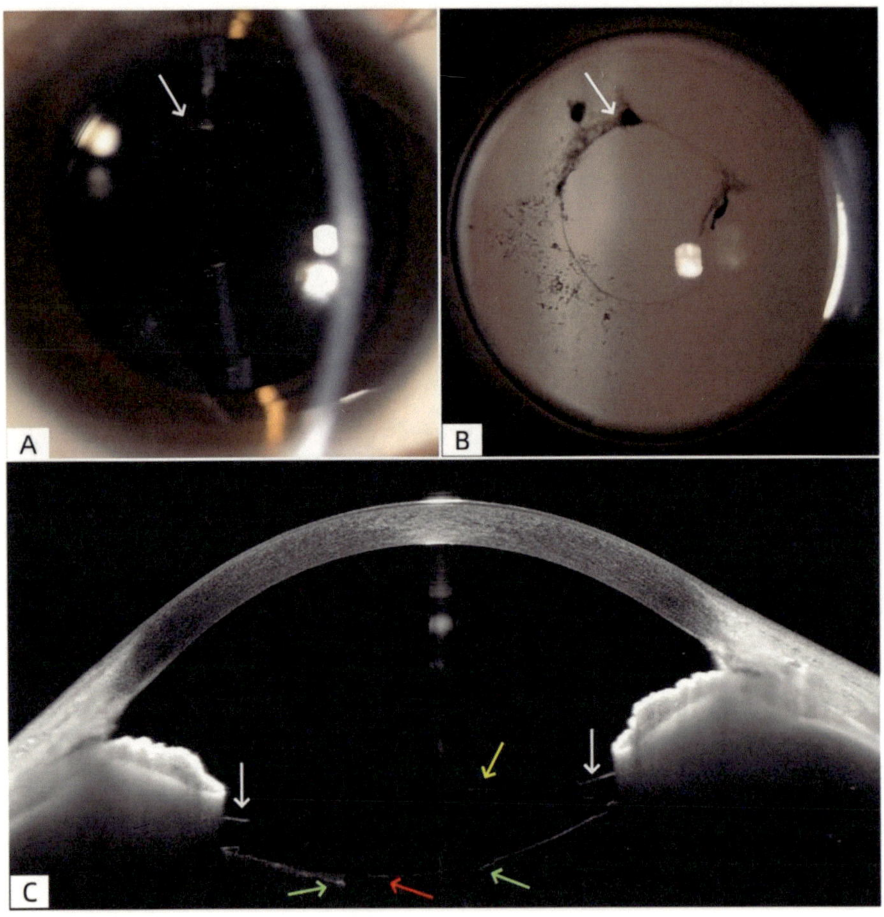

Figure 7.
Postoperative slit-lamp and SS-OCT images of posterior lenticonus. (A) The side illumination slit-lamp examination indicated that the central area of the posterior capsule had been excised (white arrow), (B) while retro-illumination revealed the area of the capsule defect to be nearly circular (white arrow). (C) SS-OCT scans clearly displayed the tear in the anterior and posterior capsules (white and green arrows), with the IOL positioned within the capsular bag. The anterior and posterior surfaces of the IOL optical zone were clearly visible (C, yellow and red arrows).

types [11]. Its defining characteristic is a congenital thinning or defect in the posterior lens capsule, making it susceptible to intraoperative complications such as posterior capsule rupture and vitreous prolapse [12]. Therefore, early and accurate preoperative diagnosis is essential to enhance surgical safety and optimize outcomes.

Case presentation: A 62-year-old male presented with a 2-year history of progressively reduced vision in the left eye. Slit-lamp examination revealed a disk-shaped, gray-white opacity firmly adhered to the posterior pole of the lens capsule.

OCT images and comments: The SS-OCT reveals a subtle posterior bulge at the posterior pole of the lens, characterized by nodular, dense, high-reflective signals. The integrity of the posterior lens capsule at this location remains questionable. During phacoemulsification cataract surgery, a rupture of the posterior capsule was identified, underscoring the critical importance of assessing the lens capsule's integrity through preoperative OCT evaluation (**Figure 8**).

2.7 Retinitis pigmentosa complicated by cataract

Overview: Retinitis pigmentosa complicated by cataract is a specific type of cataract primarily characterized by subcapsular cortical opacification that typically begins in the central area of the posterior lens capsule. Therefore, individuals affected by this type of cataract often experience a more significant impact on their visual function. Additionally, some patients may experience relaxation of the lens zonules, which increases the relative surgical risk.

Case presentation: A 38-year-old male presented with blurry vision in his right eye for over 2 years, along with a history of retinitis pigmentosa. A slit-lamp examination revealed subcapsular cortical opacification in the right eye.

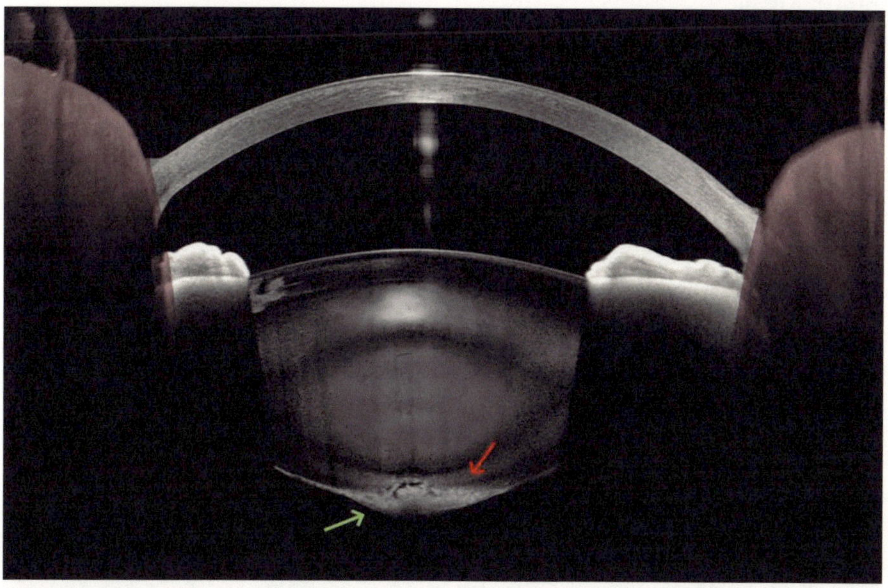

Figure 8.
The SS-OCT scan highlights a localized, highly reflective, subcapsular dense opacity at the posterior pole of the lens (indicated by the red arrow), which closely adheres to the posterior capsule and protrudes into the vitreous chamber (denoted by the green arrow), raising concerns regarding the integrity of the posterior lens capsule in this area.

The clinical diagnosis was right eye cataract complicated by retinitis pigmentosa, which led to the decision to perform cataract surgery through phacoemulsification and IOL implantation. During the surgery, it was noted that the zonules were relaxed, resulting in localized rupture of the posterior capsule. The IOL was ultimately implanted in the ciliary sulcus.

OCT imaging and comments: SS-OCT indicated that high-reflectivity signals were observed in both the anterior subcapsular and posterior cortical areas of the right eye (**Figure 9**). One day postoperatively, the OCT images showed a notch at the pupillary margin near the main and side corneal incisions (**Figure 10A** and **B**), along with vitreous incarceration and noticeable tilt of the IOL (**Figure 10C** and **D**). One week following the initial surgery, a second procedure was performed to relieve vitreous incarceration and do the IOL optic capture. One month postoperatively, the shape of the pupil appeared normal (**Figure 11A**), with no vitreous incarceration at the incision site and a relatively stable IOL (**Figure 11B** and **C**).

2.8 Posterior capsule opacification (PCO)

Overview: The clouding resulting from the proliferation of residual cortical or lens epithelial cells following cataract surgery is known as PCO. It is one of the leading causes of visual deterioration and a common long-term complication of cataract surgery [13]. Currently, Nd:YAG laser posterior capsulotomy is the primary clinical treatment for PCO [14–16].

Case presentation: A 62-year-old male, with a medical history of cataract surgery in his left eye 5 years ago, reported a decline in vision for over 3 months. A slit-lamp examination revealed a grayish-white opacity on the posterior capsule of the lens. The diagnosis was PCO and the patient underwent Nd:YAG laser posterior capsulotomy to address this issue.

OCT images and comments: SS-OCT provides a visual assessment of the type and severity of PCO. After pupil dilation, the OCT images displayed a dense, high-reflective abnormal band signal between the posterior lens capsule and IOL. Following the Nd:YAG laser capsulotomy, a defect in the central posterior capsule was visible, along with the laser-created opening in the posterior capsule (**Figure 12**).

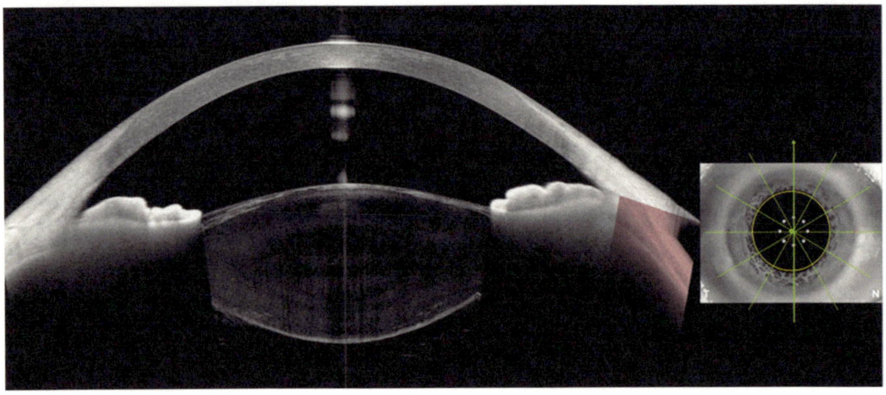

Figure 9.
SS-OCT image of a patient with retinitis pigmentosa complicated by cataract. High-reflectivity signals were observed in both the anterior and posterior subcapsular cortex.

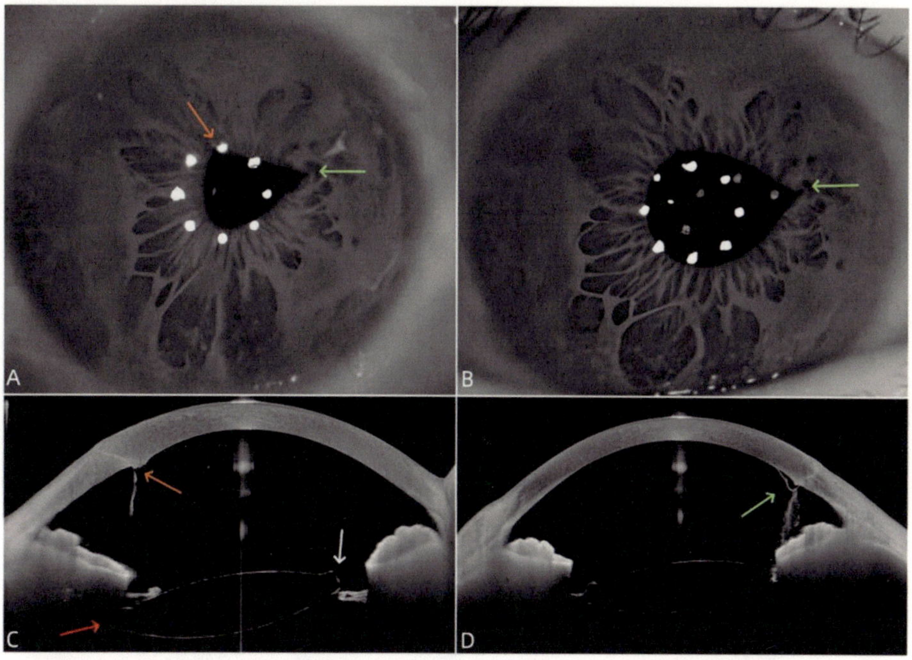

Figure 10.
SS-OCT images 1 day post-surgery. (A) Infrared images reveal notches at the pupillary margin at the 11:00 and 3:00 positions (yellow arrow; green arrow); (B) a notch at the 3:00 position remains visible even after pupil dilation (green arrow). (C) OCT images indicated vitreous incarceration at the main incision (yellow arrow), with IOL significantly tilt (red arrow and white arrow). (D) OCT images showed vitreous incarceration at the side port accompanied by localized Descemet membrane detachment (green arrow).

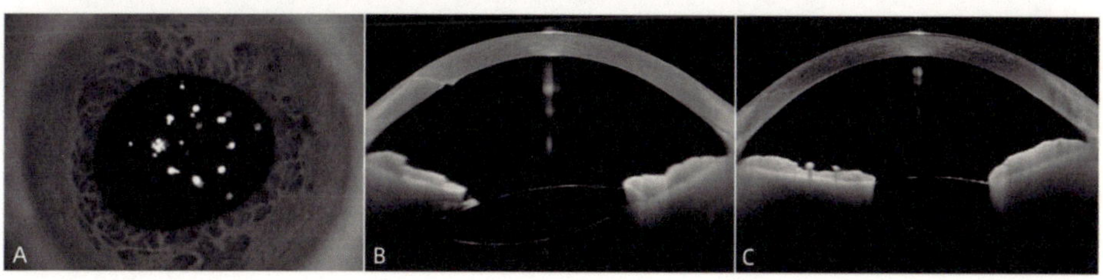

Figure 11.
SS-OCT images 1 month after the second surgery. (A) The infrared image reveals a nearly round pupil after pupil dilation; (B, C) OCT images indicate no vitreous incarceration at the main and side incisions.

2.9 IOL dislocation

Overview: IOL dislocation is a rare but serious complication following cataract surgery [17], with multiple mechanisms contributing to its occurrence. The IOL can dislocate into the anterior chamber, the pupil area, the posterior chamber, or the vitreous cavity. Based on the timing of occurrence, IOL dislocation can be classified into early and late types [18]. Early dislocation occurs within 3 months after cataract surgery, while late dislocation occurs after 3 months. In 1993, Davison first reported spontaneous late-onset IOL dislocation due to capsular contraction [19]. Although the incidence of late IOL dislocation is lower than that of early IOL dislocation, the

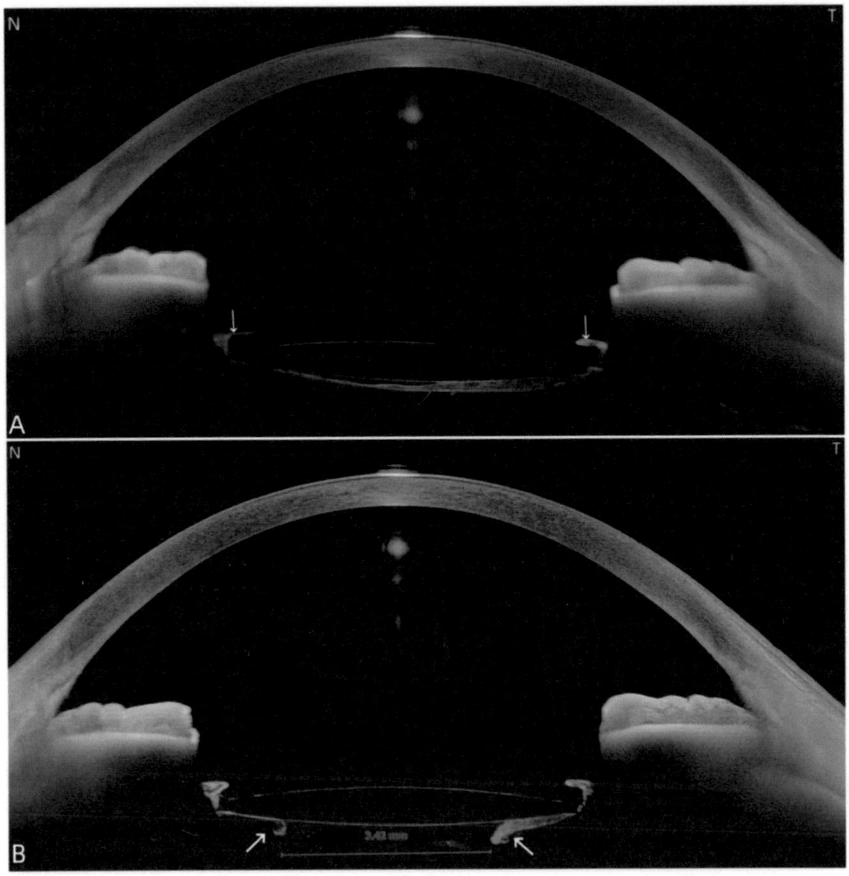

Figure 12.
SS-OCT image of PCO. (A) The SS-OCT examination revealed a high-reflective signal at the anterior capsule opening margin (white arrow). A dense, high-reflective, irregular band signal was observed between the posterior surface of IOL and the posterior lens capsule (A, red arrow). After performing Nd:YAG laser posterior capsulotomy, a defect in the central posterior lens capsule was noted, with a circular opening approximately 3.42 mm in diameter. (B) The edges of the laser opening in the posterior lens capsule exhibited curling (white arrow).

consequences are often severe, and the prognosis is typically poor [20]. Common treatment options include IOL repositioning, IOL fixation, and IOL replacement surgery.

2.9.1 Case presentations

Case 1: A 55-year-old male presented with blurred vision for 2 weeks with a medical history of right eye cataract surgery 7 years ago. A slit-lamp examination revealed that the IOL had dislocated to the iris surface, accompanied by a ruptured posterior capsule and vitreous prolapse.

OCT images and comments: The IOL had dislocated into the anterior chamber, resting on the iris surface with vitreous prolapse (**Figure 13**).

Case 2: A 53-year-old male presented with blurred vision for 2 weeks with medical history of cataract surgery in his left eye 3 years ago. A slit-lamp examination revealed

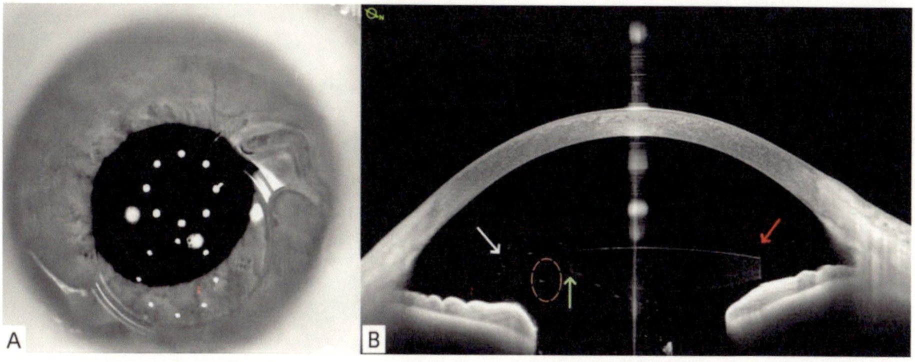

Figure 13.
SS-OCT image of IOL dislocation in Case 1. (A) The infrared image showed the IOL in the anterior chamber, with the optical zone displaced downward. The end of the IOL haptic was in contact with the anterior chamber angle. (B) The SS-OCT revealed that the IOL's optical zone was located on the iris surface (green and red arrows), accompanied by vitreous prolapse (white arrow). A low-reflective zone was observed between the IOL optical edge and the pupil margin (A, orange-dashed line).

downward displacement of the IOL and the capsule complex, with the optical zone of the IOL visible in the upper part of the pupil area. The clinical diagnosis was IOL-capsular bag complex dislocation in the left eye.

OCT images and comments: The IOL had shifted posteriorly, significantly increasing the distance from the iris plane. The IOL-capsular bag complex was floating or dislocated into the vitreous cavity. In the pupil area, downward displacement of the IOL-capsular bag complex was visible (**Figure 14**).

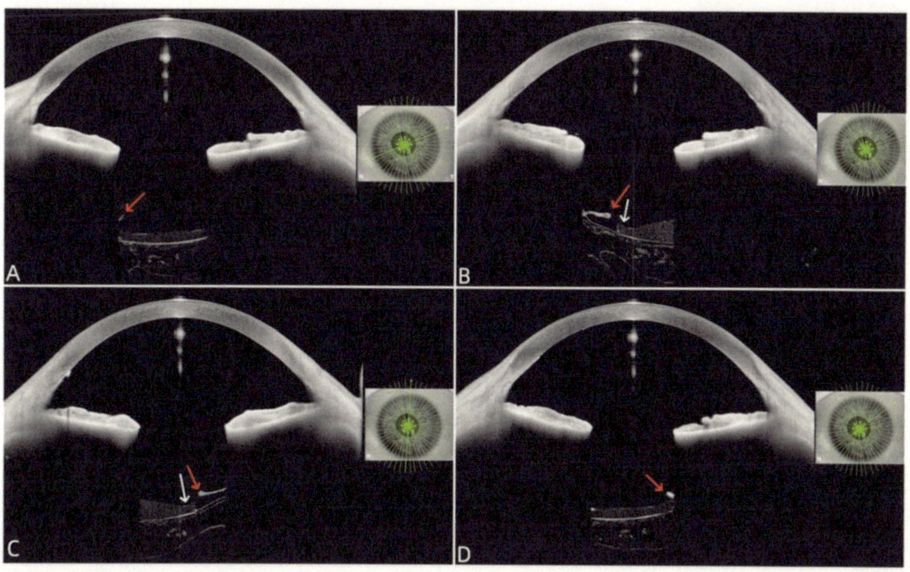

Figure 14.
SS-OCT image of IOL dislocation in Case 2. The distance between IOL and the iris was significantly widened. High-reflective signals of the anterior capsule were observed at the 8:00, 10:00, 12:00, and 2:00 o'clock positions at the pupil margin (A–D, red arrows), along with the edges of the IOL (B, C, white arrows).

2.10 IOL opacification

Overview: IOL opacification refers to the decrease in transparency of the IOL postoperatively due to various causes. Reports of opacification have been documented for IOLs made from different materials [21–24]. A slit-lamp examination reveals multiple manifestations depending on the location of the opacification. Different types of IOL opacification exhibit varying appearances on OCT images. Currently, IOL replacement surgery is the primary treatment for IOL opacification.

2.10.1 Case presentation

Case 1: A 57-year-old male underwent right eye cataract surgery 7 years ago. Over the past 2 years, he reported experiencing blurred vision. A slit-lamp examination revealed a frosted glass-like opacification on the surface of the IOL (**Figure 15A**). The clinical diagnosis was right eye IOL opacification, and the patient underwent IOL replacement surgery.

OCT images and comments: The OCT images clearly depict the position and morphology of the IOL opacification. In this patient, the reflective signal on the anterior surface of the right eye IOL was enhanced, with normal echogenicity within the IOL optical zone (**Figure 15B**).

Case 2: A 79-year-old female underwent left eye cataract surgery 3 years ago. Over the past year, she has experienced significant blurred vision in her left eye. A slit-lamp examination revealed diffuse, champagne-like opacification on the IOL (**Figure 16A**). The clinical diagnosis was left eye IOL opacification, and the patient underwent IOL replacement surgery.

OCT images and comments: The OCT images of the left eye demonstrated diffuse enhancement of the internal echogenicity within the optical zone, appearing as a uniform, consistent, diffuse punctate opacification. A dense, high-reflective band-like structure was observed between the posterior surface of the IOL and the posterior lens capsule (**Figure 16B**).

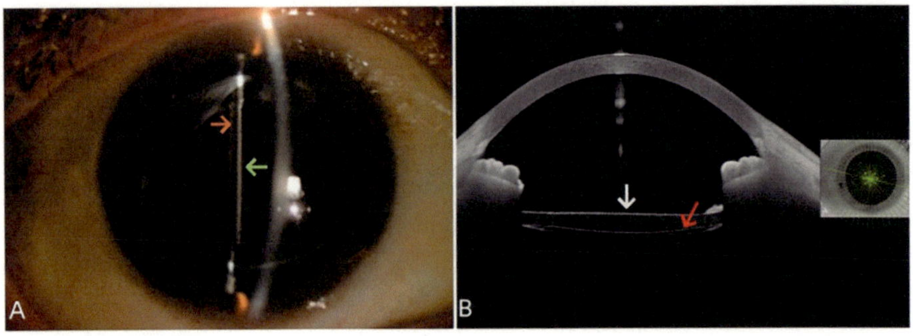

Figure 15.
Slit-lamp and SS-OCT images in Case 1. (A) The slit-lamp examination revealed a frosted glass-like opacification on the IOL anterior surface (green arrow), with the internal optical zone remaining transparent. The degree of opacification on the IOL posterior surface was slightly less than that on the anterior surface (orange arrow). (B) The OCT image demonstrated a uniformly high-reflective signal on the anterior surface of the IOL (white arrow), with low echogenicity within the optical zone, and the signal intensity on the IOL posterior surface was intermediate between the two (red arrow).

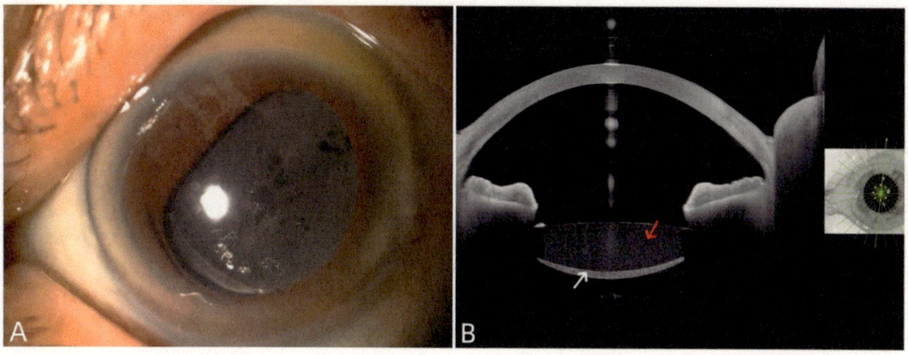

Figure 16.
Slit-lamp and SS-OCT images in Case 2. (A) The slit-lamp examination showed diffuse champagne-like opacification on the IOL. (B) The SS-OCT image revealed uniform, consistent, diffuse punctate enhancement of the echogenicity within the optical zone (red arrow), with a dense, high-reflective band observed between the IOL posterior surface and the posterior lens capsule (white arrow).

2.11 Capsular block syndrome (CBS)

Overview: CBS is a relatively rare complication [25]. It can occur intraoperatively, in the early postoperative period, or even years after surgery. This condition is related to the closure of the anterior capsular opening and the anterior surface of IOL, leading to the accumulation of opacified fluid between the IOL and the posterior lens capsule. This accumulation may result in IOL movement anteriorly, alterations of the eye refractive status, shallower anterior chamber depth, and secondary glaucoma, etc. Currently, Nd:YAG laser capsulotomy is one of the effective treatments for early

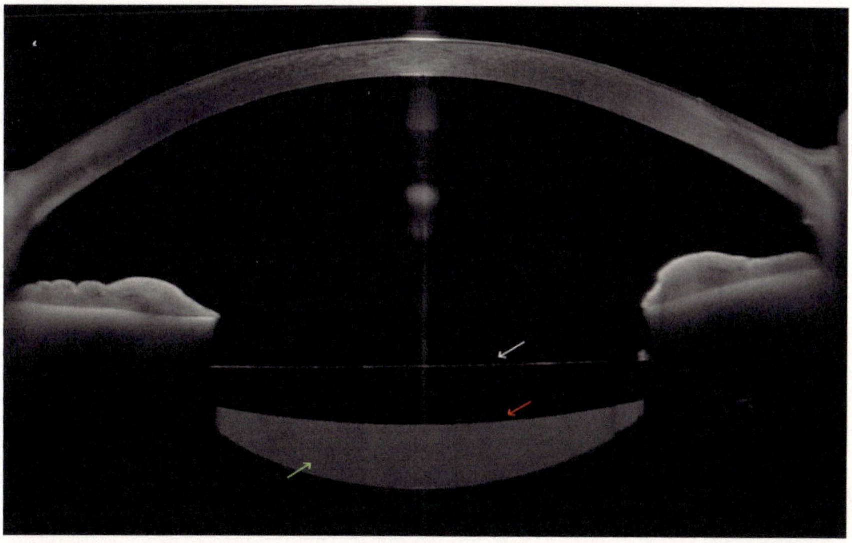

Figure 17.
SS-OCT image of CBS. The SS-OCT image clearly shows the anterior and posterior surface of the IOL (white arrow and red arrow), demonstrating a uniform high-reflective signal indicative of fluid retention between the IOL posterior surface and the posterior lens capsule. The thickness of the IOL in the central region was approximately equal to the thickness of the fluid accumulation.

capsular block syndrome; reoperation may also be conducted to remove the accumulated opacified fluid, lens cortex, and fibrotic anterior lens capsule [26].

Case presentation: A 76-year-old female underwent left eye cataract surgery 5 years ago and reported experiencing blurred vision for the past 2 months. A slit-lamp examination revealed a significant accumulation of grayish-white fluid between the IOL and the posterior lens capsule. The clinical diagnosis was CBS in the left eye.

OCT images and comments: In patients with CBS, SS-OCT imaging provides a clear visualization of the IOL morphology and the fluid accumulation within the capsular bag. It accurately quantifies the distance between the posterior surface of the IOL and the posterior lens capsule, thereby reducing the risk of misdiagnosing CBS as IOL opacification (**Figure 17**).

3. Conclusions

The above case examples illustrate that SS-OCT, as a non-invasive imaging tool, provides a significant reference value for the clinical diagnosis and treatment of anterior segment diseases. Its precise data measurement and analysis can offer evidence for changes before and after the treatment of various anterior segment pathologies. In the future, SS-OCT is expected to have even broader applications in assessing anterior segment diseases and may become a golden standard for some conditions.

Acknowledgements

All the cases mentioned in this chapter are real clinical cases.

Author details

Feiyan Chai and Xiaogang Wang*
Shanxi Eye Hospital Affiliated to Shanxi Medical University, Taiyuan, Shanxi Province, China

*Address all correspondence to: movie6521@163.com

References

[1] Aggarwal S, Al Bayyat G, Karp CL. Nonclearing corneal edema after phacoemulsification and intraocular lens implantation. Journal of the American Medical Association Ophthalmology. 2021;**139**:480-481. DOI: 10.1001/jamaophthalmol.2020.4660

[2] Sharma N, Singhal D, Nair SP, et al. Corneal edema after phacoemulsification. Indian Journal of Ophthalmology. 2017;**65**:1381-1389. DOI: 10.4103/ijo.IJO_871_17

[3] Gogaki E, Tsolaki F, Tiganita S, et al. Iridoschisis: Case report and review of the literature. Clinical Ophthalmology. 2011;**5**:381-384. DOI: 10.2147/OPTH.S17269

[4] Ben Aoun S, Hachicha I, Bouraoui R, et al. Atypical presentation of bilateral iridoschisis with abnormal visibility of iris vessels: Role of anterior segment optical coherence tomography. European Journal of Ophthalmology. 2024;**34**:NP38-NP42. DOI: 10.1177/11206721231206792

[5] Loewenstein A, Foster J. Iridoschisis with multiple purpose of stromal threads. The British Journal of Ophthalmology. 1945;**29**:277-282

[6] Schoneveld PG, Pesudovs K. Iridoschisis. Clinical & Experimental Optometry. 1999;**82**:29-33. DOI: 10.1111/j.1444-0938.1999.tb06784.x

[7] Mansour AM. A family with iridoschisis, narrow anterior chamber angle, and presenile cataract. Ophthalmic Paediatrics and Genetics. 1986;**7**:145-149. DOI: 10.3109/13816818609004131

[8] Gueudry J, Muraine M. Anterior uveitis. Journal Français d'Ophtalmologie. 2018;**41**:e11-e21. DOI: 10.1016/j.jfo.2017.11.003

[9] Gibbs ML, Jacobs M, Wilkie AO, et al. Posterior lenticonus: Clinical patterns and genetics. Journal of Pediatric Ophthalmology and Strabismus. 1993;**30**:171-175. DOI: 10.3928/0191-3913-19930501-10

[10] Khalil M, Saheb N. Posterior lenticonus. Ophthalmology. 1984;**91**:1429-1430, 43A. DOI: 10.1016/s0161-6420(84)34132-x

[11] Kapoor G, Seth S, Ahluwalia TS, Dhar SK. Posterior polar cataract: Minimizing risks. Medical Journal, Armed Forces India. 2016;**72**(3):242-246. DOI: 0.1016/j.mjafi.2016.04.004

[12] Osher RH, Yu BC, Koch DD. Posterior polar cataracts: A predisposition to intraoperative posterior capsular rupture. Journal of Cataract and Refractive Surgery. 1990;**16**(2):157-162. DOI: 10.1016/s0886-3350(13)80724-9

[13] Wormstone IM. Posterior capsule opacification: A cell biological perspective. Experimental Eye Research. 2002;**74**:337-347. DOI: 10.1006/exer.2001.1153

[14] Apple DJ, Peng Q, Visessook N, et al. Eradication of posterior capsule opacification: Documentation of a marked decrease in Nd:YAG laser posterior capsulotomy rates noted in an analysis of 5416 pseudophakic human eyes obtained postmortem. Ophthalmology. 2001;**108**:505-518. DOI: 10.1016/s0161-6420(00)00589-3

[15] Ursell PG, Dhariwal M, O'Boyle D, et al. 5 year incidence of YAG capsulotomy and PCO after cataract

surgery with single-piece monofocal intraocular lenses: A real-world evidence study of 20,763 eyes. Eye (London, England). 2020;**34**(5):960-968. DOI: 10.1038/s41433-019-0630-9

[16] Chambless WS. Neodymium: YAG laser posterior capsulotomy results and complications. Journal - American Intra-Ocular Implant Society. 1985;**11**:31-32. DOI: 10.1016/s0146-2776(85)80111-7

[17] Lorente R, de Rojas V, Vazquez de Parga P, et al. Management of late spontaneous in-the-bag intraocular lens dislocation: Retrospective analysis of 45 cases. Journal of Cataract and Refractive Surgery. 2010;**36**:1270-1282. DOI: 10.1016/j.jcrs.2010.01.035

[18] Davis D, Brubaker J, Espandar L, et al. Late in-the-bag spontaneous intraocular lens dislocation: Evaluation of 86 consecutive cases. Ophthalmology. 2009;**116**:664-670. DOI: 10.1016/j.ophtha.2008.11.018

[19] Davison JA. Capsule contraction syndrome. Journal of Cataract and Refractive Surgery. 1993;**19**:582-589. DOI: 10.1016/s0886-3350(13)80004-1

[20] Vaiciuliene R, Jasinskas V. Corneal endothelial status in different grades of late spontaneous in-the-bag IOL dislocation. International Ophthalmology. 2021;**41**:1625-1634. DOI: 10.1007/s10792-021-01702-7

[21] Apple DJ, Peng Q, Arthur SN, et al. Snowflake degeneration of polymethyl methacrylate posterior chamber intraocular lens optic material: A newly described clinical condition caused by unexpected late opacification of polymethyl methacrylate. Ophthalmology. 2002;**109**:1666-1675. DOI: 10.1016/s0161-6420(02)01122-3

[22] Elgohary M, Zaheer A, Werner L, et al. Opacification of array SA40N silicone multifocal intraocular lens. Journal of Cataract and Refractive Surgery. 2007;**33**:342-347. DOI: 10.1016/j.jcrs.2006.09.034

[23] Gurabardhi M, Häberle H, Aurich H, et al. Serial intraocular lens opacifications of different designs from the same manufacturer: Clinical and light microscopic results of 71 explant cases. Journal of Cataract and Refractive Surgery. 2018;**44**:1326-1332. DOI: 10.1016/j.jcrs.2018.07.026

[24] Fernández-Vigo JI, Macarro-Merino A, De Moura-Ramos JJ, et al. Comparative study of the glistening between four intraocular lens models assessed by OCT and deep learning. Journal of Cataract and Refractive Surgery. 2024;**50**:37-42. DOI: 10.1097/j.jcrs.0000000000001316

[25] Davison JA. Capsular bag distension after endophacoemulsification and posterior chamber intraocular lens implantation. Journal of Cataract and Refractive Surgery. 1990;**16**:99-108. DOI: 10.1016/s0886-3350(13)80883-8

[26] Kanclerz P, Wang X. Postoperative capsular bag distension syndrome - Risk factors and treatment. Seminars in Ophthalmology. 2019;**34**:409-419. DOI: 10.1080/08820538.2019.1640750

Chapter 7

Optical Coherence Tomography in Strabismus: Innovations and Clinical Applications

Emine Tinkir Kayitmazbatir

Abstract

Strabismus, a visual disorder involving eye misalignment, presents significant diagnostic and treatment challenges. Optical coherence tomography (OCT) has transformed the management of strabismus by providing high-resolution imaging of ocular tissues, which aids in accurate diagnosis and management. Continuous advancements in OCT technology, including anterior segment OCT (AS-OCT) and OCT-angiography (OCT-A), enhance preoperative planning, postoperative monitoring, and evaluation of associated conditions such as thyroid ophthalmopathy and amblyopia. This chapter aims to provide a comprehensive overview of OCT's role in strabismus management, highlight technological advancements, and discuss the integration of OCT tools in clinical practice. It will explore current research trends and future directions in the application of OCT for strabismus and amblyopia.

Keywords: anterior segment OCT, clinical applications, ocular imaging, OCT-angiography, optical coherence tomography, strabismus, amblyopia

1. Introduction

1.1 Overview of strabismus

1.1.1 Definition and types

Strabismus, commonly known as "crossed eyes" or "squint," is a condition where the eyes do not properly align with each other when looking at an object. Strabismus, or misalignment of the eyes, can be classified based on several key factors. Heterophoria is a latent misalignment, while heterotropia is a visible, consistent deviation. Ocular alignment refers to proper positioning of the eyes, with deviations such as esotropia (inward), exotropia (outward), hypertropia (upward), and hypotropia (downward). Comitant strabismus involves a constant angle of deviation in all gaze directions, whereas incomitant strabismus varies depending on gaze direction, often due to muscle weakness or paralysis. Strabismus can be constant or intermittent, depending on whether the deviation is always present or occurs only under specific conditions. Vergence classifications describe the difference in alignment at near or far distances, with conditions such as convergence excess or divergence insufficiency. Fixation habits also play a role, distinguishing between nonalternating (one eye always fixates) and alternating strabismus (both eyes alternate). The onset of strabismus can be congenital (present at birth) or acquired later in life, influenced by trauma, nerve issues, or other conditions. Paralytic strabismus occurs when there is nerve damage affecting the extraocular muscles, leading to a loss or reduction in muscle function. Restrictive (mechanical) strabismus results from structural abnormalities, such as muscle fibrosis or scarring, that physically restrict normal eye movement. Orbital strabismus arises from anatomical abnormalities in the orbit or surrounding facial structures, such as craniofacial dysostosis or hydrocephalus, which cause the eyes to misalign due to altered bone or tissue structures [1].

1.1.2 Epidemiology and prevalence

Strabismus affects around 3–4% of the population, making it one of the most common visual disorders in both children and adults [2]. It can occur at any age, though it often manifests in early childhood. In congenital cases, the incidence is reported to be higher, with esotropia being more common than exotropia in these early cases. However, in some populations, exotropia may be more prevalent, particularly in Asia and other regions.

In terms of gender distribution, no significant gender predilection exists for strabismus as a whole [3]. However, some studies have shown that specific types of strabismus, such as intermittent exotropia, may occur slightly more frequently in females in certain demographics [4].

1.1.3 Clinical significance and impact on patients

Strabismus is not merely a cosmetic concern; it can significantly affect visual function and quality of life. Amblyopia, commonly known as "lazy eye," is a frequent complication, occurring when the brain suppresses the image from the misaligned eye, leading to reduced vision in that eye. Strabismus can also impair binocular vision, affecting depth perception and leading to issues with coordination and spatial awareness.

The psychosocial impact of strabismus on patients, especially children, can be profound [5]. Children with noticeable eye misalignment may face social stigma, bullying, and self-esteem issues. In adults, strabismus can impact professional and social interactions, leading to difficulties in maintaining eye contact or performing tasks requiring precise vision, such as driving or reading. Early detection and intervention are critical in preventing long-term complications, especially in children, where therapies such as patching or strabismus surgery can significantly improve outcomes.

1.1.4 Extraocular muscles: Location and functions

Strabismus is closely linked to the function and coordination of the extraocular muscles that are responsible for controlling eye movements. There are six extraocular muscles in each eye that work in unison to move the eye in different directions. These muscles are innervated by three cranial nerves: the oculomotor nerve (cranial nerve III), the trochlear nerve (cranial nerve IV), and the abducens nerve (cranial nerve VI).

1. The medial rectus is located on the inner (nasal) side of the eye. Its primary function is to move the eye inward toward the nose (adduction). It is innervated

by the oculomotor nerve (cranial nerve III), and its insertion point is approximately 5.5 mm from the limbus.

2. The lateral rectus, positioned on the outer (temporal) side of the eye, moves the eye outward, away from the nose (abduction). It is innervated by the abducens nerve (cranial nerve VI) and inserts approximately 6.9 mm from the limbus.

3. The superior rectus is located on the top of the eye. It primarily elevates the eye (moves it upward), with the additional roles in slight inward rotation (intorsion) and inward turning (adduction). This muscle is innervated by the oculomotor nerve (cranial nerve III), and it inserts approximately 7.7 mm from the limbus.

4. The inferior rectus is situated on the bottom of the eye. It primarily depresses the eye (moves it downward), while also contributing to slight outward rotation (extorsion) and inward turning (adduction). It is also innervated by the oculomotor nerve (cranial nerve III), and its insertion point is approximately 6.5 mm from the limbus.

5. The superior oblique originates at the back of the eye socket, loops through the trochlea (a pulley-like structure), and attaches to the top of the eyeball. Its primary function is to move the eye downward and outward (depression and abduction), with an additional role in inward rotation (intorsion). It is innervated by the trochlear nerve (cranial nerve IV). The superior oblique does not insert directly near the limbus but functions through the trochlea system.

6. The inferior oblique originates from the front part of the orbital floor and runs beneath the eye, attaching to the bottom of the eyeball. It primarily elevates the eye and moves it outward (elevation and abduction), while also causing outward rotation (extorsion). The muscle is innervated by the oculomotor nerve (cranial nerve III) and, like the superior oblique, does not have a direct insertion near the limbus.

1.1.5 Coordination of eye movements and strabismus

For normal binocular vision, the extraocular muscles must work in a highly coordinated fashion to align both eyes on the same target. The movements of both eyes must be synchronized, allowing them to track objects, focus, and move in parallel across different directions of gaze. This coordination is controlled by the brainstem and cerebellum that process information from the visual system and the vestibular system (balance and spatial orientation). When the extraocular muscles do not work together properly or if there is an issue with the cranial nerves supplying these muscles, strabismus occurs. Understanding the function and anatomy of these muscles is essential in diagnosing and managing different forms of strabismus.

1.2 Optical coherence tomography (OCT)

1.2.1 History and development of OCT

Optical coherence tomography (OCT) is a non-invasive imaging technique that provides high-resolution cross-sectional images of biological tissues. It was first introduced in the early 1990s by a group of researchers led by Dr. David Huang and

Dr. James Fujimoto at the Massachusetts Institute of Technology (MIT) [6]. Initially developed for use in ophthalmology, OCT has since expanded into other medical fields, including cardiology, dermatology, and oncology.

The early versions of OCT, such as time-domain OCT (TD-OCT), provided foundational advancements by allowing the visualization of retinal layers in unprecedented detail. However, its relatively slow acquisition speed and limited resolution prompted the development of newer technologies. In the early 2000s, the introduction of spectral-domain OCT (SD-OCT) revolutionized the field. By utilizing Fourier transformation of interference patterns, SD-OCT significantly improved image resolution and acquisition speed. More recently, the development of swept-source OCT (SS-OCT) has further enhanced depth penetration and speed, allowing for more detailed imaging of deeper structures, such as the choroid and the optic nerve head.

1.2.2 Basic principles and technology

OCT is based on the principle of low-coherence interferometry. It works similar to ultrasound, but instead of sound waves, OCT uses light waves (typically near-infrared light) to generate images. The system directs a beam of light onto the tissue, and the light that reflects back from different layers of the tissue is captured. By measuring the time delay and intensity of the reflected light, OCT creates a detailed, cross-sectional image of the tissue.

The light used in OCT has a short coherence length, which allows it to achieve high axial resolution, typically on the order of microns (micrometers). The resolution depends on the wavelength and bandwidth of the light source, and OCT can differentiate between various layers of the retina, from the inner-limiting membrane to the retinal pigment epithelium (RPE). The depth and resolution make it particularly suitable for diagnosing and managing retinal diseases.

Modern OCT devices employ spectral-domain or swept-source technologies to capture images rapidly and with high resolution. SD-OCT uses a broadband light source and a spectrometer to detect light reflected at different depths simultaneously, while SS-OCT employs a tunable laser and a photodetector to scan the tissue, providing enhanced penetration and faster imaging [7].

1.2.3 Advantages of OCT in ophthalmology

OCT has revolutionized ophthalmology, particularly in the diagnosis and management of retinal and optic nerve diseases. Its advantages include the following:

1. Non-invasive and fast: OCT provides high-resolution images without the need for any contact with the eye or use of contrast agents. Imaging can be completed within seconds, making it highly convenient for both patients and clinicians.

2. High-resolution imaging: The ability to visualize retinal layers in great detail allows clinicians to detect and monitor subtle structural changes, which is especially valuable for early diagnosis and treatment of diseases such as macular degeneration, diabetic retinopathy, and glaucoma.

3. Quantitative analysis: OCT not only provides images but also offers precise quantitative measurements, such as retinal thickness, nerve fiber layer thickness, and

the size of macular lesions. These measurements help track disease progression and response to treatments.

4. Real-time monitoring: OCT allows for real-time imaging, enabling immediate assessment of therapeutic interventions, such as in cases of retinal laser therapy or intravitreal injections.

5. Wide range of applications: While initially developed for retinal imaging, OCT has applications in anterior segment imaging, corneal disease assessment, glaucoma management, and strabismus and even in surgical planning. Its versatility makes it a valuable tool in comprehensive ophthalmic care.

6. Guidance in clinical decision making: OCT has become indispensable in clinical practice for its ability to guide treatment decisions. For example, it is essential in determining the need for anti-VEGF (vascular endothelial growth factor) therapy in patients with neovascular age-related macular degeneration (AMD) or diabetic macular edema (DME).

2. Clinical applications of OCT in strabismus

2.1 Assessment of extraocular muscles, retinal, and optic nerve changes

OCT has become an indispensable tool in the evaluation of various ocular structures and conditions. In the context of strabismus, OCT plays a crucial role in assessing the health and integrity of extraocular muscles, the macula, and the retinal nerve fiber layer (RNFL), offering valuable insights into both functional and structural changes in the eye.

2.1.1 Extraocular muscles

While OCT is primarily used for imaging the retina and anterior segment, it has also been applied to assess extraocular muscles, especially in cases of strabismus (**Figure 1**). Imaging the extraocular muscles can provide valuable information about their structure, size, and possible atrophy or hypertrophy, which is crucial in the diagnosis and management of strabismus. In patients with strabismus, abnormalities in extraocular muscles may contribute to or result from the misalignment. For instance, in thyroid eye disease, extraocular muscle enlargement is common and may exacerbate or even cause strabismus due to muscle fibrosis or restrictions. In these cases, OCT can offer adjunctive imaging when combined with MRI or CT to provide a detailed assessment of muscle changes. Although OCT's ability to directly visualize the extraocular muscles is limited, its value lies in its ability to complement other imaging modalities for a comprehensive evaluation of strabismus cases involving muscle pathology.

2.1.2 Macular evaluation

Macular assessment with OCT is critical in patients with strabismus, especially in those with long-standing or untreated strabismus. The macula is responsible for central vision, and any abnormalities or misalignments in the eye can lead to macular

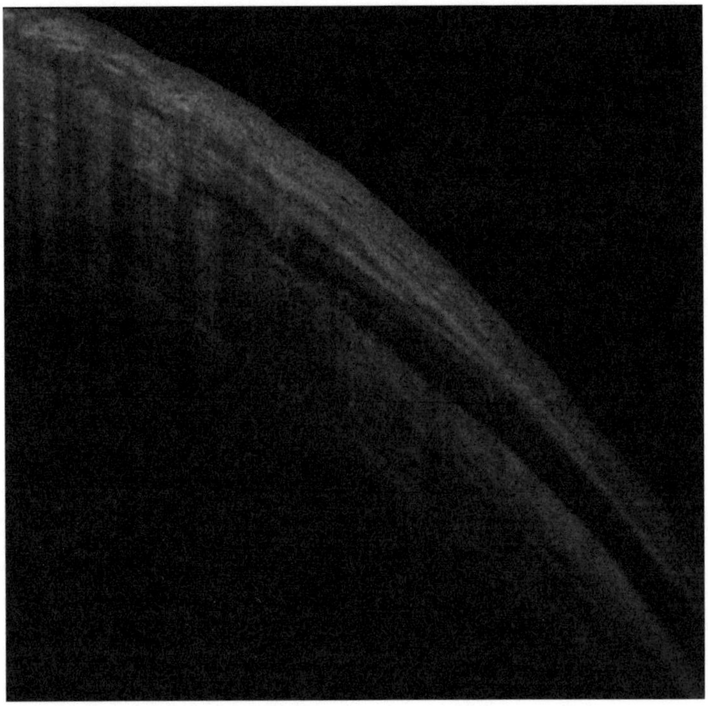

Figure 1.
Anterior segment optical coherence tomography (AS-OCT) image showing the cross-sectional view of the extraocular muscle insertion site. The image illustrates the muscle-tendon interface in the scleral region, highlighting the thickness, structural integrity, and anterior insertion point of the muscle.

changes over time. In patients with strabismic amblyopia, OCT can reveal subtle macular abnormalities, such as thinning or thickening of the retinal layers, which may not be detectable through clinical examination alone. Additionally, the presence of macular pathology, such as macular edema or macular holes, may affect the treatment plan for patients with strabismus, particularly in surgical planning. Preoperative OCT evaluation of the macula ensures that any underlying retinal pathology is addressed, optimizing the outcomes of strabismus surgery (**Figure 2**).

Optical coherence tomography angiography (OCTA) is a non-invasive imaging technique that allows detailed visualization of retinal and choroidal blood flow. It captures high-resolution images of the microvasculature, making it invaluable in diagnosing and monitoring various eye conditions. Preoperative and postoperative changes in the vascular network can also be evaluated by using OCT angiography (**Figure 3**).

Amblyopia, particularly in children, can lead to changes in the macular structure. OCTA has proven valuable in examining the microvascular changes associated with amblyopia, often present in patients with strabismus. In a study involving amblyopic children, OCTA revealed a larger foveal avascular zone (FAZ) in amblyopic eyes compared to non-amblyopic eyes. This was associated with reduced vessel density, suggesting that amblyopia may involve not just functional impairment but also structural changes in the retinal vasculature [8]. In another study involving 32 children with anisometropic myopic amblyopia, OCTA was used to assess changes in vessel density (VD) before and after treatment. Results showed significant improvements in visual acuity and VD, suggesting that OCTA is not only useful in evaluating treatment efficacy but also in tracking progress during amblyopia management and follow-up care [9].

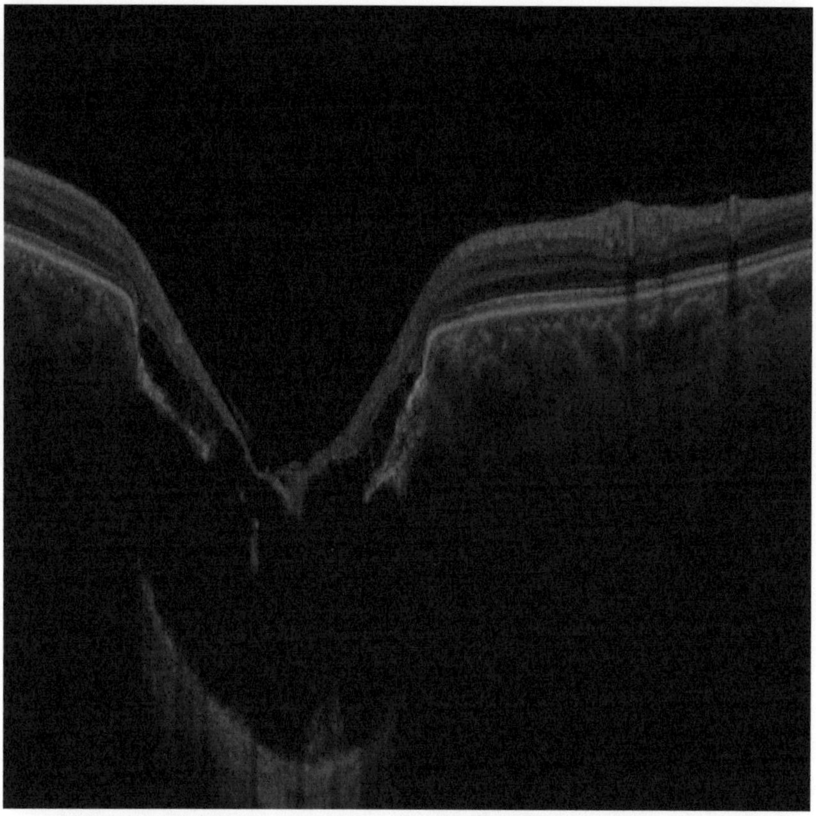

Figure 2.
Preoperative optical coherence tomography (OCT) image of the right eye showing macular scar. The scan highlights the scarring in the macular region, which is associated with reduced visual acuity in the affected eye. The patient is scheduled for surgery due to esotropia related to the visual impairment on the scarred side. The OCT image provides detailed information about the extent and location of the scar tissue.

2.1.3 Retinal nerve fiber layer analysis

OCT's ability to assess the RNFL is another valuable application in patients with strabismus. The RNFL consists of ganglion cell axons that form the optic nerve, and any damage to this layer can lead to visual impairment. OCT provides a non-invasive way to measure the thickness of the RNFL, allowing for the detection of early glaucomatous changes or optic neuropathies, In patients with strabismus, especially those with associated conditions such as optic nerve hypoplasia. RNFL analysis can help monitor the health of the optic nerve. RNFL thinning may indicate optic nerve atrophy or damage, which can affect both the treatment plan and prognosis. Additionally, in cases of congenital strabismus or amblyopia, OCT-based RNFL analysis provides insight into any subclinical optic nerve changes that could contribute to the visual dysfunction. Overall, RNFL analysis through OCT offers a detailed evaluation of optic nerve health, complementing the clinical assessment of visual function and aiding in the management of complex strabismus cases where optic nerve involvement is suspected. Patients with high myopia often present with tilted optic discs, which can complicate the diagnosis and management of associated strabismus. A study using spectral-domain OCT (SD-OCT) developed a new method for quantifying the tilt

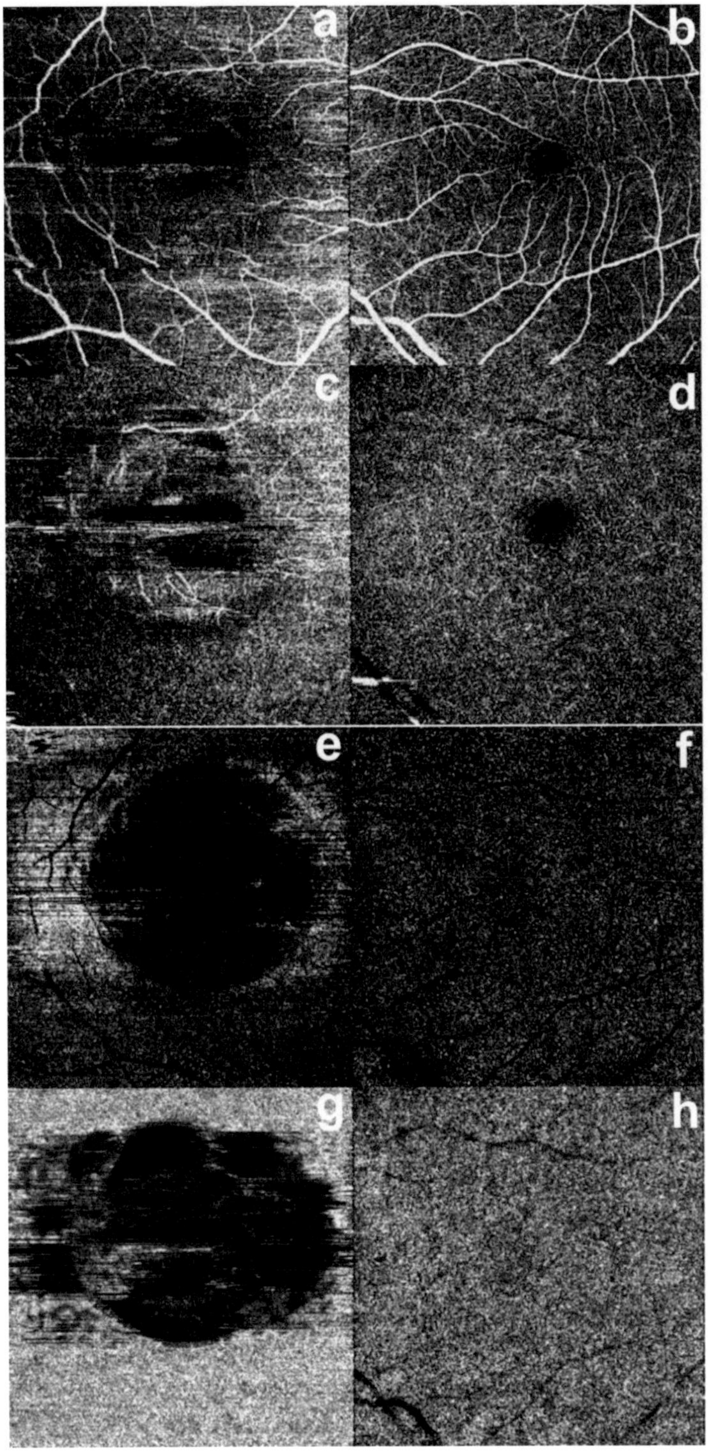

Figure 3.
OCT angiography (OCTA) images of the same patient's right and left eyes, respectively, displaying the superficial plexus (a, b), deep plexus (c, d), outer retina (e, f), and choriocapillaris (g, h). Preoperative and postoperative changes in the vascular network can also be evaluated by using OCT angiography (OCTA). In the right eye, however, shadowing caused by scar tissue is observed across all layers, making the evaluation insufficient.

angle of the optic disc. This method revealed that patients with high myopia and a greater optic disc tilt angle also had significant thinning of the RNFL, a finding that could predispose them to glaucoma [10].

2.2 Preoperative assessment

2.2.1 Identifying structural abnormalities including challenging cases like trauma and thyroid ophthalmopathy

OCT is an invaluable tool in the preoperative assessment of patients undergoing strabismus surgery, particularly in complex cases where structural abnormalities may affect surgical outcomes. By providing detailed cross-sectional images of ocular tissues, OCT helps identify hidden or subtle anatomical issues that may not be apparent during a routine clinical examination (**Figure 4**). In patients requiring reoperations for strabismus, particularly those with previous surgeries where muscle position data is no longer available, anterior segment OCT (AS-OCT) provides a highly effective way to localize extraocular muscles. A study involving 35 horizontal rectus muscles showed that AS-OCT was accurate in determining the distance between the muscle insertion and the limbus, matching intraoperative caliper measurements with a high level of agreement [11].

1. Trauma: In cases of ocular trauma, OCT is critical for evaluating both anterior and posterior segment structures before surgery. Traumatic injuries can affect multiple layers of the eye, including the cornea, lens, retina, and optic nerve. OCT can detect retinal tears, macular edema, or subclinical retinal detachment, ensuring that these issues are addressed before surgical correction of strabismus. Trauma-related changes, such as scarring or fibrosis of the extraocular muscles, may also complicate the surgical approach, making detailed imaging essential

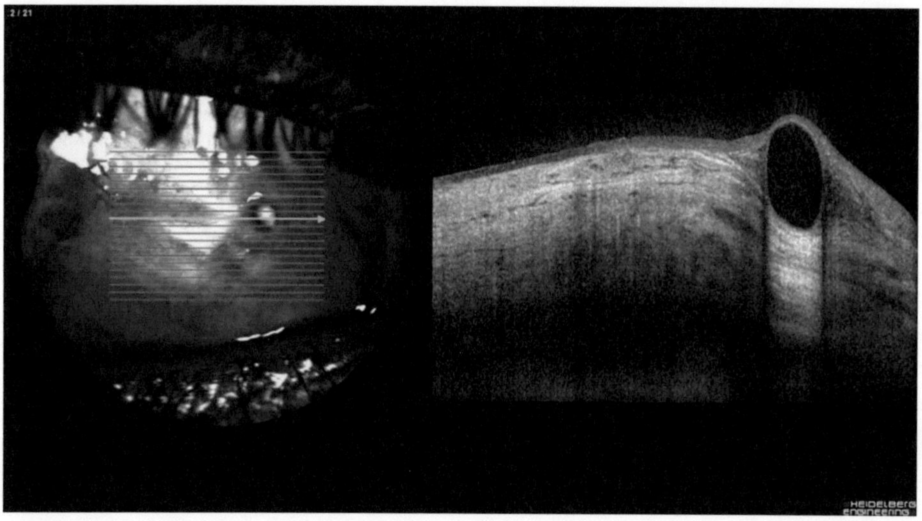

Figure 4.
Preoperative anterior segment OCT (AS-OCT) image of a patient with a history of strabismus surgery performed years ago, for which detailed surgical information is unavailable. The image reveals an inclusion cyst consistent with the possible site of the previous surgical intervention located at the region corresponding to the medial rectus muscle.

for planning. A study highlights the utility of anterior segment optical coherence tomography (AS-OCT) in managing cases of strabismus, particularly in reoperations, muscle hypoplasia, and detecting lost or slipped muscles. AS-OCT is also valuable in ocular trauma, identifying foreign bodies in extraocular muscles and differentiating their material composition. Although limited to visualizing anterior muscle segments, AS-OCT is useful in confirming muscle injury and preventing the need for MRI in some cases [12].

2. Thyroid ophthalmopathy (Graves' orbitopathy): Patients with thyroid ophthalmopathy often present with restrictive strabismus due to enlargement and fibrosis of the extraocular muscles. Preoperative OCT can assist in evaluating the integrity of the optic nerve and macula, which may be compressed by swollen orbital tissues. This is particularly important in preventing optic neuropathy, a potential complication of thyroid eye disease. Identifying early signs of optic nerve compression or macular changes *via* OCT allows for timely intervention and adjustment of surgical plans to minimize postoperative complications. Moreover, OCT can provide complementary imaging to orbital imaging techniques such as MRI and CT, especially for evaluating extraocular muscle involvement and ruling out optic nerve involvement, particularly in severe cases of thyroid ophthalmopathy. The integration of OCT findings with other imaging modalities ensures a holistic preoperative evaluation of these complex cases. In a study involving retinal perfusion variations in thyroid-associated ophthalmopathy (TAO) patients, OCT and OCTA were used to evaluate key parameters, including the FAZ and macular perfusion density (mPD). The study found that active TAO patients exhibited the lowest mPD and significant differences in retinal perfusion across stages. These findings highlight the potential of OCT and OCTA in non-invasively detecting peripapillary and macular changes, making them valuable tools for monitoring TAO progression and assessing disease severity [13].

In a study investigating extraocular rectus muscle tendons in patients with Graves' ophthalmopathy using OCT, researchers measured the medial and lateral rectus tendon thicknesses in healthy controls and patients with both inactive and active Graves' ophthalmopathy. Results showed that patients with Graves' ophthalmopathy had thicker rectus tendons compared to controls, and active disease was associated with thicker tendons than inactive disease. OCT was found to be an effective tool for assessing tendon thickness, correlating with clinical activity scores of the disease [14]. In a study evaluating the impact of conjunctiva and Tenon's capsule thickness (CTT) on strabismus surgery outcomes, researchers used swept-source anterior segment optical coherence tomography (AS-OCT) to measure the preoperative and postoperative CTT. The results revealed increased CTT on the resection side and decreased CTT on the recession side 1 year after surgery. The study also found that the corrective effect of surgery was closely correlated with preoperative CTT on the recession side, suggesting that CTT could serve as a valuable prognostic factor in strabismus surgery outcomes [15].

2.2.2 Surgical planning and customization

OCT has significantly enhanced the precision of surgical planning in strabismus cases by offering detailed insights into ocular structures. In complex cases, such as those involving trauma or restrictive strabismus, OCT enables surgeons to customize their approach to the unique anatomical characteristics of each patient.

1. Corneal topography and anterior segment imaging: In cases where anterior segment abnormalities are present, such as in trauma or post-surgical corneal scarring, OCT provides high-resolution images of the cornea and anterior chamber. This can be crucial in avoiding corneal complications during surgery and ensuring that any pre-existing anterior segment pathology does not interfere with the surgical correction of strabismus.

2. Posterior segment assessment: Preoperative OCT of the posterior segment allows for careful assessment of the retina and optic nerve, both of which are essential for visual function. In patients with previous retinal surgery, macular diseases, or optic neuropathy, OCT can help in predicting the visual outcomes of strabismus surgery. For example, patients with pre-existing macular pathology may have limited visual recovery postoperatively, and this information is vital for setting realistic expectations for both the surgeon and the patient. It is also useful in demonstrating pathologies associated with high myopia (**Figure 5**).

3. Customization of surgical approach: OCT also plays a role in tailoring the surgical technique based on the individual patient's anatomy. In cases of reoperation, OCT is useful for detecting scar tissue or muscle slippage, which may

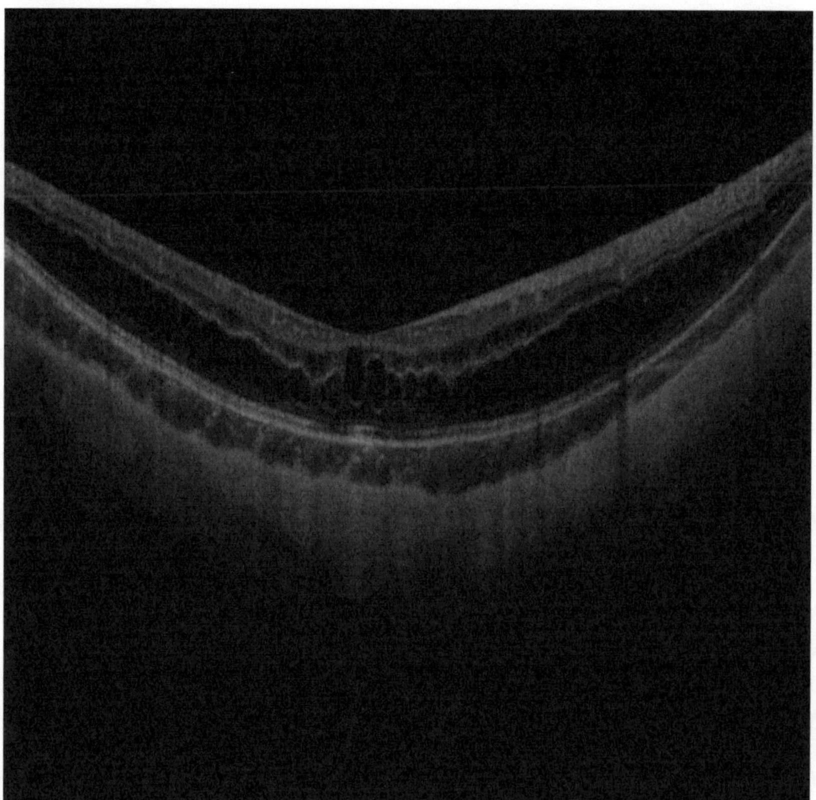

Figure 5.
Optical coherence tomography (OCT) image of the macula in a child with myopic macular retinoschisis. The scan reveals intraretinal splitting, with visible schisis cavities predominantly in the outer retinal layers.

require a more customized surgical approach. In a prospective observational study, the role of swept-source anterior segment optical coherence tomography (SS-ASOCT) in extraocular muscle imaging was evaluated in 150 subjects, covering 1104 extraocular muscles. The study included normal eyes, re-operated eyes, paralytic and non-paralytic strabismus, post-traumatic strabismus, and eyes with thyroid disease. The mean age of the subjects was 38.15 ± 16.25 years, and muscle insertion was identified in over 90% of cases. SS-ASOCT provided clinically valuable information by imaging the anterior 4–14 mm of the rectus muscles, facilitating optimal preoperative surgical planning. The tool proved especially useful in complex cases, such as traumatic muscle slippage and thyroid muscle hypertrophy, making it a reliable aid in surgical decision-making for various strabismic conditions [16].

OCT's ability to provide detailed structural images enhances preoperative planning by identifying hidden anatomical challenges and optimizing the surgical approach. This results in better patient outcomes, particularly in complex and high-risk cases where precise anatomical information is critical.

2.3 Intraoperative use: Intraoperative optical coherence tomography (iOCT)

2.3.1 Real-time imaging and guidance

The advent of intraoperative optical coherence tomography (iOCT) has marked a significant advancement in ophthalmic surgery, offering real-time, high-resolution imaging during surgical procedures. iOCT integrates OCT technology into the surgical microscope, allowing surgeons to visualize ocular structures in cross section without interrupting the surgery. This real-time imaging capability is particularly beneficial in strabismus surgery, where precise manipulation of delicate ocular tissues is crucial.

In strabismus surgery, iOCT can assist in several ways:

1. Visualization of tissue planes: iOCT provides detailed images of the sclera, Tenon's capsule, conjunctiva, and extraocular muscles. Real-time imaging helps in identifying the exact location and depth of tissues, which is essential for precise dissection and minimizing tissue damage. iOCT has brought a new level of precision to strabismus surgeries, especially in cases where tissue manipulation is complex. One study demonstrated the utility of iOCT during scleral suturing in strabismus surgeries, allowing the surgeon to visualize scleral passes in real time. This reduced the risk of deep scleral penetration or muscle misplacement, which are common causes of surgical failure in strabismus correction. iOCT ensured the precise positioning of extraocular muscles, particularly in reoperations where scarring made anatomical landmarks less visible [17].

2. Assessment of extraocular muscle insertion and pathology: During surgery, iOCT can help visualize the insertion points of extraocular muscles on the sclera. This is particularly useful in reoperations or complicated cases where scar tissue or previous surgical alterations may obscure normal anatomical landmarks. iOCT aids in identifying residual muscle tissue and any anomalous insertions or pathologies.

3. Guidance in complex cases: In cases involving restrictive strabismus, such as in thyroid ophthalmopathy or scarring from trauma, iOCT assists in visualizing fibrotic tissues and adhesions. This guidance allows for careful dissection and release of restrictive tissues, reducing the risk of inadvertent damage to surrounding structures.

4. Verification of surgical manipulations: Surgeons can use iOCT to confirm the success of muscle recessions, resections, or transpositions intraoperatively. By imaging the surgical site immediately after manipulation, any adjustments can be made on the spot, enhancing the overall outcome of the surgery.

2.3.2 Enhancing surgical precision

iOCT enhances surgical precision by providing unparalleled visualization of ocular structures at a microscopic level. This precision translates into several clinical benefits:

1. Improved outcomes: Precise surgical manipulations reduce the likelihood of residual strabismus postoperatively. iOCT allows for exact measurements and positioning of extraocular muscles, which is critical for achieving optimal ocular alignment.

2. Reduced complications: By enabling surgeons to see beneath the surface tissues, iOCT helps in avoiding inadvertent damage to underlying structures such as the sclera or intraocular contents. This is especially important when operating near thin scleral areas or previous surgical sites. In complex strabismus cases, especially those involving previous surgeries where the risk of muscle slippage is high, iOCT proved essential. In one example, examining the use of OCT for imaging rectus muscle insertions in pediatric strabismus patients, OCT was employed pre-, intra-, and post-operatively. The study compared OCT measurements with intraoperative caliper measurements, demonstrating moderate-to-good correlation. OCT proved valuable in managing strabismus, particularly in cases where muscle insertions were unclear due to previous surgeries. The use of intraoperative OCT helped enhance surgical precision, providing significant implications for improving outcomes in strabismus surgery [18].

3. Customization of surgical techniques: Each patient's anatomy can present unique challenges. iOCT allows surgeons to tailor their techniques in real time based on the intraoperative findings. For example, if iOCT reveals thinner-than-expected sclera, the surgeon might modify the placement of sutures or the extent of muscle manipulation to prevent complications like scleral perforation.

4. Educational tool: iOCT serves as an excellent educational resource for training surgeons. Real-time imaging provides immediate feedback on surgical techniques and tissue responses, facilitating learning and skill development.

5. Documentation and evaluation: Intraoperative images can be saved for postoperative analysis and documentation. This can be valuable for assessing surgical techniques and outcomes, and for medico-legal purposes.

2.3.3 Integration with surgical microscopes and navigation systems

Modern surgical microscopes equipped with iOCT seamlessly integrate imaging into the surgeon's field of view. Some systems offer heads-up displays or augmented reality overlays, allowing surgeons to see OCT images without diverting their attention from the surgical field. Additionally, combining iOCT with surgical navigation systems enhances the surgeon's ability to plan and execute precise maneuvers.

2.3.4 Limitations and future directions

While iOCT offers significant advantages, there are limitations to consider:

1. Learning curve: Surgeons must become accustomed to interpreting OCT images intraoperatively and integrating this information into their surgical decision-making process.

2. Equipment costs: The implementation of iOCT requires significant investment in specialized equipment, which may not be readily available in all surgical centers.

3. Tissue penetration: OCT imaging depth is limited, which may restrict visualization in certain cases with dense fibrosis or opacification. Future advancements may address these limitations through enhanced imaging technologies, improved user interfaces, and more widespread availability of iOCT systems.

2.4 Postoperative monitoring

2.4.1 Evaluating surgical outcomes and effects on ocular structures

Postoperative monitoring with OCT plays a pivotal role in assessing the outcomes of strabismus surgery and evaluating the effects on ocular structures. Anterior segment ischemia is a rare but serious complication of strabismus surgery. In one case, OCTA was used to monitor iris vasculature post-surgery, revealing early signs of ischemia in a patient who had undergone two rectus muscle recessions. The ability of OCTA to detect these subtle changes in blood flow allowed the surgical team to intervene early, preventing further complications and preserving visual function [19]. OCT provides high-resolution images that allow clinicians to visualize changes in both the anterior and posterior segments of the eye following surgical intervention.

1. Extraocular muscle assessment: After strabismus surgery, it is essential to ensure that the extraocular muscles are correctly positioned and functioning as intended. While OCT primarily focuses on the retinal and optic nerve structures, its indirect benefits include monitoring how well the eyes are aligned postoperatively by observing the overall functional outcomes and any secondary effects on the posterior segment.

2. Retinal and macular evaluation: OCT is crucial for detecting any changes in the retina, particularly the macula, following strabismus surgery. Strabismus can have long-term effects on retinal structures, especially in patients with amblyopia or pre-existing retinal conditions. OCT allows for the precise measurement

of macular thickness, providing insights into whether surgical realignment has contributed to improvements in visual function. In cases where strabismus surgery may inadvertently affect intraocular structures, OCT helps identify any adverse effects, such as retinal edema, subclinical retinal detachment, or macular changes. By assessing these postoperative retinal changes, clinicians can make timely interventions to prevent further complications. Postoperatively, monitoring retinal and choroidal blood flow can provide valuable insights into the healing process and long-term ocular health. In a study evaluating horizontal rectus muscle surgeries, OCTA was used to measure changes in vessel density and choroidal thickness. The results showed a significant increase in vessel density in the superficial capillary plexus (SCP) and choriocapillaris (CC) in the first week post-surgery. This indicated a transient increase in blood flow in the retina and choroid, which was normalized by 1-month post-surgery [20]. Another study compared single- and two-muscle surgeries using OCTA. Patients who underwent two-muscle surgeries exhibited more significant changes in retinal vessel density than those who had only one muscle operated on. This was particularly evident in the parafoveal region, where vessel density increased in the early postoperative period. These findings suggest that more extensive strabismus surgeries may lead to greater hemodynamic changes in the retina, requiring closer monitoring with OCTA [21].

3. Optic nerve evaluation: Although rare, strabismus surgery could have indirect effects on the optic nerve, especially in cases involving significant ocular manipulation or trauma. OCT enables the monitoring of the RNFL, helping to detect any early signs of optic nerve damage or atrophy, which may not be evident through clinical examination alone.

2.4.2 Long-term follow-up and prognosis

Long-term follow-up with OCT is essential in ensuring that the benefits of strabismus surgery are maintained over time and that any potential complications are addressed promptly. Postoperative OCT scans allow for continuous monitoring of ocular structures, offering valuable data on the stability of the surgical outcome. (1) Monitoring for recurrence or overcorrection: Strabismus surgeries may, in some cases, lead to overcorrection or recurrence of the initial misalignment. OCT can help track the functional success of the surgery and guide decisions for further corrective procedures, if needed. (2) Prognosis and visual recovery: In cases where strabismus surgery is performed on patients with associated conditions such as amblyopia, thyroid ophthalmopathy, or optic neuropathy, OCT plays a significant role in monitoring the long-term prognosis. For instance, visual improvements post-surgery may depend on the health of the retinal layers and optic nerve. OCT imaging allows for objective measurements of these structures, helping to predict long-term visual outcomes. (3) Detecting late complications: Some patients may develop late complications following strabismus surgery, including retinal detachment, macular edema, or optic nerve changes. OCT provides an ongoing monitoring tool to detect these complications early and ensure that they are managed before they result in significant vision loss. By integrating OCT into long-term postoperative care, clinicians can ensure comprehensive monitoring of both the functional and anatomical outcomes of strabismus surgery, enhancing overall patient prognosis.

3. Summary of key points

OCT and OCTA have revolutionized strabismus management, providing critical insights at each stage—preoperative, intraoperative, and postoperative. AS-OCT offers precise localization of extraocular muscles, improving surgical planning and outcomes, especially in reoperations and trauma cases. Intraoperative OCT enhances surgical precision by offering real-time feedback, minimizing complications. Postoperatively, OCTA helps monitor retinal and choroidal changes, providing early detection of issues such as ischemia and abnormal healing. OCT and OCTA also contribute significantly to the management of amblyopia, revealing vascular changes such as an enlarged FAZ in amblyopic eyes, and evaluating optic disc and retina in myopic patients.

4. Future outlook

The integration of AI with OCT, advancements in OCTA technology, and the potential for long-term monitoring of retinal health are expected to further enhance the role of OCT in strabismus management. As these technologies evolve, they will likely improve the precision and outcomes of surgeries while offering better diagnostic tools for related conditions such as amblyopia and myopia.

5. Conclusions

OCT and OCTA have become essential tools in strabismus management, offering precise preoperative planning, real-time intraoperative guidance, and effective postoperative monitoring. These technologies improve surgical precision, reduce complications, and provide valuable insights into retinal and choroidal changes. OCT and OCTA also enhance the diagnosis and treatment of related conditions such as amblyopia and myopia. As these imaging technologies continue to evolve, they promise to further optimize strabismus management, ultimately improving patient outcomes and care.

Despite their significant advantages, these technologies require both user expertise and interpreter experience, which can limit their effectiveness in centers with insufficiently trained staff. Additionally, patient cooperation plays a crucial role in obtaining accurate images. This poses a particular challenge in pediatric age groups and in patients with conditions such as restricted eye movements or nystagmus, where involuntary eye movements can lead to difficulties in imaging. Furthermore, patients with poor cooperation may result in suboptimal image quality or incomplete scans. Another important limitation is the high cost of those devices, which can be prohibitive for many centers, especially in resource-limited settings. The lack of accessibility in some institutions restricts the widespread use of these technologies.

Acknowledgements

No external funding or financial support was received for the work presented in this chapter. The author has utilized artificial intelligence in the editing of the manuscript.

Conflict of interest

The author declares no conflict of interest.

Nomenclature

OCT	optical coherence tomography
AS-OCT	anterior segment optical coherence tomography
iOCT	intraoperative optical coherence tomography
OCTA	optical coherence tomography angiography
RNFL	retinal nerve fiber layer
FAZ	foveal avascular zone
VEGF	vascular endothelial growth factor
SCP	superficial capillary plexus
CC	choriocapillaris
Scleral Pass	a surgical technique involving the placement of sutures through the sclera during strabismus surgery

Appendix

In this chapter, we explored the detailed role of optical coherence tomography (OCT) in the assessment, surgical planning, and postoperative monitoring of strabismus. We covered the application of different OCT techniques including anterior segment OCT (AS-OCT), intraoperative OCT (iOCT), and OCT angiography (OCTA). We also included several references demonstrating how these technologies are employed in real-life scenarios, providing valuable insights into extraocular muscle assessment, retinal and macular changes, and optic nerve evaluation and the utility of OCT in trauma-induced strabismus, thyroid ophthalmopathy, and amblyopia.

Author details

Emine Tinkir Kayitmazbatir
Department of Ophthalmology, Faculty of Medicine, Selcuk University, Konya, Turkiye

*Address all correspondence to: drtinkir@gmail.com

References

[1] Van Noorden GK, Campos EC. Binocular Vision and Ocular Motility: Theory and Management of Strabismus. 6th ed. St. Louis: Mosby; 2002. pp. 127-133

[2] Robaei D, Rose KA, Kifley A, Cosstick M, Ip JM, Mitchell P. Factors associated with childhood strabismus: Findings from a population-based study. Ophthalmology. 2006;**113**(7):1146-1153. DOI: 10.1016/j.ophtha.2006.01.058

[3] Laughton SC, Hagen MM, Yang W, von Bartheld CS. Gender differences in horizontal strabismus: Systematic review and meta-analysis shows no difference in prevalence, but gender bias towards females in the clinic. Journal of Global Health. 2023;**13**:4085. DOI: 10.7189/jogh.13.04085

[4] Nusz KJ, Mohney BG, Diehl NN. Female predominance in intermittent exotropia. American Journal of Ophthalmology. 2005;**140**(3):546-547. DOI: 10.1016/j.ajo.2005.03.026

[5] Buffenn AN. The impact of strabismus on psychosocial health and quality of life: A systematic review. Ophthalmology. 2009;**116**(8):1831-1837. DOI: 10.1016/j.ophtha.2009.03.036

[6] Huang D, Swanson EA, Lin CP, et al. Optical coherence tomography. Science. 1991;**254**(5035):1178-1181. DOI: 10.1126/science.1957169

[7] Aumann S, Donner S, Fischer J, Müller F. Optical coherence tomography (OCT): Principle and technical realization. In: Bille JF, editor. High Resolution Imaging in Microscopy and Ophthalmology: New Frontiers in Biomedical Optics. Cham (CH): Springer; 2019. pp. 59-85

[8] Nourinia R, Rajavi Z, Sabbaghi H, et al. Optical coherence tomography angiography in patients with amblyopia. Strabismus. 2022;**30**(3):132-138. DOI: 10.1080/09273972.2022.2097705

[9] AttaAllah HR, Abdelaziz STA, Mohamed AAM, et al. Assessment of macular microvascular changes in children following treatment of anisometropic myopic amblyopia using optical coherence tomography angiography. Graefe's Archive for Clinical and Experimental Ophthalmology. 2023;**261**:2689-2699. DOI: 10.1007/s00417-023-06055-8

[10] Li Y, Jia W, Liu X, et al. Measurement of the tilt angle of the optic disc using spectral-domain optical coherence tomography and related factors in myopia. Translational Vision Science & Technology. 2024;**13**(9):24. DOI: 10.1167/tvst.13.9.24

[11] Shoeib MI, Khafagy MM, Hassan NA, Bahgat NMM. Anterior segment optical coherence tomography for the preoperative visualization of extra-ocular muscles in adult patients with strabismus. Journal of the Egyptian Ophthalmological Society. 2022;**115**(4):145-149. DOI: 10.4103/ejos.ejos_12_22

[12] Kaur S, Bradfield Y, As V, et al. Anterior segment optical coherence tomography (AS-OCT) in strabismus following trauma. Journal of AAPOS. 2024;**28**(4):103955. DOI: 10.1016/j.jaapos.2024.103955

[13] Xu B, Wang S, Chen L, Tan J. The early diagnostic value of optical coherence tomography (OCT) and OCT angiography in thyroid-associated ophthalmopathy.

Therapeutic Advances in Chronic Disease. 2023;**14**:20406223231166802. DOI: 10.1177/20406223231166802

[14] De-Pablo-Gómez-de-Liaño L, Fernández-Vigo JI, Ventura-Abreu N, et al. Optical coherence tomography thickness measurements of the extraocular rectus muscle tendons in graves' ophthalmopathy. Journal of Pediatric Ophthalmology and Strabismus. 2018;**55**(6):356-362. DOI: 10.3928/01913913-20180802-01

[15] Miyata M, Suda K, Uji A, et al. One-year outcome predictors of strabismus surgery from anterior segment optical coherence tomography with multiple B-scan averaging. Scientific Reports. 2019;**9**:2523. DOI: 10.1038/s41598-019-39361-5

[16] Pujari A, Patil V, Chauhan N, et al. Defining the clinical role of swept-source anterior segment optical coherence tomography in eyes undergoing strabismus surgery. Clinical Ophthalmology. 2022;**16**:1449-1465. DOI: 10.2147/OPTH.S365622

[17] Kuhn J, Pihlblad MS. Integrated intraoperative optical coherence tomography during scleral pass in strabismus surgery. Journal of Binocular Vision and Ocular Motility. 2022;**72**(1):29-31

[18] Pihlblad MS, Troia A, Tibrewal S, Shah PR. Pre-, intra-, and post-operative evaluation of extraocular muscle insertions using optical coherence tomography: A comparison of four devices. Journal of Clinical Medicine. 2019;**8**(10):1732. DOI: 10.3390/jcm8101732

[19] Vanlangenaeker L, Van Aerschot J, Putcuijps K, et al. The use of optical coherence tomography angiography to measure changes in iris vasculature after strabismus surgery. Strabismus. 2023;**31**(4):244-252. DOI: 10.1080/09273972.2023.2271539

[20] Huseyinhan Z, Ozcaliskan S, Gurez C, Artunay O. Retinal and choroidal microvasculature is altered after strabismus surgery. European Journal of Ophthalmology. 2023;**33**(2):774-778. DOI: 10.1177/11206721221137156

[21] Xiao D, Cao T, Meng Y, et al. Changes in retinal and choroidal blood flow after one or two horizontal rectus muscle surgeries by optical coherence tomography angiography. Annals of Medicine. 2023;**55**(2):2261494. DOI: 10.1080/07853890.2023.2261494

Section 3

OCT and Posterior Segment Diseases

Chapter 8

Artefacts in Optical Coherence Tomography of Posterior Segment: Clinical Impact and How to Correct Them

Nikita Dash

Abstract

This chapter shall enumerate the various types of artefacts encountered while conducting optical coherence tomography imaging in a clinic. It shall also focus on how these artefacts can cause a loss in data acquisition and affect our interpretation of the image formed. Common clinical conditions that lead to poorer image quality and loss of data points shall be discussed. Methods to tackle such situations shall be enumerated. Spotlight on conditions that can lead to segmentation errors will be focused on. Technical nuances for better image acquisition during optical coherence tomography shall be discussed. Overall, the focus of this chapter will be to discuss and shed light on various artefacts and how to avoid or correct them.

Keywords: optical coherence tomography, artefacts, clinical interpretation, data interpretation, retinal diseases, glaucoma imaging

1. Introduction

Optical coherence tomography (OCT) is a noninvasive imaging modality that gives us information regarding the layers of the retina, the anatomy of the optic nerve head, and anterior segment abnormalities in various conditions [1]. It is based on the principle of optical interference and helps in obtaining real-time, *in vivo* optical sections of the tissue being scanned [2]. Previously, OCT imaging used a time-domain function that employed a mechanically moving scanning reference arm that sequentially measured the echo time delay. Later, Fourier-domain OCT came into the picture. It utilises a stationary reference arm to obtain an interference spectrum. The interference pattern obtained undergoes Fourier transformation, which allows concurrent measurements of all echo time delays. This results in faster and more efficient data acquisition [1]. Fourier-domain OCT can be classified into Spectral Domain OCT (SD-OCT) and Swept-Source OCT (SS-OCT). The SD-OCT instrument uses a near-infrared diode light source, with a centre wavelength of approximately 840 nm. It is detected by a spectrometer. On the other hand, SS-OCT uses a tunable swept laser which has a wavelength of 1050 nm and is detected by a single photodiode [3].

The data that is collected by OCT imaging can be either qualitative in nature or quantitative in nature. Qualitative data gives the clinician an about the pathology identified on the scan such as vitreomacular traction, macular holes, cystoid macular oedema, maculopathy involving photoreceptor layers, and choroidal neovascular membranes. Quantitative data such as central macular thickness is used for decision-making and tailoring treatment strategies in conditions such as diabetic macular oedema, cystoid macular oedema due to vein occlusions, and age-related macular degeneration [4–6].

However, images acquired on OCT can be subject to artefacts that can interfere with its interpretation. These artefacts can be misleading for the clinician if not identified and clinically correlated [7]. Therefore, it is important to be aware of the artefacts that can arise while acquiring images on an OCT scan. This knowledge will not only help us interpret data with caution but also employ techniques that can address the issue.

In this chapter, we shall be focusing on artefacts encountered during posterior segment OCT scans. Ray et al. were among the early researchers to classify artefacts acquired on time-domain OCT [2]. They discussed six types of artefacts associated with TD-OCT, namely misidentification of the inner retinal layer, misidentification of the outer retinal layer, out-of-register artefact, degraded image scan, cut-edge artefact and off-centre artefact [2]. Although originally reported in TD-OCT scans, they can also be detected in scans acquired on SD-OCT machines. Certain artefacts, such

Type of artefact	Description
Software-related	
Segmentation errors	Due to incorrect detection of retinal borders
Incomplete segmentation failure	Missing segmentation lines before reaching the lateral sides of the scan
Complete segmentation failure	No segmentation lines placed along retinal boundaries
Mirror/inverted artefact	The image folds on itself near the zero-delay line
Degraded images	Software unable to delineate retinal layers
Static artefact	Multiple B-scan images showing a fixed part of image
Linear artefact	Three hyper-reflective lines near the sclera-choroidal interface
Patient-related	
Blink artefact	Data loss due to blinking by the patient
Off-centre artefact	Displacement of fovea over 0.25 mm from its real location
Motion artefact	Distortion in image due to eye movement
Foveal duplication	Double fovea in OCT image of the same eye
Segmentation shift	Vertical shift in segmentation lines
PFCL-producing artefact	Distortion of structures below the PFCL bubble
Implant-producing artefact	Shadow effect due to intravitreal implant
Operator-related	
Cut-edge artefact	The edge of the scan is inappropriately illustrated
Out-of-register artefact	Vertically displaced image as a part of the inner or outer retina.

Table 1.
A summary of all the artefacts encountered on the OCT scan.

as the mirror artefact, are noted exclusively with the SD-OCT machines as a result of the technique involved in image acquisition.

Moreover, not all artefacts are software related. Some can result due to patient factor and operator-related factors. All of these artefacts are summarised in **Table 1** and will be discussed in the chapter.

2. Artefacts in posterior segment OCT imaging

2.1 Software-related artefacts

2.1.1 Segmentation errors

Segmentation errors can be defined as missing or inappropriate segmentation lines produced by incorrect detection of borders of the retinal layers as shown in **Figure 1** [8]. There can be an error in the precise positioning of the segmentation line or an absence of the segmentation line in the boundaries [9]. These errors are commonly found in TD-OCT and are less likely with SD-OCT. Retinal layer misidentification can give rise to thickness map error and misinterpretation of quantitative data of the retinal or nerve fibre layers [8].

These errors are commonly associated with outer retinal diseases such as age-related macular degeneration, cystoid macular oedema, pigment epithelial detachment, central serous chorioretinopathy, and geographic atrophy and inner retinal disorders such as vitreoretinal interface diseases [8]. Although all OCT instruments identify the internal limiting membrane as the inner retinal boundary, there is a variation in identifying the outer boundary [10]. Stratus Zeiss OCT identifies the inner–outer segment junction of the photoreceptor (ellipsoid zone) as the outer retinal boundary. The Topcon 3D OCT-1000 and the Copernicus OCT both identify the outer retinal boundary as the inner part of the retinal pigment epithelium (RPE) layer. However, the Zeiss Cirrus, the OptovueRTvue-100, and the Heidelberg Spectralis identify the outer boundary at the middle of the RPE, the outer part of the RPE, and the Bruch membrane respectively [10]. This can result in a variation of the frequency of the detected errors of segmentation.

Further classification of segmentation errors was brought about by Han and Jaffe. Depending on the proportion of retinal thickness involved, they were classified as mild (segmentation error less than one-third of retinal thickness), moderate

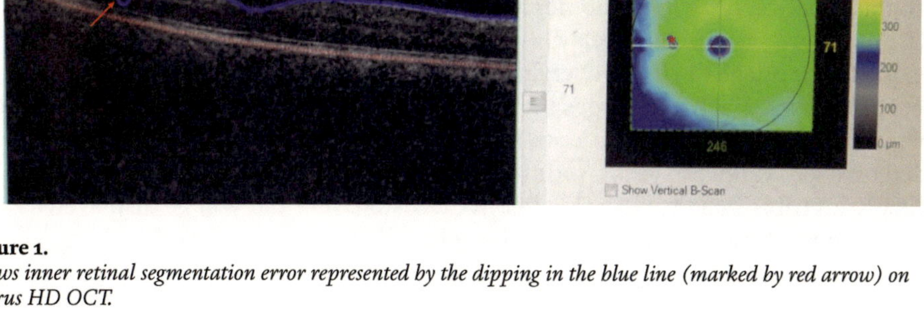

Figure 1.
Shows inner retinal segmentation error represented by the dipping in the blue line (marked by red arrow) on Cirrus HD OCT.

(between one-third and two-thirds of retinal thickness), and severe (more than two-thirds of retinal thickness) [11]. This can result in erroneous foveal thickness measurements if they are located within a 1 mm region of the central ETDRS and topographic maps [1].

Segmentation errors including the ganglion cell layer (GCL) and GCL-inner plexiform layer (GCL-IPL) can occur in various macular disorders. Since the GCL-IPL layer has an important role to play in the identification of glaucomatous and neurodegenerative conditions, it is important to identify them. Segmentation error including the GCL-IPL complex has been further classified by Alshareef et al. as mild (amount of error less than 10 μm), moderate (error between 10 and 50 μm), and severe (error >50 μm) [12]. They also observed that the frequency of these artefacts was more in eyes with macular diseases (55%) as compared to eyes with a healthy macula (26.8%) [12].

2.1.2 Incomplete segmentation errors

These errors occur when the automated segmentation lines were placed accurately by the software along retinal boundaries but stopped before reaching the lateral edges of the scan. They are more frequently encountered with the Spectralis and Cirrus OCT machines. It can also occur as a result of degradation of images toward the edges of acquisition areas.

Han et al. observed that it was a quite common artefact affecting about 80.7% of all volume scans and 33.2% of all individual scans. They rarely affect the central subfield but may alter measurements in the peripheral areas. Eyes with media opacity or disease were more likely to come across this artefact [11].

2.1.3 Segmentation failure

As described by Han et al., a segmentation failure is said to have occurred if no segmentation lines were placed along either the inner or outer retina boundaries, as shown in **Figure 2**. This is a rare artefact with a prevalence of 4.5% in Spectralis machines and 2% in the Cirrus machines. Occurrences of these errors in Spectralis machines were reported in spite of identifiable inner and outer retinal boundaries [11].

2.1.4 Mirror artefact/inverted artefact

A mirror artefact is characteristic of OCT machines employing the Fourier transformation technology, such as SD-OCT and SS-OCT, for image acquisition. This occurs when the image folds on itself around the zero-delay line in the entirety of its length or at the ends of the image. Since Fourier-domain detection is unable to distinguish between positive and negative time delays, they can produce symmetrical OCT images around the zero-delay line. Commercial OCT machines usually truncate one side of the image during processing so that an erect image is displayed on the screen. However, when the images move closer to the zero-delay line, some part of the otherwise unseen half crosses over to the visible side and appears as a mirror image folded on itself. If the image is continued to move toward the zero-delay line, the normally invisible image will cross over to the visible side and will be displayed as an inverted image, thus leading to a mirror artefact [13].

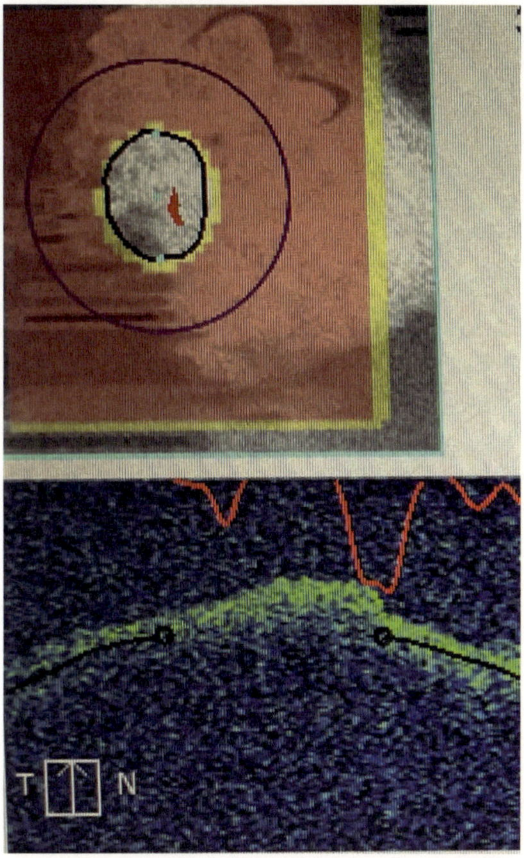

Figure 2.
Shows complete segmentation failure of OCT RNFL on Cirrus HD OCT.

Maximum sensitivity for image acquisition occurs when the instrument is adjusted with the retina near the zero-delay line. Thus, measurements are often taken with the retina near the zero-delay and this can leave a limited room for axial scan depth range. Therefore, axial eye movements during image acquisition can also result in mirror artefacts [13].

Conditions, where mirror artefacts are commonly encountered, include high myopia, posterior staphyloma, and tractional retinal detachments causing elevation of the retina at one end of the image. **Figure 3** is an example of such a mirror image due to tractional retinal detachment. Ho et al. reported that mirror artefact occurred significantly in worse visual acuity, higher axial length (26.5 mm), and more myopic refraction [13]. Han and Jaffe observed that mirror artefacts were more common in scans obtained with the Cirrus OCT machine as compared to Spectralis [11].

Mirror artefacts can also result from poor positioning of the OCT scans or extreme tilting of the OCT scan when the scan beam of the instrument is off-centre in the eye's pupil. This can result in the retina crossing the zero-delay line at the peripheral area of the scan, resulting in image inversion. These artefacts can result in segmentation breakdown in the image periphery, thus resulting in inaccuracies in quantitative OCT analysis, including volumetric and thickness analysis.

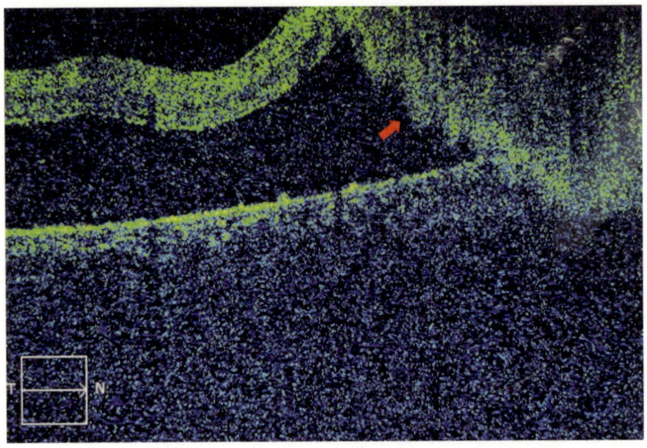

Figure 3.
Shows a mirror image artefact (red arrow) in a case of tractional retinal detachment on Cirrus HD OCT.

2.1.5 Degraded images

Degraded images are a result of poor image capture, which results when the software is unable to delineate the inner and outer retinal layers properly resulting in errors in retinal thickness map measurement. Its frequency has been noted to be about 6.7–11.7%. Media opacities may also play a role in producing this artefact [2, 12].

Since the software is unable to compensate for the acquisition errors caused by a degraded image, this results in an inaccurate foveal thickness measurement. The artefact may be resolved by refocusing on the area of interest. **Figure 4** shows a degraded image artefact with corresponding errors in the retinal thickness map [2].

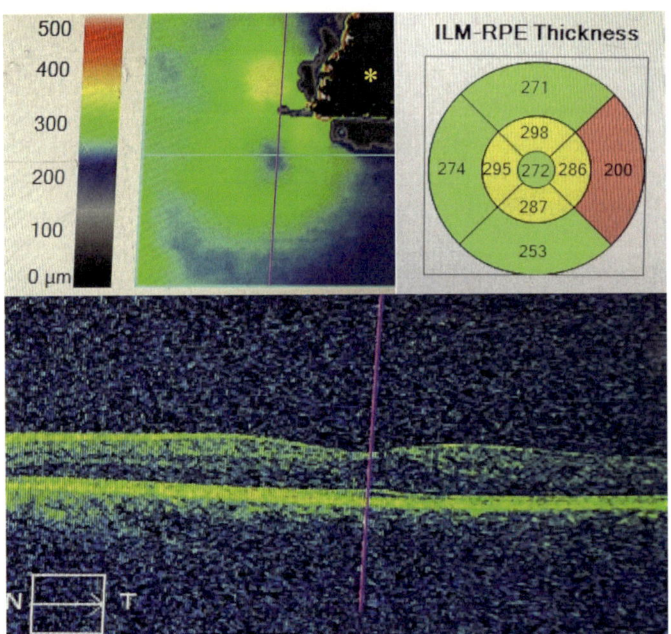

Figure 4.
Shows a degraded image (yellow asterisk) scan that has caused an erroneous estimation of the foveal thickness map.

2.1.6 Static or fixed image artefact

This is a rare artefact specific to Spectralis OCT with a frequency of 0.001–0.004%. Han and Jaffe described it as an artefact caused when a fixed part of the image of the specific scan was shown on multiple adjacent B-scans with no changes [11].

2.1.7 Linear artefact

This artefact, described by Zuo et al., is a duplication image artefact of three layers from the ellipsoid zone to the retinal pigment epithelium (RPE) layer. It is formed as three hyper-reflective lines with a stable location. With the thickness of the lines being approximately the same thickness as ellipsoid zone to the RPE. It can be misidentified as a sclera-choroidal interface causing errors in choroidal thickness measurements. It is more frequent when the media is clear [14].

2.2 Patient-related artefacts

2.2.1 Blink artefacts

This artefact is caused when the subject blinks during the process of image acquisition. This results in a loss of data in the portion of blink and can lead to erroneous estimation of thickness maps. It presents as a black, horizontal line on the red-free fundus image and as blank areas in the en-face image [7]. B-scan can reveal lost retinal data that manifests as macular thinning on the macular map and optic nerve head thinning on the RNFL map, as seen in **Figure 5**.

It is important to counsel the patient to not blink during scanning and make use of lubricants in patients with suspected dry eye disease. Blink artefact occurs less frequently in devices with better eye-tracking software and faster image acquisition [10].

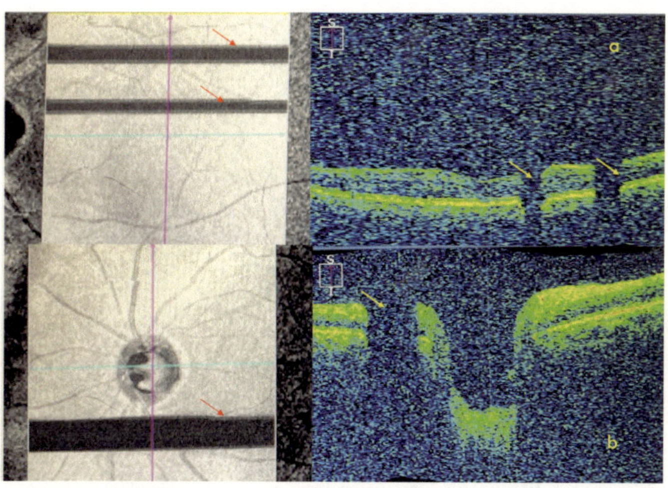

Figure 5.
Shows blink artefacts (yellow and red arrows) on (a) macular scan and (b) RNFL scan.

2.2.2 Off-centre artefact (grid-centration artefact)

This occurs when the foveal centre is displaced more than 0.25 mm from its real location in the ETDRS map. It can be attributed to fixation errors due to eccentric fixation, low vision and attention deficit. It has a prevalence of 3.7–16.7% [10]. Ho et al. found that the Cirrus machine has a lower frequency of this error due to faster scanning protocols [13]. In machines like the RT-Vue and Topcon 3D OCT 1000, the ETDRS map can be moved to the presumed location of true fovea [10].

Presence of this artefact will cause errors in thickness map, foveal thickness measurements, and retinal nerve fibre thickness.

2.2.3 Motion artefact

Motion artefacts are a result of eye movement during acquisition of images which manifests as structural distortion or doubling of the OCT image [8]. They can be caused by eye saccades, drift movements, respiratory movements, heartbeat movements, alternation in head position and poor fixation. It appears as a sharp alternation on OCT cross-section and blood vessel misalignment on red-free and en-face scans. **Figure 6** shows a motion artefact [8].

Because of distortion created, it can result in clinically significant segmentation errors, especially in the measurement of thickness of RNFL layer. Although it is commonly encountered in TD-OCT, due to greater time required for image acquisition, it can be seen in SD-OCT machines as well. It is proposed that better eye tracking, faster image acquisition and repeating the imaging can help reduce motion artefact [13, 15, 16].

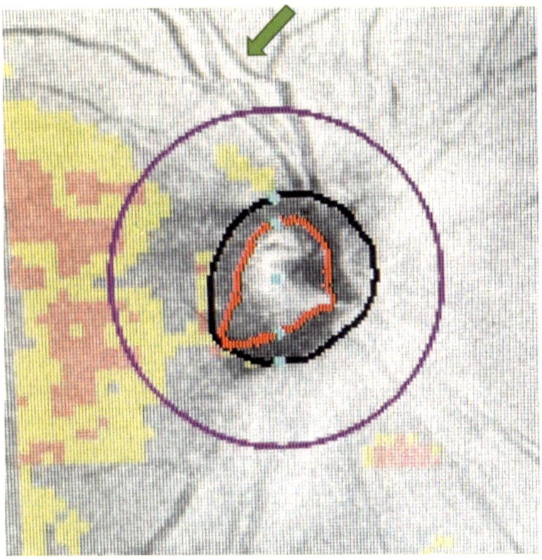

Figure 6.
Shows motion artefact on OCT RNFL with distortion of blood vessels highlighted by the green arrow.

2.2.4 Foveal duplication artefact

This is caused by transient movements of the eye and appears as double fovea on the OCT image of the scanned eye (**Figure 7**). It is the result of a double scan of the fovea of the same eye at two separate times. This was described by Baskin et al. who explained this phenomenon with the transitory micro-saccadic upward movement creating an extra image of fovea in the downward direction and then central re-fixation. It can lead to erroneous foveal thickness measurements [17].

2.2.5 Segmentation shift

Segmentation shift occurs when the position of the segmentation lines in the inner and outer borders of the retina was stable, but a vertical shift in the image formed was noted. It does not influence the thickness map due to fixed distance between the segmentation lines. Therefore, it is not clinically significant.

2.2.6 Perfluorocarbon liquid-producing artefact

Differences in refractive index of perfluorocarbon liquid (PFCL) and aqueous/vitreous humour can result in distortion of structures below the bubble. This retinal distortion occurs more at the centre of bubble than its edges. The bubble can also act as a spherical lens magnifying underlying structures. Although this has been identified with PFCL, it may also occur by other tamponading agents [18, 19].

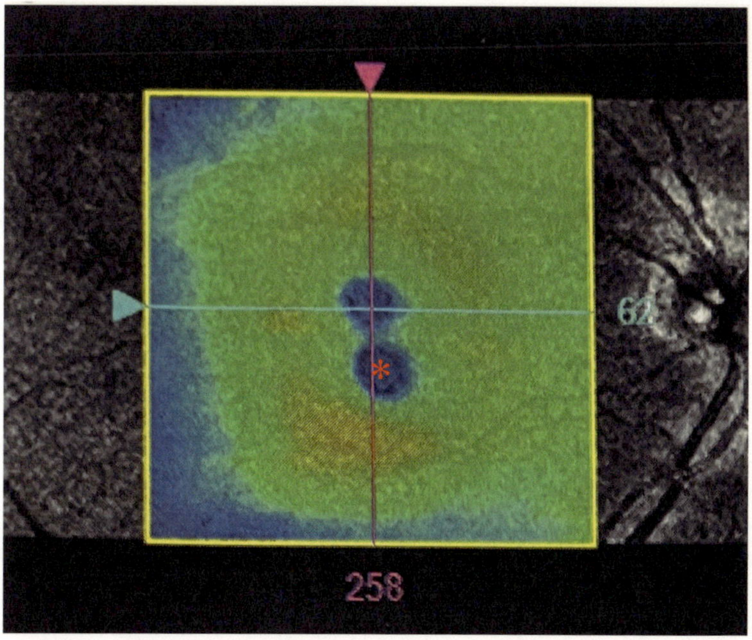

Figure 7.
Shows a foveal duplication artefact marked by the red asterisk.

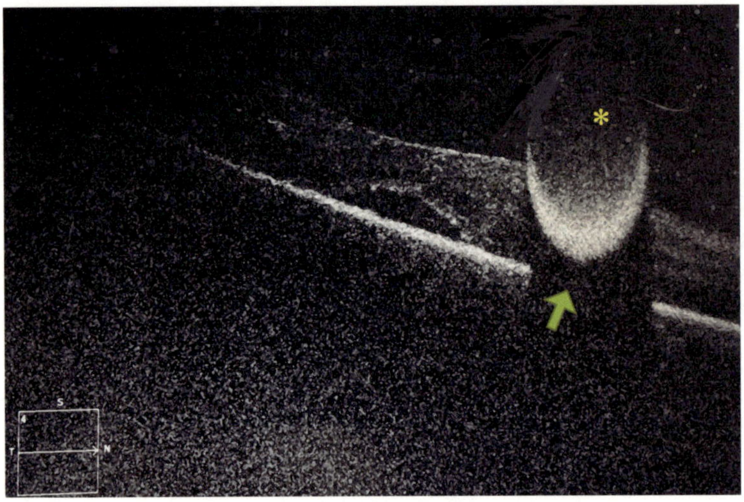

Figure 8.
Shows a shadow artefact (green arrow) caused by the intravitreal dexamethasone implant Ozurdex (yellow asterisk).

2.2.7 Artefact due to intravitreal implants

Intravitreal implants can also cause shadow artefacts and loss of data during retinal thickness evaluation. **Figure 8** shows a shadow artefact caused by dexamethasone implant Ozurdex (Allergan Inc.) as noted by the author.

2.3 Operator-related artefacts

2.3.1 Cut edge artefact

Cut-edge artefact is said to occur if the edge of the scan is truncated and is seen in 2.3–6.35% of cases [1, 7]. **Figure 9a** shows a cut-edge artefact. They are noted in the periphery of the scanned image and do not affect central retinal thickness measurements. They are seen with the same frequency in normal and diseased eyes. They are operator induced due to inappropriate technique of image acquisition. If it occurs during the first scan, it should be disregarded [20].

It can also occur in scans taken with non-dilated pupils due to iris blockage that causes vignetting and peripheral elimination of OCT signal [8].

2.3.2 Out-of-register artefact

The image is displaced vertically and appears to be vertically cut off in this artefact. **Figure 9b** shows an out-of-register artefact. This artefact has a prevalence ranging from 2.4–13% across various OCT machines. Ray et al. reported that the frequency of these artefacts can be as high as 35.7% in TD-OCT machines.

This artefact is a result of poor image acquisition and misalignment of the scan. The occurrence of these artefacts does not differ whether the eye is normal or diseased. It can cause errors in retinal thickness map reporting and GCL-IPL thickness measurements.

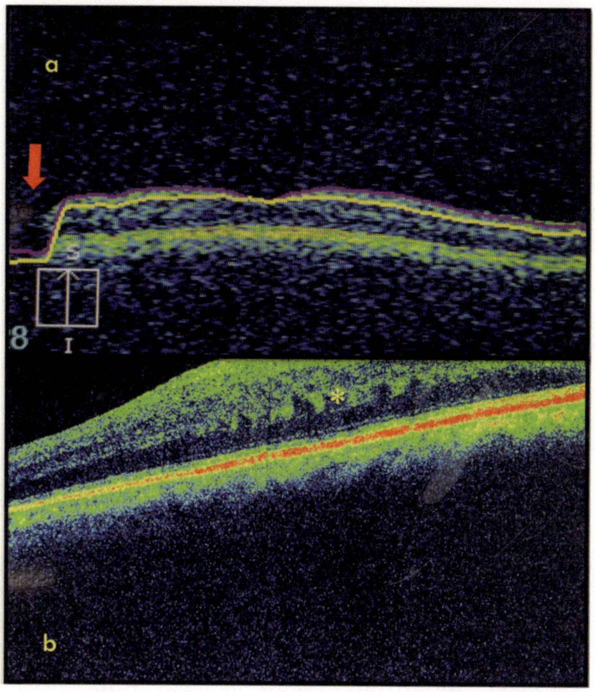

Figure 9.
Shows operator-related artefacts. (a) shows a cut-edge artefact (red arrow) and (b) shows an out-of-register artefact (yellow asterisk).

3. Clinical significance of artefacts

OCT is useful in tracking progression of disease as well as treatment response in a variety of retinal pathologic conditions such as diabetic macular oedema, uveitic cystoid macular oedema, and choroidal neovascularisation [21, 22]. Any artefact that causes segmentation errors of more than 10% of the real ETDRS centre subfield thickness (CST) is considered as clinically significant. In STRATUS TD-OCT measurements, any artefact resulting in an error of more than 50 microns is considered clinically significant. Artefacts that can cause misdiagnosis of retinal thickening or thinning are also noted as significant [23–25].

Since OCT plays a major role for quantitative thickness measurements not only in general clinical setting but also in important trials necessary for formulating newer regimens, it is therefore of utmost importance to recognise and correct artefacts associated with image acquisition promptly [25].

4. Management of artefacts

While it is known that artefacts can cause errors and inaccuracies in data interpretation and subsequent fallacies in clinical workup, it is also essential to learn to overcome these artefacts for better interpretation.

Segmentation errors by software if identified should be manually changed wherever possible. OCT machines have an option to change the inner and outer segmentation line manually. This can serve to handle errors in data interpretation due to software segmentation discrepancies. If there is a mirror artefact, we can retake the scan of interest with better axial positioning to avoid image inversion. The same goes for any degraded image scan [10, 25].

Other patient and operator-related artefacts can be handled by re-taking the scan of interest with better compliance on part of the patient.

Moreover, better tracking system, faster image acquisition, and repeating the imaging are proposed to reduce motion artefact [25]. A significantly faster scanning speed allows for higher data acquisition with lower probability of motion artefacts. In addition, instruments using higher wavelengths (1050 nm) have been developed that capture better images by reducing media opacity-related artefact [7]. It has also been found that age of the patient may be a factor in the occurrence of artefacts in SS-OCT [26].

5. Conclusion

Artefacts can occur in all OCT machines, therefore it is necessary to correctly identify artefacts before rectifying them. Scrutinising topography scans, screening individual scans, and looking at the rendered fundus image can help us identify majority of these artefacts. Once they are identified, one can proceed to correct them as described before. Newer algorithms for data acquisition and analysis may help reduce OCT artefacts in the future. Using different imaging modalities, along with the OCT, can lead to correct interpretation and definitive clinical diagnosis.

This chapter focuses on the artefacts encountered on optical coherence imaging in Ophthalmology. The various artefacts can be divided into different categories such as software-related, patient-related and operator-related. Management of the artefacts has also been provided to help recognise and correct them and aid in better OCT data interpretation.

Author details

Nikita Dash
Sir Ganga Ram Hospital, New Delhi, India

*Address all correspondence to: ndash18@gmail.com

References

[1] Ho J, Sull AC, Vuong LN, Chen Y, Liu J, Fujimoto JG, et al. Assessment of artifacts and reproducibility across spectral- and time- domain optical coherence tomography devices. Ophthalmology. 2009;**116**:1960-1970

[2] Ray R, Stinnett SS, Jaffe GJ. Evaluation of image artifact produced by optical coherence tomography of retinal pathology. American Journal of Ophthalmology. 2005;**139**:18-29

[3] Potsaid B, Baumann B, Huang D, et al. Ultrahigh speed 1050nm swept source/ fourier domain OCT retinal and anterior segment imaging at 100,000 to 400,000 axial scans per second. Optics Express. 2010;**18**:20029-20048

[4] Mitchell P, Korobelnik JF, Lanzetta P, Holz FG, Prunte C, Schmidt-Erfurth U, et al. Ranibizumab (lucentis) in neovascular age-related macular degeneration: Evidence from clinical trials. The British Journal of Ophthalmology. 2010;**94**:2-13

[5] Aiello LP, Beck RW, Bressler NM, Browning DJ, Chalam KV, Davis M, et al. Rationale for the diabetic retinopathy clinical research network treatment protocol for center-involved diabetic macular edema. Ophthalmology. 2011;**118**:e5-e14

[6] Keane PA, Sadda SR. Retinal vein occlusion and macular edema—Critical evaluation of the clinical value of ranibizumab. Clinical Ophthalmology. 2011;**5**:771-781

[7] Hee MR. Artifacts in optical coherence tomography topographic maps. American Journal of Ophthalmology. 2005;**139**:154-155

[8] Awadalla MS, Fitzgerald J, Andrew NH, Zhou T, Marshall H, Qassim A, et al. Prevalence and type of artefact with spectral domain optical coherence tomography macular ganglion cell imaging in glaucoma surveillance. PLoS One. 2018;**13**:e0206684

[9] Domalpally A, Danis RP, Zhang B, Myers D, Kruse CN. Quality issues in interpretation of optical coherence tomograms in macular diseases. Retina. 2009;**29**:775-781

[10] Bazvand F, Ghassemi F. Artifacts in macular optical coherence tomography. Journal of Current Ophthalmology. 2020;**32**(2):123-131

[11] Han IC, Jaffe GJ. Evaluation of artifacts associated with macular spectral-domain optical coherence tomography. Ophthalmology. 2010;**117**:1177-1189

[12] Alshareef RA, Goud A, Mikhail M, Saheb H, Peguda HK, Dumpala S, et al. Segmentation errors in macular ganglion cell analysis as determined by optical coherence tomography in eyes with macular pathology. International Journal of Retina and Vitreous. 2017;**3**:25

[13] Ho J, Castro DP, Castro LC, Chen Y, Liu J, Mattox C, et al. Clinical assessment of mirror artifacts in spectral-domain optical coherence tomography. Investigative Ophthalmology and Visual Science. 2010;**51**(7):3714-3720

[14] Zuo C, Mi L, Yang S, Guo X, Xiao H, Liu X. The linear artifact in enhanced depth imaging spectral domain optical coherence tomography. Scientific Reports. 2017;**7**:8464

[15] Ricco S, Chen M, Ishikawa H, Wollstein G, Schuman J. Correcting

motion artifacts in retinal spectral domain optical coherence tomography via image registration. Medical Image Computing and Computer Assistance Intervention. 2009;**12**:100-107

[16] Kraus MF, Potsaid B, Mayer MA, Bock R, Baumann B, Liu JJ, et al. Motion correction in optical coherence tomography volumes on a per A-scan basis using orthogonal scan patterns. Biomedical Optics Express. 2012;**3**:1182-1199

[17] Baskin DE, Gault JA, Vander JF, Dugan JD Jr. Double fovea artifact. Ophthalmology. 2011;**118**:429.e1

[18] Strampe MR, Kaehr MM, Carroll J, Kim JE. Intraoperative imaging of retained perfluorocarbon liquid using spectral domain optical coherence tomography. Retinal Cases and Brief Reports. 2019;**13**:381-384

[19] Langlo CS, Flatter JA, Dubra A, Wirostko WJ, Carroll J. A lensing effect of inner retinal cysts on images of the photoreceptor mosaic. Retina. 2014;**34**:421-422

[20] Sull AC, Vuong LN, Price LL, Srinivasan VJ, Gorczynska I, Fujimoto JG, et al. Comparison of spectral/fourier domain optical coherence tomography instruments for assessment of normal macular thickness. Retina. 2010;**30**:235-245

[21] Arevalo JF, Lasave AF, Arias JD, Serrano MA, Arevalo FA. Clinical applications of optical coherence tomography in the posterior pole: The 2011 Jose Manuel Espino Lecture—Part II. Clinical Ophthalmology. 2013;7:2181-2206

[22] Arevalo JF, Lasave AF, Arias JD, Serrano MA, Arevalo FA. Clinical applications of optical coherence tomography in the posterior pole: The 2011 Jose Manuel Espino Lecture—Part I. Clinical Ophthalmology. 2013;7:2165-2179

[23] Browning DJ, Fraser CM, Propst BW. The variation in optical coherence tomography-measured macular thickness in diabetic eyes without clinical macular edema. American Journal of Ophthalmology. 2008;**145**:889-893

[24] Diabetic Retinopathy Clinical Research Network, Krystolik MG, Strauber SF, Aiello LP, Beck RW, Berger BB, et al. Reproducibility of macular thickness and volume using Zeiss optical coherence tomography in patients with diabetic macular edema. Ophthalmology. 2007;**114**:1520-1525

[25] Chhablani J, Krishnan T, Sethi V, Kozak I. Artifacts in optical coherence tomography. Saudi Journal of Ophthalmology. 2014;**28**:81-87

[26] Li C, Yuan Y, Kong X, Han X, Zhang J, Xuan M, et al. Segmentation errors and off-center artifacts in SS-OCT: Insight from a population-based imaging study. Current Eye Research. 2023;**48**(10):949-955

Chapter 9

Influence of Non-Mydriasis on Optical Coherence Tomography Imaging Quality in Patients with Retinitis Pigmentosa

Salvador Pastor-Idoate, Santiago Mejía-Freire, Milagros Mateos-Olivares, Francisco Javier Valentín-Bravo, Eva Maria Sobas Abad, Ricardo Usategui Martín and José Carlos Pastor Jimeno

Abstract

This chapter examines the influence of non-mydriasis on the quality of optical coherence tomography (OCT) imaging in patients with retinitis pigmentosa (RP). The focus is on the analysis of OCT imaging quality, specifically addressing the types of artifacts that can potentially confound the interpretation of OCT and OCT angiography (OCTA) images. Common artifacts such as signal attenuation, motion artifacts, and projection artifacts are identified and discussed. The chapter also explores methods for removing these artifacts and compensation techniques applicable in clinical settings for RP cases. Findings suggest that non-mydriasis does not significantly limit the acquisition and interpretation of OCT images in patients with mild to moderate stages of RP. However, pupillary dilation may be necessary in severe stages of the disease to enhance image quality and reduce artifacts despite the potential increase in glare and photophobia for these patients. The discussion includes practical strategies for optimizing OCT imaging protocols without using mydriatic agents, improving patient comfort, and the efficiency of clinical procedures. Ultimately, this chapter aims to enhance diagnostic accuracy and patient care by addressing and mitigating the challenges associated with OCT imaging in RP patients.

Keywords: signal strength, artifacts, non-mydriasis, optical coherency tomography, retinitis pigmentosa

1. Introduction

Retinitis pigmentosa (RP) is an inherited retinal dystrophy where the degeneration of retinal photoreceptors leads to a significant and progressive loss of visual function [1–3]. RP affects approximately 167,000 individuals in Europe and has a global prevalence of 1:3000 to 1:5000 people [4, 5]. The disease usually begins with nyctalopia and a reduction in the visual field as the most frequent visual symptoms [3, 6]. Despite ongoing research, there is currently no definitive treatment to halt or cure RP, although promising therapies are being developed for some mutations (e.g., RPE65), making regular monitoring essential for managing the disease [5].

Optical coherence tomography (OCT) and OCT-angiography (OCT-A) are crucial noninvasive imaging techniques that provide detailed insights into retinal and choroidal structures and their vascularization. These imaging modalities are indispensable for tracking disease progression in RP patients [7, 8]. However, the accuracy of OCT and OCTA images can be compromised by various artifacts, which may lead to incorrect interpretations and diagnoses [9, 10].

Generally, mydriatic eye drops are recommended in all routine ophthalmic examinations to achieve satisfactory imaging quality. However, RP is a chronic and disabling disease, and over time, depending on the severity and rate of progression, central vision loss, glare, and photophobia can severely impair the patient's quality of life [11, 12]. RP patients can experience severe light adaptation and glare problems after pupil dilation, affecting their ability to cooperate with image collection and, in some cases, resulting in transient complete functional blindness [13], which limits the usefulness of all imaging techniques. This must be considered when conducting eye examinations on individuals with retinal dystrophies [14].

This chapter delves into the impact of non-mydriasis on OCT imaging quality in RP patients. It focuses on identifying and analyzing common artifacts, such as signal attenuation, motion artifacts, and projection artifacts, that can confound image interpretation. Additionally, the chapter explores strategies for artifact removal and compensation techniques applicable in clinical practice for RP cases. By employing these strategies, clinicians can improve the accuracy and reliability of OCT imaging in RP cases, leading to better patient outcomes and more effective disease management.

Our research findings indicate that non-mydriasis does not significantly impede the acquisition and interpretation of OCT images in mild to moderate stages of RP [15, 16]. However, pupillary dilation may be necessary in severe stages to improve image quality and reduce artifacts despite potential drawbacks such as increased glare and photophobia. The effect of pupil dilation on visual test performance has been previously studied. In RP, dilation did not influence visual acuity, visual field tests, or electroretinograms [17–20]. Although multiple OCT and OCT-A metrics have been extensively studied in RP [13, 21], there is very little literature on the influence of topical mydriatic eye drops on OCT parameters [11, 12], and to the best of our knowledge, this has not been previously studied in RP patients. This chapter also presents practical recommendations for optimizing OCT imaging protocols without mydriatic agents, enhancing patient comfort and clinical efficiency.

Ultimately, this chapter aims to improve diagnostic accuracy and patient care by addressing the challenges associated with OCT imaging in RP patients, ensuring more reliable and precise monitoring of this progressive retinal disease.

2. Background on retinitis pigmentosa

2.1 Overview of RP as a genetic retinal dystrophy

Retinitis pigmentosa (RP) refers to a group of inherited retinal degenerative disorders characterized by the progressive loss of photoreceptors, leading to significant visual impairment and eventual irreversible blindness [1–6]. RP is a genetically heterogeneous condition, with mutations identified in over 60 genes. These genes are responsible for the development, function, and maintenance of photoreceptors, and their mutations disrupt these processes, leading to the characteristic retinal degeneration seen in RP.

Despite ongoing research, no definitive treatment exists to halt or cure RP. However, encouraging treatments have been proposed for RP, including gene therapy (e.g., RPE65), stem cell transplantation, neurotrophic growth factors, and retinal prosthesis. These emerging treatments offer hope for mitigating the progression of RP and potentially restoring some degree of vision [22].

2.2 Epidemiology and prevalence of RP

Despite being considered a rare disease, RP is the most typical inherited retinal dystrophy, affecting approximately one in 4000 people worldwide [1–4]. In Europe, it is estimated that around 167,000 individuals are affected by this condition [1, 2, 4, 23, 24]. The prevalence of RP varies geographically and ethnically, with specific populations exhibiting higher rates due to genetic factors [23, 24].

RP can be inherited in an autosomal dominant, autosomal recessive, or X-linked manner, with autosomal recessive inheritance being the most common [25]. The condition equally affects males and females. However, as X-linked RP is expressed only in males, statistically, men may be affected slightly more than women [25]. Around 40–50% of cases are classified as sporadic or simplex, meaning only one family member is affected, and no familial history or known genetic cause is found [26]. Digenic cases of RP are exceedingly rare [27]. The disease manifests across all ethnic groups, although the severity and progression can vary significantly between individuals and families. For example, the USH3 gene, associated with type III Usher syndrome, is typically rare but occurs more frequently among Finns and Ashkenazi Jews [28, 29].

RP may also appear as part of syndromic conditions such as Usher syndrome and Bardet-Biedl syndrome [25]. Over 60 genes have been identified as being linked to RP, many of which are expressed in the retinal photoreceptors or retinal pigment epithelium (RPE) [1, 2]. Due to the variety of mutations and the potential for different mutations within the same gene to result in distinct disorders, the genetic complexity of RP complicates efforts to establish transparent genotype-phenotype relationships [28].

2.3 Pathophysiology and progression of the disease

The pathogenesis of RP is complicated and involves the progressive loss of photoreceptors, starting typically with the rods responsible for peripheral and night vision, followed by the degeneration of cones crucial for central and color vision [1, 2, 30]. Further changes in retinal ganglion cells (RGCs) and RPE, the inner retina disorganization, and the vascular supply attenuation following the outer retina damage ultimately cause vision loss [1, 2, 4, 23, 24, 26, 30].

This sequential loss leads to the characteristic symptoms of RP, including night blindness and a gradual constriction of the visual field. The exact mechanisms of photoreceptor death in RP are complex and multifactorial, involving oxidative stress, inflammation, and apoptosis [26, 30]. The disease progression can be influenced by specific genetic mutations, environmental factors, and other modifying genetic factors [1–6, 26, 30].

2.4 Common symptoms and stages of RP

RP typically manifests in adolescence, with significant visual impairment occurring by middle age (40–50 years). Early-onset forms of RP can resemble Leber congenital amaurosis, and later-onset or non-penetrant variants also exist [1, 2, 30].

The most common early symptom is nyctalopia, or difficulty seeing in low light, followed by progressive narrowing of peripheral vision. Over time, the disease may result in the loss of central vision and photopsia as it advances. Additional symptoms such as impaired color vision, fluctuating day-to-day vision, and photophobia may develop, significantly reducing the patient's quality of life and increasing their risk of stress and anxiety due to difficulties in performing daily tasks [1–6, 26, 30].

Clinical hallmarks include:

1. An abnormal fundus with bone-spicule deposits and attenuated retinal vessels.

2. Abnormal, diminished, or absent a- and b-waves in the electroretinogram (ERG).

3. Reduced visual field (VF), changing from patchy loss of peripheral VF to a ring scotoma, tunnel vision, and eventually blindness.

4. Outer retinal abnormalities, such as loss of external limiting membrane (ELM) line integrity and ellipsoid zone (EZ) line integrity. Intraretinal abnormalities include cystoid macular oedema (CME) and the presence of intraretinal hyper-reflective foci (HF). Vitreomacular interface abnormalities, such as epiretinal membrane (ERM), full-thickness macular hole (FTMH), and lamellar macular hole (LMH), are also observed.

5. Vascular dysfunction and reductions in retinal blood flow in OCTA scans.

The stages of RP can be broadly categorized as:

1. Early stage: Characterized by night blindness and mild peripheral vision loss. Central vision is typically unaffected.

2. Mid stage: Marked by a noticeable constriction of the visual field, leading to significant peripheral vision loss. Central vision may begin to be affected.

3. Late stage: Severe visual field constriction, often reducing vision to a small central island. Central vision may also be severely compromised, leading to legal blindness [1, 2, 23, 30].

These stages highlight the progressive nature of RP and underscore the importance of regular monitoring and early intervention to manage symptoms and maintain quality of life for as long as possible.

3. Importance of imaging in retinitis pigmentosa

3.1 Role of imaging techniques in diagnosing and monitoring RP

Imaging techniques are pivotal in both the diagnosis and ongoing management of RP. They provide detailed visualization of the retinal structures and allow clinicians to track changes over time, facilitating early detection, accurate diagnosis, and effective monitoring of disease progression [1, 2, 4, 23, 31].

The clinical evaluation of patients suspected of RP typically involves a thorough ophthalmic examination. This examination includes measuring best-corrected visual acuity (BCVA), checking intraocular pressure (IOP), and performing slit-lamp and fundus examinations. Additionally, perimetric tests are conducted to assess VF, retinal imaging, and electrophysiological evaluations to comprehensively assess retinal function and structure [1, 2, 4, 23, 31].

Tests such as visual acuity, contrast sensitivity, and color vision are crucial to establish a baseline and monitor the progression of dyschromatopsia, indicating cone photoreceptor involvement. Color and wide field fundus imaging are useful for documenting RP and monitoring its progression. Fundus autofluorescence (FAF) imaging often reveals a ring of increased autofluorescence around the fovea, known as the "AF ring" or Robson-Holder ring, which correlates with disease severity and progression. As RP advances, this ring contracts, indicating worsening rod and cone function. FAF also shows atrophic patches of decreased autofluorescence in the mid-periphery, representing RPE and photoreceptor cell death, which spread over time. It is important to recognize that hyperfluorescent rings are not exclusive to RP; they can also be observed in other retinal conditions, including cone-rod dystrophies [1, 2, 4, 30, 31].

Visual field assessment using kinetic perimetry is the most effective method for evaluating peripheral vision loss in RP. In the early stages of the disease, visual field testing reveals a gradual loss of the mid-peripheral visual field. As the condition progresses, a mid-peripheral ring scotoma forms, generally spreading more quickly toward the peripheral areas than the central region.

Humphrey's visual fields can assess the remaining visual field, aiding in determining visual disability. Electrophysiologic evaluations, such as full-field electroretinography (ffERG), the most common technique for diagnosing RP, are crucial for detecting early electroretinographic abnormalities, often before nyctalopia and fundoscopic changes appear. ERG helps diagnose RP, quantify disease severity, and track progression. Over time, ERG responses diminish, reflecting the extent of photoreceptor loss [1, 2, 4, 31, 32].

Microperimetry (MP), frequently used in clinical trials for inherited retinal diseases (IRDs) alongside traditional measures like visual acuity and visual fields, has proven effective in detecting changes in retinal sensitivity over relatively short periods. These changes often occur before any measurable decline in best-corrected visual acuity (BCVA), making MP a valuable complementary tool in monitoring disease progression and evaluating treatment outcomes in clinical trials [2, 31–33].

Fluorescein angiography (FA) characterizes blood-retinal barrier breakdown, retinal and choroidal blood flow abnormalities, and macular oedema in RP. OCT evaluates retinal changes, showing significant retinal thinning and disruptions in the photoreceptor layer. OCT can also identify ERM and CME, which are common in RP. OCTA is emerging as a valuable tool for visualizing retinal microvasculature changes, correlating with disease severity. Adaptive optics scanning laser ophthalmoscopy (AOSLO) provides high-resolution images of photoreceptor damage, aiding in early detection and monitoring of disease progression [1, 2, 4, 31–33].

3.1.1 Diagnosis

3.1.1.1 Confirmation of diagnosis

Imaging techniques help confirm the presence of RP by revealing characteristic structural changes in the retina. Features such as thinning of the retinal layers, bone spicule pigmentation, and atrophy of the RPE are visible through imaging.

3.1.1.2 Differentiation from other retinal disorders

Imaging can differentiate RP from other retinal dystrophies and degenerative conditions that mimic RP symptoms, which can be distinguished through detailed imaging [1, 2, 23, 30].

The differential diagnosis for RP is broad and includes various conditions such as infections, drug-induced effects (e.g., chloroquine), iatrogenic causes (e.g., laser photocoagulation), metabolic disorders (e.g., gyrate atrophy), and nutritional deficiencies (e.g., vitamin A and zinc). It also encompasses other inherited retinal dystrophies like choroideremia, congenital stationary night blindness, and Oguchi disease. Additionally, several metabolic diseases with fundus findings like RP need to be ruled out, including abetalipoproteinemia (Bassen-Kornzweig disease), ataxia with vitamin E deficiency, and adult Refsum disease [1, 2, 4, 23, 30].

3.1.2 Identification of genetic variants

Specific imaging findings can correlate with certain genetic mutations associated with RP. For example, patients with RPE65 or PRPH2 mutations often exhibit significant thinning of the outer nuclear layer (ONL), subretinal deposits or drusen-like material, and loss of the EZ [34].

Advanced imaging techniques help identify phenotypic variations that might suggest a particular genetic etiology. For instance, patients with Usher syndrome often display specific retinal changes such as CME or initially more localized EZ disruption, which are more common in Usher syndrome than in non-syndromic RP [35].

3.1.3 Monitoring disease progression

3.1.3.1 Tracking structural changes

Regular imaging allows for monitoring changes in retinal thickness, photoreceptor integrity, and other structural aspects of the retina, providing objective data on disease progression [2, 23, 30, 31].

3.1.3.2 Assessing functional impact

Imaging findings can correlate with functional assessments, such as visual field tests and visual acuity, providing a comprehensive view of disease impact. For example, changes in retinal imaging, such as the contracting autofluorescent ring (the

Robson-Holder ring) in FAF or thinning ONL in OCT scans, can help predict future visual function decline, enabling timely interventions [1, 2, 4, 23, 30].

3.1.3.3 Evaluating treatment efficacy

Imaging plays a crucial role in assessing the effectiveness of emerging treatments such as gene therapy, stem cell therapy, and retinal implants. For instance, in the case of gene therapy for RPE65-related RP, imaging techniques provide comprehensive evidence of treatment success. The observed stabilization of retinal layers, reduction in autofluorescence, and improved ERG responses collectively demonstrate the positive impact of the therapy, thereby supporting its efficacy in treating this genetic condition [2, 31, 32].

3.1.4 Guiding clinical management

Detailed imaging data inform clinical decisions regarding patient management, including the timing of interventions and adjustments to treatment plans. Imaging can help determine the necessity of therapeutic changes based on observed disease progression [2, 30, 31].

3.1.5 Research and development

3.1.5.1 Advancing understanding of RP

Imaging techniques contribute to research by providing detailed insights into the pathophysiology of RP and identifying potential biomarkers for disease progression, such as the reduced vessel density and abnormal capillary networks in patients with RPGR mutations, a common cause of XLRP [36–38]. These vascular changes offer insights into the role of blood supply and vascular health in the progression of RP, contributing to a more comprehensive understanding of the disease's impact on retinal structure and function. These biomarkers are valuable for tracking disease progression and evaluating the efficacy of new treatments [36–39].

3.1.5.2 Developing new treatments

Imaging techniques such as OCT, FAF, ERG, and OCT/OCTA provide precise metrics for evaluating the efficacy of new treatments in clinical trials. Researchers can use imaging data to refine and optimize therapeutic approaches based on observed outcomes [1, 2, 4, 8, 13, 21, 23, 30, 31].

In summary, imaging techniques are essential in diagnosing and monitoring RP. They provide critical information that aids in confirming diagnoses, tracking disease progression, evaluating treatment efficacy, and guiding clinical management. The detailed and quantitative data obtained through imaging support clinical decision-making and research efforts to understand and treat RP [2, 30, 31].

3.2 Optical coherence tomography (OCT) and OCT-angiography (OCTA) in RP

Optical coherence tomography and OCTA are invaluable noninvasive tools in clinical practice, providing detailed visualization of ocular structures and enabling quantification of various retinal and ocular parameters crucial for diagnosing and managing eye diseases [8, 13, 21, 40–42]. Optical coherence tomography has been used to assess RP, showing decreased foveal thickness, photoreceptor inner/outer segment (IS/OS) junction disruption, and markedly reduced choroidal thickness. These structural changes observed via OCT are closely associated with the progressive loss of vision [7, 8, 13, 42].

In RP, where the pathology primarily affects the outer retinal layers and photoreceptors, traditional imaging technologies may need to be revised, necessitating advanced imaging methods. One such advancement is enhanced depth imaging OCT, which allows for improved visualization of choroidal structures and applying quantitative techniques like the choroidal vascularity index. This provides deeper insights into the choroidal changes associated with RP [40, 41, 43].

Optical coherence tomography angiography is a recent technological advancement that enables the rapid, noninvasive acquisition of high-resolution, depth-resolved images of both retinal and choroidal vascular layers. With its capability to differentiate between the superficial capillary plexus (SCP), deep capillary plexus (DCP), and choriocapillaris plexus (CCP), OCTA has become widely used for the early detection of vascular abnormalities and the diagnosis of vascular pathologies in various inherited retinal diseases (IRDs), including RP.

OCTA offers comprehensive retinal information by analyzing both structural and vascular aspects through blood flow analysis, thus enhancing the utility of OCT in RP compared to conventional methods [8, 38, 40, 41, 43].

Both OCT and OCTA perform multiple scans of the exact location. In OCT, post-acquisition processing averages these scans into a single high-resolution B-scan. In contrast, OCTA interprets differences between scans as blood flow over time, enabling the mapping of vascular architecture. Consequently, OCT-A can identify numerous retinal vascular anomalies in RP, such as non-perfusion areas, closed vessels, neovascularization in previously avascular areas, increased vascularization, micro- and macro-aneurysms, capillary remodeling, and macular telangiectasia [8, 38, 40, 41, 43].

However, OCTA's capability to capture movement information over short durations limits its ability to assess changes over more extended periods, such as those caused by blood or fluid leakage [1, 2, 8, 38–41, 43]. Thus, FA remains essential for evaluating the breakdown of the blood-retinal barriers in RP. The primary advantage of OCTA over fluorescein angiography is eliminating the need for intravenous contrast dye injections and reducing the risk of complications [1–4, 42]. In summary, OCT and OCTA are critical tools in managing RP, providing detailed structural and vascular insights essential for accurate diagnosis, monitoring disease progression, and assessing the efficacy of emerging treatments.

3.3 Advantages of noninvasive imaging in RP management

Noninvasive imaging techniques offer significant benefits in managing RP, primarily by enhancing patient comfort and reducing post-examination visual disturbances [12, 15, 16, 19, 20]. Here are the key advantages:

1. Avoidance of pupil dilation and reduction of glare and light sensitivity: Without the need for dilating eye drops, patients avoid common side effects such as increased light sensitivity and glare. These effects can cause significant discomfort and hinder daily activities for several hours.

2. Enhanced patient comfort: Noninvasive imaging techniques are painless, quick, and efficient, reducing the time patients spend in the clinic and minimizing discomfort associated with prolonged examinations.

3. Immediate post-examination relief: Patients experience no visual disturbances after the procedure, allowing them to resume normal activities promptly without any discomfort.

4. Improved patient compliance: A better overall patient experience reduces anxiety and enhances compliance with follow-up visits. This is crucial for managing progressive conditions like RP, ensuring consistent monitoring and timely interventions.

Noninvasive imaging plays a vital role in effectively managing RP by minimizing patient discomfort and improving the overall examination experience [12, 15, 16, 19, 20].

4. Challenges in OCT imaging for RP patients

4.1 Common artifacts in OCT/OCA images

Artifacts in OCT images have been documented to affect image quality, analysis, and interpretation, potentially leading to incorrect diagnoses, prognoses, or staging. They can result from data acquisition methods, data processing algorithms, intrinsic properties of the eyeball, pathological alterations, or insufficient patient cooperation [7–10, 15, 16, 44–47]. Particularly, given their low vision, patients with RP often struggle to maintain adequate fixation, making them more predisposed to insufficient image quality for proper and accurate analysis [7–10, 45].

4.1.1 Signal attenuation

All OCT devices have a standard for signal intensity, which must be met to determine if an image possesses the minimum necessary quality to be considered analyzable. Signal attenuation is the failure to meet these minimum conditions. The causes of signal attenuation can be diffuse or localized:

- Diffuse: The most common cause in patients with RP is the presence of cataracts. Other causes include a deficient tear film, incorrect patient positioning, and refractive defects such as astigmatism or myopia [7–10, 44].

- Localized: These can be caused by transparent vitreous floaters that produce aberrations in the OCT light beam. If these are more pronounced, they generate shadows that prevent imaging of certain areas (**Figure 1**) [7–10, 44].

4.1.2 Projection artifacts

Also known as decorrelation tails, these artifacts occur when the OCT light beam does not reach structures such as photoreceptors or the RPE due to reflection, absorption, or scattering by the retinal blood vessels. This results in the shadows of superficial retinal blood vessels appearing in the deeper layers of the retina (**Figure 2**) [8–10, 47].

These artifacts can lead to an underestimation of parameters obtained in OCT-A and an overestimation of the severity of RP involvement.

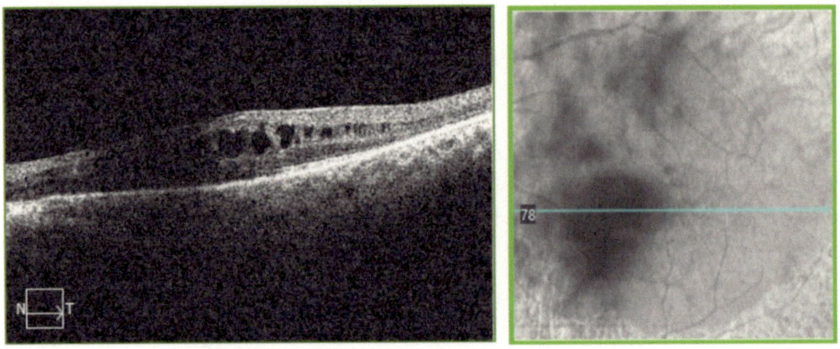

Figure 1.
Optical coherence tomography (OCT) B-scan and en-face *images of a patient with retinitis pigmentosa (RP) and cystoid macular oedema. A vitreous floater causes signal attenuation, hindering the visualization of retinal structures.*

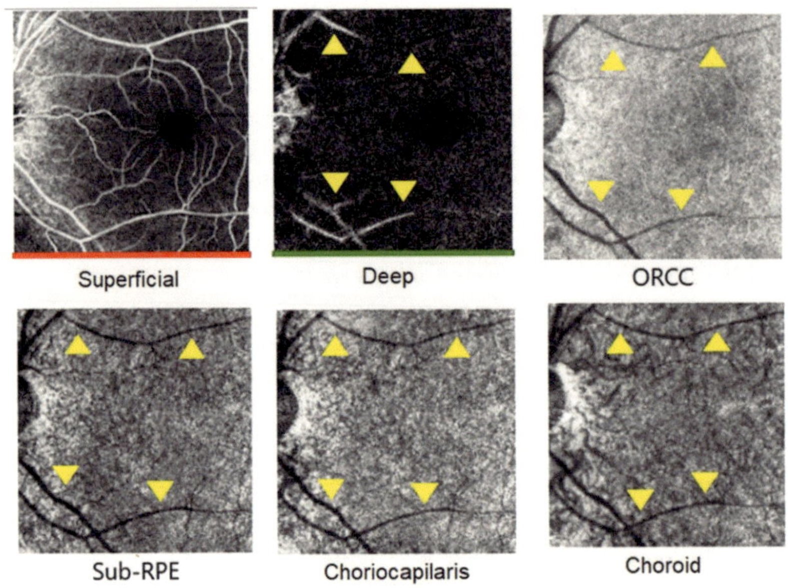

Figure 2.
Optical coherence tomographic angiography (OCT-A) with projection artifact displaying superficial vascular structures incorrectly in deeper layers (yellow arrows). ORCC: outer retina to choriocapillaris.

4.1.3 Motion artifacts

These artifacts are significant in both structural OCT and, more notably, in OCTA, which is more sensitive to motion. They can be classified into two categories:

- Large or sudden movements: These include extensive eye movements, head movements, patient movements, and microsaccades (**Figure 3**) [8–10, 45, 46].
- Axial movements (anterior-posterior): Caused by heartbeat pulsations or respiration, these movements can cause significant changes from one B-scan to the next [8–10, 44].

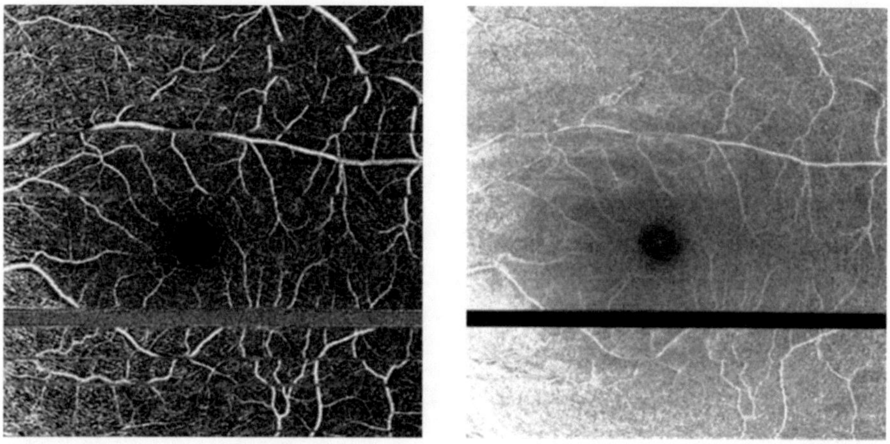

Figure 3.
Motion artifacts are observed because of eye movement, an illusory interruption, and/or displacement of the vessels.

4.2 Impact of these artifacts on image interpretation and diagnosis

Given the advances in gene therapy for the treatment of RP, proper phenotyping and genotyping, monitoring, and identification of biomarkers associated with functional outcomes are extremely important. Additionally, OCTA is an invaluable technique for complementing other imaging modalities better to characterize retinal and choroidal vascular changes in these patients.

Without adequate knowledge of these artifacts, images can lead to erroneous diagnoses and incorrect assessments of disease progression, providing inaccurate information to patients [8–10, 48]. This can result in misinformed treatment decisions and potentially ineffective or harmful interventions. Recognizing and accounting for these artifacts is essential to ensure accurate image interpretation and reliable clinical outcomes in RP patients.

4.3 Importance of recognizing and correcting artifacts

A good understanding and interpretation of artifacts enable a more precise interpretation of the images, ensuring they reflect reality. Correcting artifacts helps achieve accurate interpretation and proper staging of the disease. Among the numerous artifacts described in the literature, segmentation, projection, and masking artifacts can lead to observing abnormal structures in layers that are not indeed affected. Therefore, special attention should be paid to these artifacts when analyzing OCTA images, especially in structures intended for analysis that might be affected, such as layers beneath larger blood vessels (**Figure 4**) [7–10, 44, 47].

Each OCT device is equipped with tools to control artifacts, such as active eye tracking, which quickly measures the eye's position and makes corresponding corrections if the eye exceeds a certain movement threshold; or software-based correction, included in the devices, though unfortunately, the mechanism of its operation is proprietary to the manufacturer [46]. Additionally, to recognize artifacts, it is important to always interpret OCTA images with other complementary tests such as fundus photography, autofluorescence, and fluorescein angiography [7–10, 46].

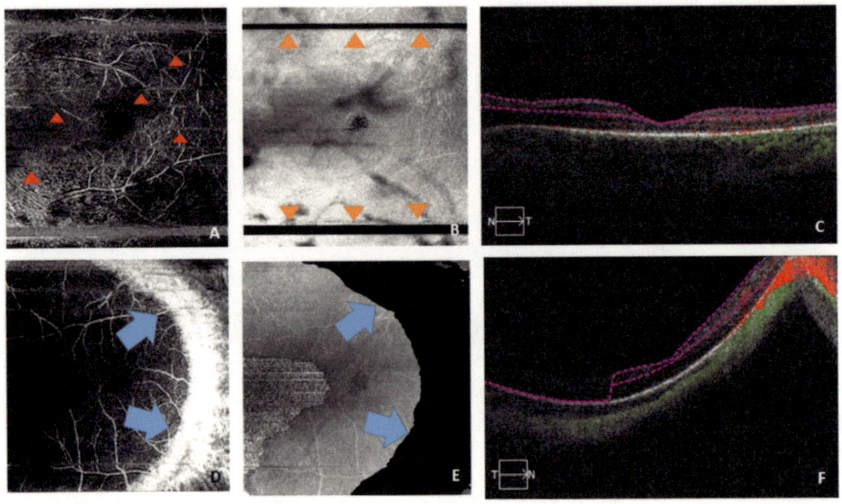

Figure 4.
Different optical coherence tomographic angiography (OCTA) artifacts. A. Banding artifact. Horizontal stripes of different brightness are observed (red arrows). B. Blink artifact. Black lines due to images were not acquired for closing eyelids (orange arrows). C. OCT B-Scan of a patient with RP without Artifacts: a clear reference image demonstrating an artifact-free scan. D–F. Out-of-window artifact. Loss of focus of the scan is observed (blue arrows) compared to C.

Finally, it is essential to emphasize that although some tools are available to minimize artifacts, the compensation effects are imperfect, and not all OCT devices have these capabilities. Therefore, knowledge and attention to detail are essential for managing artifacts in patients with RP [7–10, 44].

5. Non-mydriasis in OCT imaging

5.1 Definition and significance of non-mydriasis in ophthalmic imaging

Mydriasis is the dilation of the pupil. Tropicamide 1%, cyclopentolate 0.5, 1, 2%, and atropine 10% have an anticholinergic nature and, with variable affinity, act as antagonists of the muscarinic receptors at the iris sphincter relaxing it. Phenylephrine (2.5, 10%), by contrast, is an α1-adrenergic agonist that stimulates the iris dilator muscle when applied, producing a synergistic effect [49].

Those are the active principles commonly used as mydriatic agents for ophthalmological assessment and treatment, allowing a comprehensive exam of the lens, vitreous cavity, and fundus and facilitating diagnostic and therapeutic procedures. Tropicamide is the most used for examination purposes in adults due to its rapid action (25–30 min), duration (4–8 hours), high mydriatic power, and safeness [50].

Nevertheless, some adverse events have been linked to their use. Patients complain about stinging, light sensitivity, and blurred vision, although they are transient. They produce a certain cycloplegic action when blocking the muscarinic receptors of the ciliary body, which allows their use with therapeutical intention too, but is inconvenient when the aim is the examination [50]. Moreover, for anatomical reasons, all of them can produce a drug-induced angle closure, mainly in patients with a shallow anterior chamber (3% of the general population), although the risk in the clinical setting has been estimated to be around 3 out of 10,000 patients [51, 52].

Last but not least, as with every medication, either the active principles or the accompanying excipients can cause hypersensitivity reactions in predisposed patients and, given their anticholinergic nature when absorbed into the bloodstream, they can have systemic side effects such as hives, breathing difficulties, high blood pressure, heart arrhythmias, flushing and dryness, and swelling of the face, lips, tongue, or throat [49–51]. In addition, disorientation and unusual behavior have been described as linked to the use of cyclopentolate and atropine in children [53].

In large population studies, such as diabetic retinopathy screening programs, the possibility of non-mydriasis in ophthalmic imaging has already been studied, maintaining high sensitivity and specificity levels [54, 55]. In agreement with ETDRS, the classic seven conventional 35-mm slide photographs were considered the gold standard in imaging for diabetic screening [56]. However, the available means have changed, and with them, new, comparable in efficacy, and more cost-effective methods of retinal imaging have emerged, such as non-mydriatic cameras of 45 degrees and Ultra-widefield cameras and lasers that cover up to 200° [57–59]. Classic ones used to require pupil dilation, and a skilled photographer as compared to new devices that have an interface kinder to the user, do not require mydriasis and are less dependent on media transparency [58].

Given this situation, imaging technology has allowed the avoidance of compulsory mydriasis for diabetic screening in some regions, and patients are the most benefited since they can return to their normal lives after the screening visit improving compliance among patients [60].

This could be extended to patients with RP since the new imaging techniques allow the visualization in detail of the peripheral retina, an area of high interest in those patients [61]. They also allow us to study fundus autofluorescence (FAF) that can show different patterns according to the genotype, the degree of outer retinal, and retinal pigmentary epithelium atrophy and evaluate the rate of progression by the AF ring which forms between functional and dysfunctional retina [62–64].

5.2 Benefits of avoiding mydriatic agents in RP patients

While dilation of the pupil for diagnostic purposes can be time-consuming and uncomfortable for everyone, in RP patients, photophobia and light sensitivity are among the most common symptoms reported, and these worsen significantly under mydriasis conditions.

Due to their photoreceptor degeneration, RP patients' retinas cannot adapt to bright environments, changes in light conditions, and scattering, even slight ones, the more challenging, the more advanced stage of the disease [65, 66]. Glare can cause discomfort because of the difficulties in light adaptation, but it can also be disabling when contrast sensitivity decreases [65, 67]. Moreover, they have a higher prevalence of posterior subcapsular cataracts that produce light scattering too [68]. Therefore, it is significantly more complicated for them to recover from those caused pharmacologically.

They also experience bright and glimmering lights, called photopsia, usually reported at the edges of the visual field scotomas. These are thought to be linked to the aberrant signals sent from the dying photoreceptors [64]. These photopsia and glare and constricted visual field can make their lives very difficult, affect their reading and long-distance vision, and even their mobility [69].

Considering that RP is a chronic disease, patients need to be monitored. This can be done annually or even more often if they are included in an essay or clinical trial or suffering from any concomitant eye problem or complication related to the disease. Therefore, all patients with RP will have quite a few appointments in ophthalmology clinics throughout their lives and, consequently, frequent pharmacological mydriasis, so their problems with it are not trivial.

5.3 Review of literature on non-mydriatic OCT imaging in RP and other retinal conditions

First-time-domain (TD) OCT scans were highly dependent on media transparency, mydriasis, and fixation [70]. Nowadays, with spectral domain (SD), swept-source (SS), confocal scanning OCT technology, and technological development in general, they have improved enormously in speed, definition, and registration, constituting an indispensable instrument for ophthalmological examination [71].

Pupil dilation does not affect macular thickness measurements when assessing diabetic macular oedema, nor does diagnostic accuracy, sensitivity, or specificity, so there is no reason to think that it would affect the measurements and diagnosis of macular oedema in patients with RP. Only segmentation errors and signal intensity improved under mydriasis [15, 16, 72].

Regarding OCTA, some published studies have shown differences in artifact incidence and some parameter measures, such as peripapillary vessel density and choroidal thickness measured with SD-OCTs, especially if both tropicamide and phenylephrine at 0.5% concentrations were used, could affect uveal structure and regulation [12, 73, 74].

No differences were found in some important values in retinal perfusion, such as foveal density and foveal avascular zone at the superficial and deep capillary plexus [12]. SS-OCT scan measurements in mydriatic conditions noted a slight increase in retinal thickness in some retinal sectors [73]. All studies agreed that non-mydriasis does not affect OCTA usefulness when studying retinal structure and vascularization in diabetic patients, branch retinal vein occlusion, or age-related macular degeneration [73, 75, 76].

6. Our research findings

6.1 Methodology of the study on non-mydriasis and OCT imaging quality in RP

For detailed information on the methodology for these RP patients, please refer to our group's prior publications [77, 78]. Briefly, 76 out of 78 patients with a prior RP diagnosis, along with 30 healthy controls, were included in our cross-sectional study conducted between January 2020 and June 2023. All participants were examined at the Department of Ophthalmology, Hospital Clínico Universitario de Valladolid, and the Instituto de Oftalmobiología Aplicada (IOBA), University of Valladolid, Valladolid, Spain.

It is important to note that the decision to perform imaging without mydriasis was based on previously published studies showing that high-quality imaging can be obtained in RP patients without inducing pharmacological mydriasis. This approach was chosen to avoid potential side effects of mydriatic agents and to ensure patient comfort, especially given that repeated imaging sessions were required.

6.2 Patient selection and criteria

Detailed information on the inclusion and exclusion criteria and RP grading in these patients can be found in a previous publication by our group [77, 78].

All patients were part of the "Retinitis Pigmentosa Castilla y León" association (RECyL). The study also included 30 healthy volunteers without ocular diseases. All participants underwent a comprehensive ophthalmic examination, including refraction, BCVA, SD-OCT, visual field test, anterior segment examination, and fundus examination without using mydriatic drops. RP patients were graded into severity disease groups based on the criteria by Smith et al. [79]. The inclusion criteria for the RP group were an RP diagnosis, age between 18 and 60, and Caucasian ethnicity. Exclusion criteria for all groups included patients with ≥6 diopters spherical equivalent, dense cataracts, corneal opacities, nystagmus, or other retinal diseases.

We want to highlight that the exclusion criteria were specifically chosen to avoid factors that could compromise the quality of OCT and OCTA imaging. For instance, high refractive errors (≥6 diopters) and media opacities such as cataracts could affect the ability to obtain clear images, thus impacting the validity of our findings.

6.3 Imaging protocols and parameters used

Structural OCT imaging was conducted with the SD-OCT Zeiss Cirrus Plex Elite 5000® (Carl Zeiss Meditec, Dublin, CA, USA), which has an A-scanner speed of 68,000 scans/second with 5 microns of axial resolution and a scan depth of 2 mm. The instrument uses a wavelength of light of 840 nm, an area of 6 × 6 millimeters for the angiography, and 512 × 128 for the cube images of the macular area. AngioPlex ™ software (AngioPlex software, version 10.0; Carl Zeiss Meditec) incorporated in the device was used for OCTA analysis. In addition, the AngioPlex incorporated the FastTrac retinal tracking technology to minimize motion artifacts.

The same operator performed all the scans. The macula area and optic disc were imaged using the macular cube 200 × 200 scan mode protocol to analyze central retinal thickness (CRT), ganglion cell inner plexiform layer (GCIPL) thickness, outer retinal layer thickness (ORT), central choroidal thickness (CCT), and retinal nerve fiber layer thickness (RNFLT).

An expert examiner performed OCTA imaging in two sessions for each patient under the same conditions in the same location. The scanning protocol was macular 6 × 6 mm scan mode for quantitative flow parameters and 3 × 3 for FAZ measurements. All patients were rested for at least 10 minutes before the second imaging session, as recommended by Alnawaiseh et al. [80].

We chose to perform imaging across two sessions to ensure the reproducibility of the OCTA data and minimize the potential for artifacts due to patient fatigue or eye movement. The 10-minute rest period between imaging sessions is an essential factor incorporated based on previous studies to ensure consistency in flow measurements. This adds robustness to the data and minimizes any variability that could arise from imaging fatigue or physiological changes during long examination periods.

The SCP, DCP, and choriocapillaris (CC) flow density data were analyzed using the Cirrus OCTA software. VD (defined as the total length of the perfused vasculature per unit area in the region of measurement) and PD (defined as the total area of the perfused vasculature per unit area in the region of measurement) of the SCP according to the ETDRS subfields were measured automatically. The area of the foveal avascular zone (FAZ) in mm^2 was calculated in the SCP automatically. In cases of error in the automated measurement of FAZ (**Figure 5**), it was manually calculated by a retina specialist, drawing the border of the FAZ manually.

In cases where automated measurements were unreliable, a trained retina specialist manually corrected the FAZ borders to ensure precision. This manual adjustment is

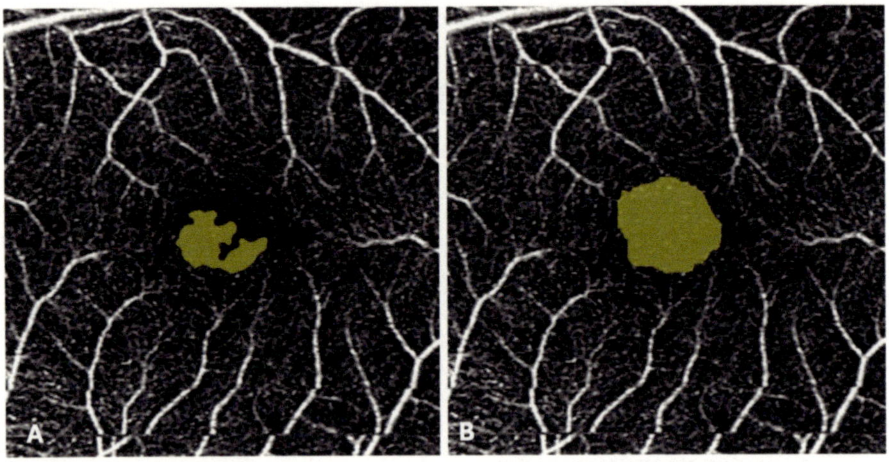

Figure 5.
Manual calculation of the foveal avascular zone (FAZ). *A. Optical coherence tomographic angiography (OCT-A) automated measurement of the FAZ performed by the optical coherence tomography (OCT) device. B. FAZ manually measured by the operator.*

essential to mitigate any inaccuracies that could arise from algorithmic errors, documented in prior studies involving OCTA imaging.

6.4 Presentation of research findings on the influence of non-mydriasis on OCT imaging quality and impact on imaging artifacts and overall image quality

Overall, 106 individuals (76 patients and 30 controls) were enrolled in this study since 13 patients excluded from the quantitative analysis could not be photographed with acceptable quality. The sociodemographic and basal characteristics of the study population are presented in **Table 1**.

Table 2 describes quantitative parameters measured in the OCT and OCT-A in patients compared to controls. FAZ could not be determined on 10 OCT-A images due to their poor image quality.

	Patients	Controls	p-value* CI (95%)
n (men/women)	78 (47/31)	30 (12/18)	0.04‡
Eyes (OR/OS)	78 (44/34)	60 (30/30)	0.606‡
Age (years) (mean ± SD)	51.59 (±13.40)	34.27 (± 9.75)	0.059*
BCVA (VAR) (mean ± SD)	43.03 (±30.43)	100 (±0.00)	**<0.001***
Visual field (MD) (mean ± SD)	−26.97 (±7.22)	−0.05 (±1.78)	**<0.001****
RP severity score (mean ± SD)	7.27/16 ± 2.46	—	—
Severity (*n*) Mild–moderate (0–10) Severe (11–16)	26 (33%) 52 (67%)	—	—

*n: number of individuals; OR: right eye; OS: left eye; BCVA: best-corrected visual acuity. VAR: Visual Acuity Range; SD: standard deviation; MD: mean deviation. Statistically significant p-values are marked in bold. *t-test for independent samples.*
‡Chi-square test.
***U-test.*

Table 1.
Study population characteristics.

Parameter	Patients (mean ± SD)	Controls (mean ± SD)	p-value* CI (95%)
Vessel density (mm/mm²)			
Central	5.60 (±4.73)	8.86 (±3.09)	**<0.001**
Internal	11.10 (±−4.53)	16.55(±2.30)	**<0.001**
External	10.96 (±3.46)	17.17 (±1.45)	**<0.001**
Complete	10.83 (±3.50)	16.81 (±1.61)	**<0.001**
Perfusion density (%)			
Central	12.86 (±11.48)	19.99 (±7.41)	**<0.001**
Internal	26.50 (±11.48)	40.26 (±5.85)	**<0.001**
External	26.11 (±9.01)	43.50 (±3.92)	**<0.001**
Complete	25.79 (±8.98)	42.11 (±4.25)	**<0.001**
FAZ, automatic			
FAZ area (mm²)	0.31 (±0.23)	0.20 (±0.09)	**0.001**
FAZ, manual correction			
FAZ area (mm²)	0.36 (±0.27)	0.22 (±0.11)	**<0.001**
Signal strength	7.86 (±1.79)	8.68 (±1.03)	**0.002**
Macular thickness (μm)			
Central	223.82 (±63.48)	266.70 (±17.18)	**<0.001**
Superior inner	268.92 (± 48.36)	330.17 (±17.46)	**<0.001**
Temporal inner	257 (±38.76)	317.48 (±14.62)	**<0.001**
Inferior inner	271.53 (±46.39)	327.75 (±13.22)	**<0.001**
Nasal inner	280.15 (±52.30)	333.33 (±13.60)	**<0.001**
Superior outer	235.30 (±44.44)	287.95 (±12.82)	**<0.001**
Temporal outer	213.62 (±35.55)	269.90 (±14.17)	**<0.001**
Inferior outer	233.66 (±48.33)	274.78 (±12.27)	**<0.001**
Nasal outer	261.67 (±42.38)	306.35 (±13.14)	**<0.001**
Ganglion cells layer	51.74 (±22.27)	84.92 (±5.39)	**<0.001**
Choroidal thickness	192.09 (±74.03)	294.07 (±42.15)	**<0.001**

*SD: standard deviation; FAZ: Foveal avascular zone; μm: microns. *: t-test for independent samples. Statistically significant p-values are marked in bold.*

Table 2.
Comparison of parameters measured in OCT-A and OCT in the patients and control group.

Artifacts were found in 47 of 60 (78.33%) of the eyes of the control group and 76 of 78 (96.2%) in the patient group. The projection was the most frequent artifact in both groups (patients: 66 [83.5%]; control 39 [65%]), followed by masking (21 [26.6%]) and band defect (18 [22.8%]) in the patient's group.

Regarding the number of artifacts found in the same image, one or two different ones were found in 59 images (74.68%) and three or four in 17 images (21.5%) of the patient's group. Due to poor image quality, the quantitative parameters of OCT and OCT-A images of patients with four artifacts could not be measured.

Respecting the distribution of artifacts between disease severity grades, in the mild-moderate group, the greatest part of the images, 54 (87.9%), had less than three compared to the severe disease group, where most of the images (14 [82.35%]) had more than four artifacts. Moreover, three patients from the mild-moderate group had no artifacts in their images, unlike the severe stage group, in which all had at least one artifact. These findings were not only clinically but also statistically significant ($p < 0.001$, *u* Mann-Whitney test).

In agreement with the secondary objectives of this study, it was decided to use all the variables analyzed and compare them to discover whether there exists or not a correlation between structural and functional parameters in RP patients. BCVA and vessel density were, even weakly, positively correlated ($r = 0.26$; $p = 0.02$), as well as perfusion density ($r = 0.28$; $p = 0.013$) and central ($r = 0.25$, $p = 0.028$) and inner macular quadrants thickness. Choroidal thickness was more strongly correlated with BCVA ($r = 0.43$; $p < 0.001$), and there was a negative and moderate correlation between FAZ and BCVA ($r = -0.32$; $p = 0.009$). In addition, the severity grade of disease was negatively but weakly correlated with central macular thickness (CMT) ($r = -0.29$ $p = 0.01$) and inner retinal thickness at superior ($r = -0.23$; $p = 0.04$) and nasal quadrants ($r = -0.25$; $p = 0.02$) as well as with choroidal thickness ($r = -0.23$; $p = 0.04$).

6.5 Discussion of our research findings

Several authors have reported the usefulness of OCT and OCT-A in monitoring patients with RP despite the challenges posed by their diminished visual function, fixation difficulties, and complications at advanced stages of the disease, such as disorganization of retinal layers and loss of ocular media transparency [13, 81–83].

Regarding the comparative structural parameters of thickness and vascular distribution between patients and controls, our findings align with the literature. Patients exhibited significantly reduced measurements in superficial and deep capillary plexus vessel densities [8, 15, 84–86], macular thickness [87, 88], ganglion cell layer thickness [87, 89], and choroidal thickness [90–92]. Notably, the FAZ area was significantly larger in RP patients, likely due to photoreceptor degeneration and reduced blood supply needs as part of RP pathogenesis [93]. These changes are consistent with the arteriolar thinning and vascular attenuation observed in advanced disease stages [7, 13]. Our findings agree with other published studies [13, 83, 94].

One important parameter in OCT devices is signal strength, which ranges from 0 to 10, with a threshold value determining whether an OCT image is acceptable [95]. In our study, the RP patient group had a signal strength approximately 10% lower than the control group yet still above the acceptable threshold, indicating that while image quality was slightly worse, it remained acceptable for clinical use.

The primary aim of our study was to determine the impact of non-mydriasis on OCT image quality in RP patients since pharmacological mydriasis can exacerbate glare and impair visual function in these patients [65]. Although no studies have directly addressed this issue in RP patients, its effects have been studied in other retinal diseases with mixed results. For example, Brücher et al. found that the motion artifact score (MAS) was higher without mydriasis in patients with AMD, suggesting worse OCT image quality. This may be due to miosis producing an insufficient fundoscopic image for the OCTA instrument tracker [12]. Conversely, Medina et al. did not find a significant effect of non-mydriasis on the accuracy of different OCT-SD devices in detecting diabetic macular oedema [72]. Wang et al. reported that as long as the pupillary size was over 2–3 mm, mydriasis did not affect the accuracy of OCT-SD devices in measuring CMT [96]. In all these studies, visual function was better preserved than in our RP patients, who had a mean BCVA of approximately 43 VAR. Additionally, Lam et al. found no significant effect of mydriasis on the VF area in Goldmann perimetry in RP patients [19].

Artifact distribution differed between patients and controls. RP patients had 16% more artifacts per image, with more artifacts in advanced disease stages. Approximately 60% of patients had more than two artifacts per image, compared to only one in 60% of the control group. The most common artifact in both groups was a projection, consistent with findings by Enders et al. in various retinal diseases [44]. In contrast, Ghasemi et al. found banding artifacts to be the most common, followed by segmentation and motion artifacts, likely due to the different OCT devices used [9]. Algorithms to suppress projection artifacts, such as the Projection-Resolved OCTA (PR-OCTA) algorithm applied by Hagag et al., can improve image interpretation in RP patients [97]. Increasing image acquisition speed, tracking the fundus during OCT, and developing new computer programs can also reduce artifacts, as described by Chen et al. [10].

Several studies have attempted to correlate clinical findings with quantitative OCT and OCT-A values to identify objective progression markers in RP. In our research, BCVA showed a weak but direct correlation with vascular density, perfusion of inner retinal layers, and macular thickness, supporting the notion that better visual function and retinal structure are associated with earlier disease stages [93]. Choroidal thickness had a stronger correlation with BCVA, likely for the same reason. Other studies, such as Alnawaiseh et al., reported similar findings but with more robust correlation indices, particularly between BCVA in LogMAR and foveal vascular density. They also found a strong correlation between vascular density measured by OCT-A and VF and multifocal electroretinogram [8].

6.6 Limitations and conclusions of our research findings

The primary limitation of our study is the need for a control group of RP patients who underwent mydriasis. Healthy subjects were dilated to obtain the highest-quality images possible (ideal condition), while RP patients were not. This poses a challenge in isolating the effect of non-mydriasis when capturing OCT and OCTA images of RP patients. However, using mydriasis in RP patients could lead to increased glare, further blurring their already diminished vision and limiting their immediate activities, which is why it was avoided.

Despite this, we found it noteworthy that in patients with mild to moderate RP, there were no significant differences in the images obtained without dilation compared to those of dilated healthy subjects. This reinforces the idea that mydriasis may not be necessary for ophthalmic examinations in these patients. Additionally, this study's absence of genetic characterization of RP patients prevented comparisons between genetic variants and structural and functional tests. Future studies should include this aspect, as it may help explain the significant heterogeneity of the disease.

This study analyzes images of RP patients and healthy controls, and its results cannot be extrapolated to patients with retinal diseases other than RP. Moreover, patients with poor gaze fixation or media opacities that did not allow for images of acceptable quality were excluded, which likely underrepresents the final stages of RP in this study. Additionally, the OCT device used in this study allowed the measurement of a limited number of parameters, excluding automatic measurement of the ellipsoid zone and FAZ area of deeper layers. These parameters should be considered for further investigations since they are important for the follow-up and assessment of disease stages in RP patients.

In conclusion, non-mydriasis was not a limiting factor for the proper acquisition and interpretation of OCT and OCTA images in patients with mild to moderate stages of RP. Conversely, in advanced stages, pupillary dilation could help improve image quality and reduce the presence of artifacts. Identifying artifacts allows for better interpretation of OCT and OCTA images, preventing diagnostic errors in RP diagnosis and follow-up. Quantitative structural parameters acquired by OCT and OCTA correlate with functional parameters such as BCVA and disease severity. OCT and OCTA techniques are useful, reliable, and readily available ancillary tests that allow for comprehensive qualitative and quantitative exploration of the pathophysiological changes and altered retinal structures in RP patients.

7. Practical strategies and recommendations for clinicians

7.1 Techniques for artifact removal and compensation in clinical settings

7.1.1 Projection artifacts

One simple method for removing projection artifacts in OCT imaging is slab subtraction, where the signal from superficial layers is subtracted from deeper angiograms [7, 10]. This technique effectively eliminates projection artifacts but also has drawbacks, such as removing true flow signals coinciding with the artifacts, potentially leading to underestimating vessel density in the DCP and affecting other OCTA metrics, particularly vessel connectivity. Slab subtraction is best suited for measurements in avascular regions, although it can disrupt other features, such as choroidal neovascularization (CNV) morphology [97, 98]. Additionally, it is limited to en-face images and cannot remove projection artifact tails in cross-sectional images [97, 98]. Accurate slab segmentation is crucial but challenging, especially in pathological eyes, making slab subtraction prone to including flow signals unrelated to superficial layers [97, 98].

A more advanced approach is PR-OCTA [97], which leverages structural OCT signals to differentiate true in situ flow from projection artifacts, effectively suppressing the latter across the volume. This method removes artifacts from en-face images and cross-sectional views, yielding cleaner volumes [97]. While PR-OCTA generally produces better results than slab subtraction, it can retain some residual artifacts in low-quality scans and does not disrupt the morphology of pathological vessels [97]. PR-OCTA's ability to distinguish CNV types based on lesion depth and its effectiveness in detecting vascular connections between the choroidal and retinal circulations enhance its utility in diagnosing conditions like macular telangiectasia and retinal angiomatous proliferation [97]. Despite its proven utility in ophthalmology, its application in other tissues remains unverified. Additionally, commercial OCTA instruments now include proprietary projection artifact removal algorithms, but it remains essential to inspect OCTA images for any residual artifacts [97].

7.1.2 Eye motion

Both hardware and software solutions can effectively mitigate eye motion artifacts in OCT imaging. Real-time tracking of microsaccades during OCTA acquisition allows for detecting and rescanning affected areas, ensuring clearer images. Alternatively, the software can omit scans affected by microsaccadic signals, or multiple volumes can be registered and merged to recover lost B-frames, eliminating the need for rescanning. This is often achieved by scanning separately along each lateral axis (x-fast and y-fast scanning schemes). Real-time tracking, which may rely on auxiliary technologies like scanning laser ophthalmoscope or solely on OCTA data, can also remove microsaccadic artifacts altogether. However, it may slightly extend the duration of imaging sessions [7, 10, 99].

Ocular pulsation and drift are other common sources of bulk motion artifacts in OCTA imaging. These disruptions, while sometimes slow enough not to compromise vessel contrast, can introduce phase noise, particularly problematic for complex- and phase-based OCTA processing. To address this, methods estimate bulk motion contribution by analyzing the flow signal statistics across avascular voxels [99]. Approaches include using histograms of phase-shift values between line scans or averaging phase changes along line scans [99]. Applying suitable thresholds to remove phase noise and avoid underestimates is crucial. Phase wrapping, introduced as OCTA moved to measure motion contrast between cross-sectional scans, can also be resolved using standard-deviation-based approaches or iterated averaging to ensure accurate phase contrast measurements and remove bulk motion noise effectively [99].

7.1.3 Signal attenuation

Signal strength in OCTA is closely tied to reflectance magnitude, impacting both direct measurements (e.g., reflectance/complex amplitude-based approaches) and indirect measurements (e.g., correlation or ratio-based approaches). Commercial instruments often quantify overall signal intensity using the Signal Strength Index (SSI) [7, 10, 99, 100]. Variations in signal intensity can influence OCTA metrics, necessitating compensation to prevent biased measurements. Signal loss across an entire image, often due to defocus, can severely affect OCTA measurements that depend on flow signal intensity. For instance, vessel density can vary by 10% within clinically acceptable scans of the same eye under different signal strengths. Defocus reduces the contrast between vessels and the background and broadens vessel width, leading to artificial variations in vessel density. While traditional image processing techniques are sensitive to such variations, modern machine learning-based quantification can mitigate the effects of defocus, ensuring more accurate measurements despite the frequent inclusion of defocused scans in OCTA datasets [10, 99]. Other common causes of global signal attenuation include cataracts and tear film breakup, with the latter affecting the focusing power of the eye and leading to dimmer images [10, 99, 100].

Local signal loss in OCTA imaging often results from severe attenuation beneath hyperreflective materials along the beam path. Hyperreflective foci in the retina, such as those observed in diabetic retinopathy, and materials outside the retina, like vitreous floaters, can cause shadowing. Vignetting is another common source of signal dropout. Depending on the extent of signal loss, it may be impossible to recover certain information, such as vessel density in specific regions of the OCTA image [10, 99, 100]. Local signal loss can suppress the global vessel density value and mimic real capillary dropout, presenting a significant challenge for traditional hand-crafted image processing algorithms. However, modern deep learning-based algorithms have shown the ability to distinguish between shadowing artifacts and real pathology, enhancing the accuracy of OCTA measurements despite these local signal losses [99, 100].

7.2 Guidelines for managing glare and photophobia in RP patients during imaging

Managing glare and photophobia in patients with RP during imaging procedures is crucial to ensure patient comfort and the accuracy of diagnostic results. Here are some guidelines that can be followed:

1. Pre-examination preparation
   - Educate the patient: Before the imaging, explain the procedures to them to help them understand what to expect, including any potential discomfort from light exposure.
   - Schedule strategically: Consider scheduling imaging sessions during times when the patient's photophobia may be less severe if they have any daily fluctuation in sensitivity.
2. Environment adaptation
   - Control ambient lighting: Keep the examination room dimly lit to help acclimate the patient's eyes before exposure to bright lights.
   - Use adjustable lighting: Equip imaging devices with adjustable lighting settings so the intensity can be increased gradually.
3. Equipment modification
   - Use filters: Apply specially selected wavelength filters on imaging equipment to reduce the intensity and harshness of the light. Filters that absorb wavelengths below 550 nm, often with an orange tonality, are particularly effective. These filters improve vision quality by reducing light dispersion and chromatic aberration, thereby enhancing retinal image contrast and reducing light adaptation recovery time.
   - Modify the equipment: Consider using diffusers on light sources to spread the light more evenly and reduce its intensity.
4. During the procedure
   - Gradual exposure: Gradually increase light exposure to allow the patient's eyes to adapt slowly.
   - Allow breaks: Provide frequent breaks during the procedure to give the patient's eyes time to rest from the light exposure.
   - Use topical agents: In some cases, topical anesthetic or anti-inflammatory eye drops can be used to reduce discomfort caused by light.
5. Patient comfort
   - Provide eye protection: Offer sunglasses or other protective eyewear (tinted contact lenses) after the procedure to help manage sensitivity as the patient's eyes readjust to normal lighting.

- Support and reassurance: Maintain verbal contact during the procedure to reassure the patient and monitor their comfort level.

- Introduce Assistive Technology: As part of managing RP patients' visual discomfort after imaging, it is beneficial to discuss and recommend assistive technologies that can aid in their daily activities. Technologies such as screen readers (e.g., JAWS, NVDA, Apple's VoiceOver, Android Talkback), Braille displays, and speech recognition software can significantly enhance accessibility and independence. These tools help mitigate challenges posed by decreased vision and heightened light sensitivity, enabling patients to better manage transitions in lighting conditions.

6. Post-exertion care

- Offer post-care advice: Advice on using lubricating eye drops or artificial tears to alleviate discomfort following the imaging session.

Implementing these strategies can significantly improve the experience for RP patients undergoing imaging, leading to better cooperation and higher-quality diagnostic images.

8. Areas for future research and emerging technologies

8.1 Areas for future research on non-mydriatic OCT imaging in RP

There are several areas where future research could significantly enhance understanding and clinical application. Here are some key areas for future research:

1. Technological advancements

- High-resolution imaging: Research on improving the resolution of non-mydriatic OCT devices to detect early microstructural changes in the retina.

- Portable and accessible devices: Development of more portable and cost-effective OCT devices for broader accessibility, especially in remote or underserved areas.

- AI and machine learning: Integration of advanced AI algorithms for automated detection and analysis of retinal changes, improving diagnostic accuracy and consistency.

2. Longitudinal studies

- Disease progression: Long-term studies using non-mydriatic OCT are conducted to observe the progression of RP, providing insights into the natural history of the disease.

- Response to treatment: Monitoring the effectiveness of emerging treatments (e.g., gene therapy, stem cell therapy) over time using non-mydriatic OCT.

3. Clinical applications

- Early diagnosis: Exploring the potential of non-mydriatic OCT for early diagnosis of RP, even before symptoms become apparent.

- Screening programs: Evaluating the feasibility and effectiveness of using non-mydriatic OCT in large-scale screening programs for early detection of RP and other retinal diseases.

4. Comparative studies

- Comparative effectiveness: Comparing the diagnostic accuracy and effectiveness of non-mydriatic OCT with traditional mydriatic OCT and other imaging modalities.

- Inter-device comparisons: Assessing the performance and reliability of different non-mydriatic OCT devices from various manufacturers.

5. Patient-centric research

- Patient comfort and compliance: Studying patient comfort, compliance, and preferences related to non-mydriatic OCT compared to traditional methods.

- Quality of life impact: Investigating how early and accurate diagnosis using non-mydriatic OCT affects the quality of life and psychological well-being of RP patients.

6. Molecular and genetic correlations

- Genotype-phenotype correlations: Researching correlations between OCT imaging findings and specific genetic mutations associated with RP.

- Biomarker identification: Identifying potential biomarkers on OCT that correlate with disease severity or progression, aiding in personalized treatment approaches.

7. Educational and training program

- Training for clinicians: Developing comprehensive training programs for clinicians on the use and interpretation of non-mydriatic OCT in RP.

- Patient education: Creating educational materials to help patients understand the role and benefits of OCT imaging in managing their condition.

8. Interdisciplinary approaches

- Integration with other modalities: Combining OCT data with other imaging techniques (e.g., fundus photography, AF) to provide a more comprehensive assessment of retinal health.

- Collaborative research: Encouraging interdisciplinary collaboration between ophthalmologists, geneticists, and bioengineers to drive innovation and improve outcomes.

8.2 Emerging technologies and advancements in retinal imaging

With the advancement of technology, several new imaging techniques have emerged to improve the diagnosis, monitoring, and treatment of RP. These innovations provide more detailed and accurate insights into retinal structure and function, facilitating better patient management.

8.2.1 Polarization-sensitive optical coherence tomography (PS-OCT)

The RPE is essential for the survival and function of photoreceptors. It contains three major pigments: lipofuscin, melanin, and melanolipofuscin. AF imaging is commonly used to evaluate the RPE, with short-wavelength AF (SW-AF) detecting lipofuscin and near-infrared AF (NIR-AF) detecting melanin. In RP patients, hyperautofluorescent rings are often observed, correlating with disease progression and retinal function [101, 102]. Evaluating melanin in the RPE is crucial for understanding RP progression.

Polarization-sensitive optical coherence tomography (PS-OCT) extends traditional OCT by measuring the polarization properties of tissues, particularly useful for imaging melanin in the RPE [101, 102]. PS-OCT provides detailed visualization of melanin distribution, aiding in early detection, monitoring disease progression, and complementing other imaging techniques. This technique offers significant potential for improving the diagnosis and management of RP [101, 102].

Potential applications in RP:

- Using PS-OCT for melanin imaging in RP patients offers several advantages.

- Detailed visualization: PS-OCT provides high-resolution images of the RPE, allowing for the detailed study of melanin distribution and structural changes.

- Early detection: Changes in melanin distribution can be an early indicator of RPE dysfunction and photoreceptor degeneration. PS-OCT can help detect these changes before they become apparent with standard OCT.

- Monitoring disease progression: By regularly imaging the RPE and melanin content, clinicians can more accurately monitor the progression of RP. This can help evaluate the effectiveness of therapeutic interventions aimed at preserving or restoring visual function.

- Complementary to other imaging techniques: PS-OCT can be used alongside other imaging modalities, such as fundus photography and OCT-A, to provide a comprehensive assessment of retinal health. This multimodal approach can improve diagnostic accuracy and patient management.

Recent studies have demonstrated the utility of PS-OCT in imaging the RPE and melanin in RP patients [101, 102]: PS-OCT has been shown to effectively visualize the melanin distribution in the RPE, providing insights into the extent of RPE damage and the corresponding impact on photoreceptors. Research has indicated that PS-OCT can detect subtle changes in melanin content that correlate with disease severity and progression, offering a potential biomarker for monitoring RP [101, 102].

8.2.2 Hyperspectral imaging (HSI)

Changes in how the retina reflects and absorbs light are central to diagnosing various ocular diseases. Traditional retinal imaging typically captures monochromatic or trichromatic (red, green, and blue) light. Still, hyperspectral imaging (HSI) can go further, collecting information across many wavelengths to create a "hyperspectral cube"—a four-dimensional dataset representing spatial data, wavelength bands, and corresponding light absorption or reflection intensities [103].

HSI collects data from tens to hundreds of narrow wavelength bands, allowing for a detailed spectral analysis of retinal tissue [103]. This additional spectral information provides several advantages:

- Early detection of metabolic changes in retinal cells.
- Differentiation of various retinal pathologies based on their spectral signatures.
- Monitoring the biochemical effects of therapeutic interventions.

In ophthalmology, HSI technology enables the evaluation of chromophores like cytochrome C and the assessment of hemoglobin's metabolic status, particularly regarding retinal blood oxygenation. This makes it a valuable tool for diagnosing and tracking the progression of various eye diseases, such as age-related macular degeneration (AMD), glaucoma, diabetic retinopathy, and retinal dystrophies [103].

8.2.3 Advanced machine learning and artificial intelligence (AI)

Artificial intelligence (AI) and machine learning (ML) are increasingly being utilized to aid in the early and accurate diagnosis of RP through image processing. These technologies leverage advanced algorithms to analyze retinal images, offering significant potential to enhance diagnostic accuracy and efficiency [104]. Machine learning and AI algorithms are increasingly being integrated into retinal imaging to:

- Automatically detect and quantify retinal lesions and abnormalities.
- Predict disease progression based on imaging data.
- Assist clinicians in making informed decisions regarding patient management.

Recent studies have demonstrated the effectiveness of AI in diagnosing and monitoring RP:

- Chen et al. [105] developed a deep learning (DL) model to detect RP using color fundus photographs. Their model achieved an accuracy of 96.00%, comparable to that of ophthalmologists examining the same images. This high level of accuracy demonstrates the potential for AI to support clinical diagnosis.

- Nagasato et al. [106] evaluated five DL models—Visual Geometry Group-16 (VGG-16), Residual Network-50 (ResNet-50), Inception V3, DenseNet121, and EfficientNetB0—to estimate visual function in RP patients. Using ultra-wide-field fundus autofluorescence images from 695 patients, these models accurately estimated visual acuity and central sensitivity ($p < 0.001$), showcasing the ability of AI to predict functional outcomes in RP.

- Liu et al. [107] trained their DL algorithm to predict visual impairment in RP patients. Testing their model against two different patient datasets, they achieved an area under the curve (AUC) of 0.83 and 0.78, respectively. This predictive capability highlights the potential of AI to forecast disease progression and visual outcomes.

- Arsalan et al. [108] developed an RP segmentation network (RPS-Net) for accurately detecting pigment in color images, achieving an accuracy of 99.5%. This high accuracy in segmentation tasks underscores the capability of AI in detailed image analysis and diagnostic support.

These examples illustrate how AI and ML can significantly enhance the diagnostic process for RP, providing tools that offer high accuracy and predictive power. By integrating these advanced technologies, clinicians can improve early diagnosis, monitor disease progression more effectively, and personalize treatment strategies, ultimately leading to better patient outcomes [104].

Emerging technologies and advancements in retinal imaging are revolutionizing the diagnosis and management of RP. These innovative tools offer greater resolution, more detailed insights, and improved accuracy in detecting and monitoring retinal changes. As these technologies continue to evolve, they hold the promise of significantly enhancing patient care and outcomes in RP.

9. Example of managing glare and photophobia in an RP patient during OCT imaging

9.1 Preparation

Before the procedure, the medical staff explains what to expect during the OCT scan. They emphasize the importance of keeping the patient's eyes open during the scan despite the bright light used in the imaging process.

9.2 Adjustment of environment and equipment

Ambient lighting: The examination room lighting is dimmed as patients arrive, allowing their eyes to gradually adjust to the lower light levels before the actual imaging begins.

9.3 Filter use

Specialized CPF-550 filter lenses can be used (**Figure 6**). These filters are designed to block wavelengths specifically below 550 nm. They effectively reduce glare and

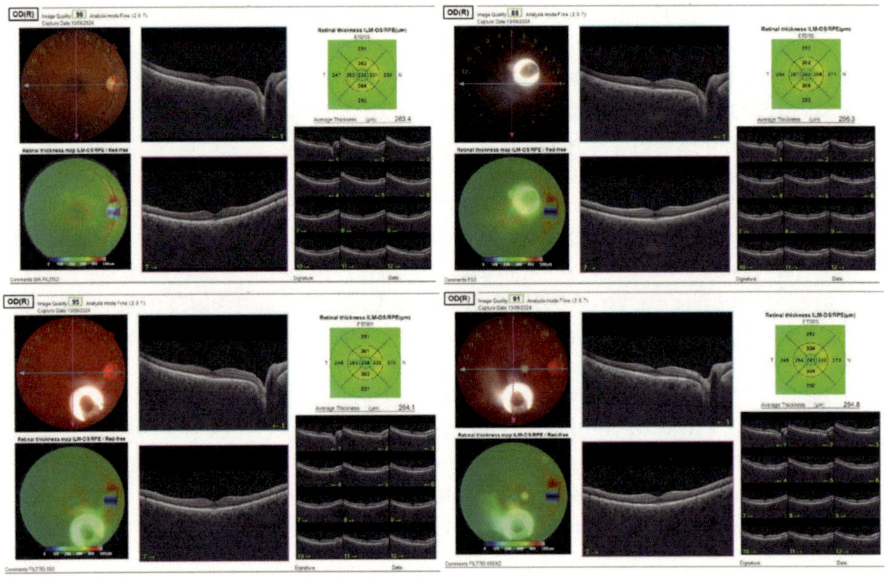

Figure 6.
Optical coherence tomography (OCT) scans without mydriasis in an asymptomatic carrier patient. A. OCT-B scan image without filter and mydriasis. B–D. Images with filters (F60, CPF 550, and CPF 550XD) and without mydriasis. CPF filters do not directly interfere with the light used in OCT imaging and improve the visibility of hyperreflective foci.

enhance visual comfort by filtering out the shorter wavelengths of visible light that are often most troubling for individuals with light sensitivity, such as those with RP. Regarding OCT machines, they use near-infrared light, typically ranging from 800 to 1300 nm for imaging. This range is well beyond the visible spectrum, which ends around 700 nm. Consequently, the light used in OCT does not intersect with the light wavelengths CPF filters are designed to block. Therefore, CPF filters do not directly interfere with the light used in OCT imaging, as this light is in a different part of the electromagnetic spectrum.

9.4 During the procedure

Gradual exposure: The intensity of the OCT machine's light slowly increases, allowing patients' eyes time to adapt to the brightness.

Comfort breaks: Short breaks are given during the procedure to let patients rest their eyes, reducing the risk of overwhelming photophobia.

Verbal guidance: Throughout the procedure, the technician maintains clear, calm communication, guiding the patient and providing reassurance, which helps reduce anxiety and ensure cooperation.

9.5 Post-procedure care

After the scan, patients are led to a dimly lit recovery area where they are given time to readjust to normal lighting. They are provided with post-care instructions, including lubricating eye drops to alleviate any discomfort caused by prolonged exposure to light.

9.6 Follow-up

The ophthalmologist reviews the OCT images with the patient, discussing the findings and ensuring that the adaptations made for the procedure effectively manage their photophobia and glare. Plans are made to use similar adjustments for future imaging sessions.

9.7 Outcome

Patients report a significantly more comfortable experience during the OCT procedure than past experiences. They appreciate the tailored approach to managing their photophobia and are pleased with the staff's care and consideration in accommodating their condition.

This example illustrates how a thoughtful, patient-centric approach to managing RP during imaging procedures can significantly enhance patient comfort and cooperation, ultimately leading to better diagnostic outcomes.

10. Conclusions

10.1 Summary of key findings on the impact of non-mydriasis on OCT imaging quality in RP

1. Image quality: Non-mydriasis does not significantly limit the acquisition and interpretation of OCT images in patients with mild to moderate stages of RP. Despite a slight reduction in signal strength, the image quality remains within acceptable limits for clinical use.

2. Artifact incidence: RP patients exhibited a higher incidence of artifacts than controls, with a 16% increase in the number of artifacts per image. The projection artifact was the most common in both groups, but RP patients, especially in advanced stages, experienced more artifacts overall.

3. Correlations with functional parameters: Quantitative structural parameters acquired by OCT and OCTA show correlations with functional parameters such as BCVA and disease severity. For example, choroidal thickness strongly correlated with BCVA, indicating its potential as a marker for disease progression.

10.2 Implications for clinical practice and patient care

1. Patient comfort and compliance: Non-mydriatic OCT imaging significantly enhances patient comfort by avoiding the discomfort associated with pupil dilation, such as increased light sensitivity and glare. This improvement in comfort can lead to better patient compliance, which is crucial for the regular monitoring required in RP management.

2. Clinical efficiency: Non-mydriatic imaging reduces the overall time required for examinations, eliminating the need for pupil dilation and the associated recovery period. This can increase patient throughput in clinical settings and enhance operational efficiency.

3. Enhanced diagnostic accuracy: While non-mydriatic OCT imaging provides good-quality images for mild to moderate stages of RP, clinicians should be aware of the increased incidence of artifacts in advanced stages. Identifying and accounting for these artifacts can prevent diagnostic errors and improve the reliability of monitoring disease progression.

10.3 Final thoughts on improving diagnostic accuracy and monitoring in RP patients

1. Artifact management: Developing and implementing advanced algorithms to detect and correct artifacts can significantly improve image quality and diagnostic accuracy. Techniques like Projection-Resolved OCTA (PR-OCTA) and faster image acquisition can help reduce the presence of artifacts.

2. Technological advancements: Continued innovation in OCT technology, such as higher resolution imaging and enhanced depth imaging, can provide better visualization of retinal structures, aiding in the early detection and monitoring of RP.

3. Patient-centric approaches: Tailoring imaging protocols to minimize discomfort and accommodate the specific needs of RP patients can improve the overall patient experience. This includes using non-mydriatic techniques and managing glare and photophobia during imaging sessions.

4. Research and development: Future studies should explore the impact of non-mydriasis across different stages of RP and other retinal diseases. Longitudinal studies and the integration of genetic data can provide deeper insights into disease progression and treatment efficacy.

5. Clinical guidelines: Establishing clear guidelines for using non-mydriatic OCT imaging in RP, including recommendations for managing artifacts and optimizing image quality, can standardize practices and improve patient outcomes across clinical settings.

By addressing these areas, clinicians can enhance the accuracy and reliability of OCT imaging, leading to better diagnosis, monitoring, and management of RP.

Acknowledgements

We thank the patients with retinitis pigmentosa from the Retina Castilla y León (ReCYL) and Federation of Associations of Hereditary Retinal Dystrophies in Spain, Valladolid, Spain.

Funding

PID2020-114585RA-I00, RD21/0002/0017 funding by MICIU/AEI/10.13039/501100011033 and GRS 2744/A1/2023.

Grant PDC2023-145857-100 funded by MICIU/AEI/10.13039/501100011033 and, as appropriate, by 'ERDF A way of making Europe,' 'ERDF/EU,' 'the European Union,' or 'the European Union NextGenerationEU/PRTR.'

Conflict of interest

The authors declare no conflict of interest.

Appendices and nomenclature

OCT	optical coherence tomography
RP	retinitis pigmentosa
OCTA	OCT angiography
RPE	retinal pigment epithelium
RGCs	retinal ganglion cells
ERG	electroretinogram
VF	visual field
ELM	external limiting membrane
EZ	ellipsoid zone
CME	cystoid macular oedema
HF	hyperreflective foci
ERM	epiretinal membrane
FTMH	full-thickness macular hole
LMH	lamellar macular hole
BCVA	best-corrected visual acuity
IOP	intraocular pressure
FAF	fundus autofluorescence
ffERG	full-field electroretinography
MP	microperimetry
FA	fluorescein angiography
AOSLO	adaptive optics scanning laser ophthalmoscopy
ONL	outer nuclear layer
IS/OS	photoreceptor inner/outer segment junction
SCP	superficial capillary plexus
DCP	deep capillary plexus
CCP	choriocapillaris plexus
SD	spectral domain OCT
SS	swept-source OCT
CRT	central retinal thickness
GCIPL	ganglion cell inner plexiform layer thickness
CCT	central choroidal thickness
RNFLT	retinal nerve-fiber layer thickness
MAS	motion artifact score
PR-OCTA	projection-resolved OCTA
CNV	choroidal neovascularization
SSI	Signal Strength Index
PS-OCT	polarization-sensitive optical coherence tomography extends
SW-AF	short-wavelength AF

NIR-AF	near-infrared AF
HSI	hyperspectral imaging
ARMD	age-related macular degeneration
AI	artificial intelligence
ML	machine learning
DL	deep learning
AUC	area under the curve

Author details

Salvador Pastor-Idoate[1,2,3,4*], Santiago Mejía-Freire[2], Milagros Mateos-Olivares[1,5], Francisco Javier Valentín-Bravo[1,6,7], Eva Maria Sobas Abad[1,4,8], Ricardo Usategui Martín[1,4,9] and José Carlos Pastor Jimeno[1,3,4]

1 Institute of Applied Ophthalmobiology (IOBA), University of Valladolid, Valladolid, Spain

2 Department of Ophthalmology, Clinical University Hospital of Valladolid, Spain

3 European Reference Network dedicated to Rare Eye Diseases, ERN-EYE, Spain

4 Networks of Cooperative Research Oriented to Health Results, RICORS-REI, National Institute of Health Carlos III, Madrid, Spain

5 Department of Ophthalmology, Moorfields Eye Hospital NHS Foundation Trust, London, United Kingdom

6 Department of Ophthalmology, Germans Trias i Pujol Hospital, Badalona, Spain

7 Institut Catalá de la Retina (ICR), Barcelona, Spain

8 Nursing School, University of Valladolid, Valladolid, Spain

9 Department of Cell Biology, Genetics, Histology and Pharmacology, Faculty of Medicine, University of Valladolid, Valladolid, Spain

*Address all correspondence to: spastor@saludcastillayleon.es

References

[1] O'Neal T, Luther E. Retinitis Pigmentosa [Internet]. 2021. Available from: https://www.ncbi.nlm.nih.gov/books/NBK519518/

[2] Menghini M, Cehajic-Kapetanovic J, MacLaren RE. Monitoring progression of retinitis pigmentosa: Current recommendations and recent advances. Expert Opinion on Orphan Drugs. 2020;**8**(2-3):67-78

[3] Verbakel SK, van Huet RAC, Boon CJF, den Hollander AI, Collin RWJ, Klaver CCW, et al. Non-syndromic retinitis pigmentosa. Progress in Retinal and Eye Research. 2018;**66**(November 2017):157-186

[4] Chawla H, Vohra V. Retinal dystrophies. [Updated 2023 Mar 16]. In: StatPearls [Internet]. Treasure Island (FL): StatPearls Publishing. p. 2024. Available from: https://www.ncbi.nlm.nih.gov/books/NBK564379/

[5] Vaidya P, Vaidya A. Retinitis Pigmentosa: Disease encumbrance in the Eurozone. International Journal of Ophthalmology and Clinical Research. 2015;**2**(4):2-3

[6] Liu G, Du Q, Keyal K, Wang F. Morphologic characteristics and clinical significance of the macular-sparing area in patients with retinitis pigmentosa as revealed by multicolor imaging. Experimental and Therapeutic Medicine. 2017;**14**(6):5387-5394

[7] Spaide RF, Fujimoto JG, Waheed NK, Sadda SR, Staurenghi G. Optical coherence tomography angiography. Progress in Retinal and Eye Research. 2018;**63**:1-55

[8] Alnawaiseh M, Schubert F, Heiduschka P, Eter N. Optical coherence tomography angiography in patients with retinitis pigmentosa. Retina. 2019;**39**(1):210-217

[9] Ghasemi Falavarjani K, Al-Sheikh M, Akil H, Sadda SR. Image artefacts in swept-source optical coherence tomography angiography. British Journal of Ophthalmology. 2017;**101**(5):564-568

[10] Chen FK, Viljoen RD, Bukowska DM. Classification of image artefacts in optical coherence tomography angiography of the choroid in macular diseases. Clinical and Experimental Ophthalmology. 2016;**44**(5):388-399

[11] Cheng J, Yu J, Jiang C, Sun X. Phenylephrine affects peripapillary retinal vasculature-An optic coherence tomography angiography study. Frontiers in Physiology. 2017;**8**(Dec):1-7

[12] Brücher VC, Storp JJ, Kerschke L, Nelis P, Eter N, Alnawaiseh M. Influence of mydriasis on optical coherence tomography angiography imaging in patients with age-related macular degeneration. PLoS One. 2019;**14**(10):1-11

[13] Oh JK, Nuzbrokh Y, Lima de Carvalho JR, Ryu J, Tsang SH. Optical coherence tomography in the evaluation of retinitis pigmentosa. Ophthalmic Genetics [Internet]. 2020;**41**(5):413-419. Available from:. DOI: 10.1080/13816810.2020.1780619

[14] Elliott DB. Clinical Procedures in Primary Eye Care. 3rd ed. Elsevier; 2007. 29-81 p. DOI: 10.1016/B978-0-7506-8896-3.X5001-9. ISBN 978-0-7506-8896-3

[15] Pastor S, Sobas-Abad EM, Bravo FJV, Arlanzon P, Coco-Martin R, Pastor J-C.

Influence of non-mydriasis on optical coherence tomography imaging quality in patients with Retinitis Pigmentosa. Investigative Ophthalmology & Visual Science. 2020;**61**(7):5288

[16] Mejia-Freire S, Mateos-Olivares M, Bravo FJV, Sobas Abad EM, Martin RU, Pastor J-C, et al. Optical coherence tomography imaging quality in patients with retinitis pigmentosa without mydriatic eye drops. Investigative Ophthalmology & Visual Science. 2022;**63**(7):4482-F0269

[17] Sandberg MA, Weigel-DiFranco C, Rosner B, Berson EL. The relationship between visual field size and electroretinogram amplitude in retinitis pigmentosa. Investigative Ophthalmology & Visual Science. 1996;**37**(8):1693-1698

[18] Grover S, Fishman GA, Gilbert LD, Anderson RJ. Reproducibility of visual acuity measurements in patients with retinitis pigmentosa. Retina. 1997;**17**:33-37

[19] Lam BL, Fishman GA, Anderson RJ, Smith DA, Alexander KR. Effect of mydriasis on visual field area in retinitis pigmentosa. Ophthalmology. 1992;**99**:1724-1727

[20] Hirasawa K, Shoji N, Kobashi C, Yamanashi A. Effects of mydriasis and miosis on kinetic perimetry findings in normal participants. Graefe's Archive for Clinical and Experimental Ophthalmology. 2015;**253**(8):1341-1346. DOI: 10.1007/s00417-015-3048-5. Epub 2015 May 19

[21] Liu G, Liu X, Li H, Du Q, Wang F. Optical coherence tomographic analysis of retina in retinitis pigmentosa patients. Ophthalmic Research. 2016;**200072**:111-122

[22] Nguyen XT, Moekotte L, Plomp AS, Bergen AA, van Genderen MM, Boon CJF. Retinitis pigmentosa: Current clinical management and emerging therapies. International Journal of Molecular Sciences. 2023;**24**(8):7481. DOI: 10.3390/ijms24087481

[23] Hartong DT, Berson EL, Dryja TP. Retinitis pigmentosa. The Lancet. 2006;**368**(9549):1795-1809. DOI: 10.1016/S0140-6736(06)69740-7

[24] Cross N, van Steen C, Zegaoui Y, Satherley A, Angelillo L. Retinitis pigmentosa: Burden of disease and current unmet needs. Clinical Ophthalmology. 2022;**16**:1993-2010. DOI: 10.2147/OPTH.S365486

[25] Daiger SP, Sullivan LS, Bowne SJ. Genes and mutations causing retinitis pigmentosa. Clinical Genetics. 2013;**84**(2):132-141. DOI: 10.1111/cge.12203

[26] Pagon RA. Retinitis pigmentosa. Survey of Ophthalmology. 1988;**33**(3):137-177. DOI: 10.1016/0039-6257(88)90079-5

[27] Kajiwara K, Berson EL, Dryja TP. Digenic retinitis pigmentosa due to mutations at the unlinked peripherin/RDS and ROM1 loci. Science. 1994;**264**(5165):1604-1608. DOI: 10.1126/science.8202715

[28] Stone EM. Leber congenital amaurosis—A model for efficient genetic testing of heterogeneous disorders: LXIV Edward Jackson memorial lecture. American Journal of Ophthalmology. 2007;**144**(6):791-811. DOI: 10.1016/j.ajo.2007.08.022

[29] Joensuu T, Hämäläinen R, Yuan B, Johnson C, Tegelberg S, Gasparini P, et al. Mutations in a novel gene with transmembrane domains underlie Usher syndrome type 3. American Journal of Human Genetics. 2001;**69**(4):673-684. DOI: 10.1086/323632

[30] Fahim AT, Daiger SP, Weleber RG. Nonsyndromic retinitis pigmentosa overview. 2000 [Updated 2023 Apr 6]. In: Adam MP, Feldman J, Mirzaa GM, et al., editors. GeneReviews® [Internet]. Seattle (WA): University of Washington, Seattle; 1993-2024. Available from: https://www.ncbi.nlm.nih.gov/books/NBK1417/

[31] Berni A, Arrigo A, Bianco L, Antropoli A, Saladino A, Mansour AM, et al. New insights in the multimodal imaging of retinitis pigmentosa. European Journal of Ophthalmology. 2024;**34**(2):357-366. DOI: 10.1177/11206721231172863. Epub 2023 Apr 27

[32] Öner A, Kahraman NS. Evaluation of full-field stimulus threshold test results in retinitis pigmentosa: Relationship with full-field electroretinography, multifocal electroretinography, optical coherence tomography, and visual field. Turkish Journal of Ophthalmology. 2024;**54**(1):23-31. DOI: 10.4274/tjo.galenos.2023.58485

[33] Iftikhar M, Kherani S, Kaur R, Lemus M, Nefalar A, Usmani B, et al. Progression of retinitis pigmentosa as measured on microperimetry: The PREP-1 study. Ophthalmology Retina. 2018;**2**(5):502-507. DOI: 10.1016/j.oret.2017.09.008. Epub 2017 Nov 9

[34] Jacobson SG, Aleman TS, Sumaroka A, Cideciyan AV, Schwartz SB, Roman AJ, et al. Retinal alterations in RPE65-associated Leber congenital amaurosis: Persistence of photoreceptors as assessed by optical coherence tomography and implications for gene therapy. Human Gene Therapy. 2003;**14**(4):347-359. DOI: 10.1089/104303403321031043

[35] Lenassi E, Vincent A, Li Z, Saihan Z, Moore AT, Bhattacharya SS, et al. Clinical and molecular genetic findings in autosomal recessive retinitis pigmentosa in the UK. Investigative Ophthalmology & Visual Science. 2015;**56**(5):3072-3081. DOI: 10.1167/iovs.14-15942

[36] Toto L, Mastropasqua R, Di Antonio L, D'Aloisio R, Carpineto P, Borrelli E. Multimodal imaging in a case of retinitis pigmentosa: Vascular and structural evaluation by means of optical coherence tomography angiography and optical coherence tomography. Retina. 2016;**36**(11):S174-S176. DOI: 10.1097/IAE.0000000000001293

[37] Battu R, Khanna H, Rani A. Molecular understanding and gene therapy for retinitis pigmentosa: Challenges and future directions. Acta Ophthalmologica. 2015;**93**(3):203-213. DOI: 10.1111/aos.12588

[38] Nesper PL, Scarinci F, Fawzi AA. Adaptive optics microvascular imaging of the parafoveal capillary network in retinitis pigmentosa. Investigative Ophthalmology & Visual Science. 2017;**58**(10):4612-4619. DOI: 10.1167/iovs.17-21831

[39] Talbot JF, Cox TA. Vascular changes in retinitis pigmentosa: Implications for potential therapeutic strategies. Eye. 2019;**33**(2):244-248. DOI: 10.1038/s41433-018-0178-6

[40] Diaconita V, Kassotis A, Ngo WK. Optical coherence tomography angiography (OCTA) findings in retinitis pigmentosa. Methods in Molecular Biology. 2023;**2560**:101-109. DOI: 10.1007/978-1-0716-2651-1_9

[41] Ling L, Gao F, Zhang Q, He T, Zhao Y, Xing Y, et al. Optical coherence tomography angiography assessed retinal and choroidal microvasculature features in patients with retinitis pigmentosa: A meta-analysis. BioMed Research

International. 2019;**2019**:6723917. DOI: 10.1155/2019/6723917

[42] Kamde SP, Anjankar A. Retinitis pigmentosa: Pathogenesis, diagnostic findings, and treatment. Cureus. 2023;**15**(10):e48006. DOI: 10.7759/cureus.48006

[43] Yilmaz AC, Durukan AH. Evaluation of retina and choroid perfusion with optical coherence tomography angiography in patients with retinitis pigmentosa. Photodiagnosis and Photodynamic Therapy. 2023;**44**:103755. DOI: 10.1016/j.pdpdt.2023.103755. Epub 2023 Aug 22

[44] Enders C, Lang GE, Dreyhaupt J, Loidl M, Lang GK, Werner JU. Quantity and quality of image artifacts in optical coherence tomography angiography. PLoS One. 2019;**14**(1):1-9

[45] Lauermann JL, Woetzel AK, Treder M, Alnawaiseh M, Clemens CR, Eter N, et al. Prevalences of segmentation errors and motion artifacts in OCT-angiography differ among retinal diseases. Graefe's Archive for Clinical and Experimental Ophthalmology. 2018;**256**(10):1807-1816

[46] Lauermann JL, Treder M, Heiduschka P, Clemens CR, Eter N, Alten F. Impact of eye-tracking technology on OCT-angiography imaging quality in age-related macular degeneration. Graefe's Archive for Clinical and Experimental Ophthalmology. 2017;**255**(8):1535-1542

[47] Zhang M, Hwang TS, Campbell JP, Bailey ST, Wilson DJ, Huang D, et al. Projection-resolved optical coherence tomographic angiography. Biomedical Optics Express. 2016;**7**(3):816

[48] Lee JJ, Lee JE, Sadda SR, Park SW, Byon I. Impact of signal strength on quantitative retinal and choriocapillaris flow measurement from optical coherence tomography angiography. Scientific Reports. 2022;**12**(1):4692

[49] Park JH, Lee YC, Lee SY. The comparison of mydriatic effect between two drugs of different mechanism. Korean Journal of Ophthalmology. 2009;**23**:40-42. DOI: 10.3341/kjo.2009.23.1.40

[50] Hong D, Tripathy K. Tropicamide. 2023 Aug 25. In: StatPearls [Internet]. Treasure Island (FL): StatPearls Publishing; Jan 2024

[51] Yang MC, Lin KY. Drug-induced acute angle-closure glaucoma: A review. Journal of Current Glaucoma Practice. 2019;**13**:104-109. DOI: 10.5005/jp-journals-10078-1261

[52] Bonomi L, Marchini G, Marraffa M, Bernardi P, De Franco I, Perfetti S, Varotto A. Epidemiology of angle-closure glaucoma: prevalence, clinical types, and association with peripheral anterior chamber depth in the Egna-Neumarket Glaucoma Study. Ophthalmology. May 2000;**107**(5):998-1003. DOI: 10.1016/s0161-6420(00)00022-1. PMID: 10811096

[53] Contreras-Salinas H, Orozco-Ceja V, Romero-López MS, Barajas-Virgen MY, Baiza-Durán LM, Rodríguez-Herrera LY. Ocular Cyclopentolate: A Mini Review Concerning Its Benefits and Risks. Clin Ophthalmol. 15 Nov 2022;**16**:3753-3762. DOI: 10.2147/OPTH.S388982

[54] Pearce E, Sivaprasad S. A Review of Advancements and Evidence Gaps in Diabetic Retinopathy Screening Models. Clinical Ophthalmology. 14 Oct 2020;**14**:3285-3296. DOI: 10.2147/OPTH.S267521

[55] Aptel F, Denis P, Rouberol F, Thivolet C. Screening of diabetic

retinopathy: Effect of field number and mydriasis on sensitivity and specificity of digital fundus photography. Diabetes & Metabolism. 2008;**34**:290-293. DOI: 10.1016/j.diabet.2007.12.007

[56] Photocoagulation for diabetic macular edema: Early treatment diabetic retinopathy study report number 1 early treatment diabetic retinopathy study research group. Archives of Ophthalmology. 1985;**103**:1796-1806. DOI: 10.1001/ARCHOPHT.1985.01050120030015

[57] Tripathy K, Chawla R, Vohra R. Evaluation of the fundus in poorly dilating diabetic pupils using ultrawide field imaging. Clinical and Experimental Optometry. Nov 2017;**100**(6):735-736. DOI: 10.1111/cxo.12484. Epub 2016 Oct 5

[58] Kernt M, Hadi I, Pinter F, Seidensticker F, Hirneiss C, Haritoglou C, et al. Assessment of diabetic retinopathy using nonmydriatic ultra-widefield scanning laser ophthalmoscopy (Optomap) compared with ETDRS 7-field stereo photography. Diabetes Care. 2012;**35**:2459-2463. DOI: 10.2337/dc12-0346

[59] Hansen AB, Sander B, Larsen M, Kleener J, Borch-Johnsen K, Klein R, et al. Screening for diabetic retinopathy using a digital non-mydriatic camera compared with standard 35-mm stereo colour transparencies. Acta Ophthalmologica Scandinavica. 2004;**82**:656-665. DOI: 10.1111/j.1600-0420.2004.00347.x

[60] Murgatroyd H, MacEwen C, Leese GP. Patients' attitudes towards mydriasis for diabetic eye disease screening. Scottish Medical Journal. Nov 2006;**51**(4):35-37. DOI: 10.1258/RSMSMJ.51.4.35

[61] Talib M, Boon CJF. Retinal Dystrophies and the Road to Treatment: Clinical Requirements and Considerations. Asia-Pacific Journal of Ophthalmology (Phila). May-Jun 2020;**9**(3):159-179. DOI: 10.1097/APO.0000000000000290

[62] Dysli C, Schürch K, Pascal E, Wolf S, Zinkernagel MS. Fundus autofluorescence lifetime patterns in retinitis pigmentosa. Investigative Ophthalmology & Visual Science. 2018;**59**:1769-1778. DOI: 10.1167/IOVS.17-23336

[63] Dowd-Schoeman TJ, Rosenbloom J, Ameri H. Patterns of autofluorescence in common genotypes of retinitis pigmentosa. Ophthalmic Surgery, Lasers & Imaging Retina. 2021;**52**:426-431. DOI: 10.3928/23258160-20210727-03

[64] Shintani K, Shechtman DL, Gurwood AS. Review and update: Current treatment trends for patients with retinitis pigmentosa. Optometry. 2009;**80**:384-401. DOI: 10.1016/j.optm.2008.01.026

[65] Herse P. Retinitis pigmentosa: visual function and multidisciplinary management. Clinical and Experimental Optometry. Sep 2005;**88**(5):335-350. DOI: 10.1111/j.1444-0938.2005.tb06717.x

[66] Prem Senthil M, Khadka J, Pesudovs K. Seeing through their eyes: Lived experiences of people with retinitis pigmentosa. Eye (Basingstoke). 2017;**31**:741-748. DOI: 10.1038/eye.2016.315

[67] Gawande AA, Donovan WJ, Ginsburg AP, Marmor MF. Photoaversion in retinitis pigmentosa. British Journal of Ophthalmology. Feb 1989;**73**(2):115-120. DOI: 10.1136/bjo.73.2.115

[68] Heckenlively J. The frequency of posterior subcapsular

cataract in the hereditary retinal degenerations. American Journal of Ophthalmology. 1982;**93**:733-738. DOI: 10.1016/0002-9394(82)90469-X

[69] Rundquist J. Low vision rehabilitation of retinitis pigmentosa. Journal of Visual Impairment & Blindness. 2004;**98**(11):718-724. DOI: 10.1177/0145482X0409801107

[70] Ripandelli G, Coppé AM, Capaldo A, Stirpe M. Optical Coherence Tomography. Seminars in Ophthalmology. W.B. Saunders; 1998. pp. 199-202. DOI: 10.3109/08820539809056053

[71] Leitgeb R, Placzek F, Rank E, Krainz L, Haindl R, Li Q, et al. Enhanced medical diagnosis for doctors: A perspective of optical coherence tomography. Journal of Biomedical Optics. Oct 2021;**26**(10):100601. DOI: 10.1117/1.JBO.26.10.100601

[72] Medina FJL, Callén CI, Rebolleda G, Muñoz-Negrete FJ, Callén MJI, Del Valle FG. Use of nonmydriatic spectral-domain optical coherence tomography for diagnosing diabetic macular edema. American Journal of Ophthalmology. 2012;**153**:536-543.e1. DOI: 10.1016/j.ajo.2011.08.008

[73] Zhang F, Li Y, Du Z, Sun H, Xie L, Liang Y, et al. Effect of mydriasis on macular and peripapillary metrics in swept-source optical coherence tomography angiography. Front Endocrinol (Lausanne). 28 Feb 2024;**15**:1292255. DOI: 10.3389/fendo.2024.1292255

[74] Wei X, Wei X, Hormel TT, Guo Y, Jia Y, Jia Y. 75-degree non-mydriatic single-volume optical coherence tomographic angiography. Biomedical Optics Express;**10**(12):6286-6295. DOI: 10.1364/BOE.10.006286

[75] Imai A, Toriyama Y, Iesato Y, Hirano T, Murata T. En face swept-source optical coherence tomography detecting thinning of inner retinal layers as an indicator of capillary nonperfusion. European Journal of Ophthalmology. 2014;**25**:153-158. DOI: 10.5301/ejo.5000514

[76] Salti HI, Antonios RS, Haddad SS, Hamam RN, Bashshur ZF, Ghazi NG. Combined nonmydriatic spectral-domain optical coherence tomography and nonmydriatic fundus photography for the detection of age-related macular degeneration changes. Ophthalmic Surgery, Lasers & Imaging Retina. 2015;**46**:531-537. DOI: 10.3928/23258160-20150521-04

[77] Mateos-Olivares M, Sobas EM, Puertas-Neyra K, Peralta-Ramírez MI, González-Pérez R, Martín-Vallejo J, et al. Hair cortisol level as a molecular biomarker in retinitis pigmentosa patients. Experimental Eye Research. 2022;**219**:109019. DOI: 10.1016/j.exer.2022.109019. Epub 2022 Mar 6

[78] Mateos-Olivares M, Pastor-Idoate S, Martín-Vallejo J, García-Vazquez C, Pastor JC, Usategui-Martín R, et al. Stress and sleep deprivation-related biomarkers in saliva in patients with retinitis pigmentosa. PLoS One. 2024;**19**(6):e0304261. DOI: 10.1371/journal.pone.0304261

[79] Smith HB, Chandra A, Zambarakji H. Grading severity in retinitis pigmentosa using clinical assessment, visual acuity, perimetry and optical coherence tomography. International Ophthalmology. 2013;**33**:237-244. DOI: 10.1007/s10792-012-9678-2.Spielberger

[80] Alnawaiseh M, Lahme L, Treder M, Rosentreter A, Eter N. Short-term effects of exercise on optic nerve and macular

perfusion measured by optical coherence tomography angiography. Retina. 2017;**37**(9):1642-1646. DOI: 10.1097/IAE.0000000000001419

[81] Hariri AH, Yang Zhang H, Ho A, Francis P, Weleber RG, Birch DG, et al. Quantification of ellipsoid zone changes in retinitis pigmentosa using en face spectral domain-optical coherence tomography group information: The principal investigators for the trial of oral valproic acid for retinitis pigmentosa group include Paul HHS. Retina Foundation of the Southwest. 2016;**134**(6):628-635

[82] Jauregui R, Park KS, Duong JK, Mahajan VB, Tsang SH. Quantitative progression of retinitis pigmentosa by optical coherence tomography angiography. Scientific Reports. 2018;**8**(1):1-7

[83] Garcia-Martin E, Pinilla I, Sancho E, Almarcegui C, Dolz I, Rodriguez-Mena D, et al. Optical coherence tomography in retinitis pigmentosa: Reproducibility and capacity to detect macular and retinal nerve fiber layer thickness alterations. Retina. 2012;**32**(8):1581-1591

[84] Toto L, Borrelli E, Mastropasqua R, Senatore A, Di Antonio L, Di Nicola M, et al. Macular features in retinitis pigmentosa: Correlations among ganglion cell complex thickness, capillary density, and macular function. Investigative Ophthalmology and Visual Science. 2016;**57**(14):6360-6366

[85] Inooka D, Ueno S, Kominami T, Sayo A, Okado S, Ito Y, et al. Quantification of macular microvascular changes in patients with retinitis pigmentosa using optical coherence tomography angiography. Investigative Ophthalmology and Visual Science. 2018;**59**(1):433-438

[86] Rezaei KA, Zhang Q, Chen CL, Chao J, Wang RK. Retinal and choroidal vascular features in patients with retinitis pigmentosa imaged by OCT based microangiography. Graefe's Archive for Clinical and Experimental Ophthalmology. 2017;**255**(7):1287-1295

[87] Liu G, Li H, Liu X, Xu D, Wang F. Structural analysis of retinal photoreceptor ellipsoid zone and postreceptor retinal layer associated with visual acuity in patients with retinitis pigmentosa by ganglion cell analysis combined with OCT imaging. Medicine (United States). 2016;**95**(52):1-9

[88] Hara A, Nakazawa M, Saito M, Suzuki Y. The qualitative assessment of optical coherence tomography and the central retinal sensitivity in patients with retinitis pigmentosa. PLoS One. 2020;**15**(5):1-15

[89] Hood DC, Lin CE, Lazow MA, Locke KG, Zhang X, Birch DG. Thickness of receptor and post-receptor retinal layers in patients with retinitis pigmentosa measured with frequency-domain optical coherence tomography. Investigative Ophthalmology and Visual Science. 2009;**50**(5):2328-2336

[90] Arrigo A, Bordato A, Romano F, Aragona E, Grazioli A, Bandello F, et al. Choroidal patterns in retinitis pigmentosa: Correlation with visual acuity and disease progression. Translational Vision Science and Technology. 2020;**9**(4):1-14

[91] Sabbaghi H, Ahmadieh H, Jalili J, Behnaz N. Choroidal thickness in different types of inherited retinal dystrophies. Journal of Ophthalmic and Vision Research. 2020;**15**(3):351-361

[92] Sodi A, Lenzetti C, Murro V, Caprorossi O, Mucciolo DP, Bacherini D,

et al. EDI-OCT evaluation of choroidal thickness in retinitis pigmentosa. European Journal of Ophthalmology. 2018;**28**(1):52-57

[93] Jones BW, Pfeiffer RL, Ferrell WD, Watt CB, Marmor M, Marc RE. Retinal remodeling in human retinitis pigmentosa. Experimental eye research. 2016;**150**:149-165

[94] Oishi A, Otani A, Sasahara M, Kurimoto M, Nakamura H, Kojima H, et al. Retinal nerve fiber layer thickness in patients with retinitis pigmentosa. Eye. 2009;**23**(3):561-566

[95] Zeiss. CIRRUS HD-OCT User Manual – Models 500, 5000. 2015

[96] Wang XG, Peng Q, Wu Q. Comparison of central macular thickness between two spectral-domain optical coherence tomography in elderly non-mydriatic eyes. International Journal of Ophthalmology. 2012;**5**(3):354-359

[97] Hagag AM, Wang J, Lu K, Harman G, Weleber RG, Huang D, et al. Projection-resolved optical coherence tomographic angiography of retinal plexuses in retinitis pigmentosa. American Journal of Ophthalmology. 2019;**204**:70-79

[98] Zhang Q, Zhang A, Lee CS, Lee AY, Rezaei KA, Roisman L, et al. Projection artifact removal improves visualization and quantitation of macular neovascularization imaged by optical coherence tomography angiography. Ophthalmology Retina. 2017;**1**(2):124-136. DOI: 10.1016/j.oret.2016.08.005

[99] Hormel TT, Huang D, Jia Y. Artifacts and artifact removal in optical coherence tomographic angiography. Quantitative Imaging in Medicine and Surgery. 2021;**11**(3):1120-1133. DOI: 10.21037/qims-20-730

[100] Wang J, Hormel TT, Bailey ST, Hwang TS, Huang D, Jia Y. Signal attenuation-compensated projection-resolved OCT angiography. Biomedical Optics Express. 2023;**14**(5):2040-2054. DOI: 10.1364/BOE.483835

[101] Pircher M, Hitzenberger CK, Schmidt-Erfurth U. Polarization sensitive optical coherence tomography in the human eye. Progress in Retinal and Eye Research. 2011;**30**(6):431-451. DOI: 10.1016/j.preteyeres.2011.06.003. Epub 2011 Jun 26

[102] Baumann B. Polarization sensitive optical coherence tomography: A review of technology and applications. Applied Sciences. 2017;7:474. DOI: 10.3390/app7050474

[103] Lemmens S, Van Eijgen J, Van Keer K, Jacob J, Moylett S, De Groef L, et al. Hyperspectral imaging and the retina: Worth the wave? Translational Vision Science & Technology. 2020;**9**(9):9. DOI: 10.1167/tvst.9.9.9

[104] Parmar UPS, Surico PL, Singh RB, Romano F, Salati C, Spadea L, et al. Artificial intelligence (AI) for early diagnosis of retinal diseases. Medicina. 2024;**60**:527. DOI: 10.3390/medicina60040527

[105] Chen T-C, Lim WS, Wang VY, Ko M-L, Chiu S-I, Huang Y-S, et al. Artificial intelligence–assisted early detection of retinitis pigmentosa—The most common inherited retinal degeneration. Journal of Digital Imaging. 2021;**34**:948-958

[106] Nagasato D, Sogawa T, Tanabe M, Tabuchi H, Numa S, Oishi A, et al. Estimation of visual function using deep learning from ultra-widefield fundus images of eyes with retinitis Pigmentosa. JAMA Ophthalmology. 2023;**141**:305

[107] Liu TYA, Ling C, Hahn L, Jones CK, Boon CJ, Singh MS. Prediction of visual impairment in retinitis pigmentosa using deep learning and multimodal fundus images. The British Journal of Ophthalmology. 2023;**107**:1484-1489

[108] Arsalan M, Baek NR, Owais M, Mahmood T, Park KR. Deep learning-based detection of pigment signs for analysis and diagnosis of retinitis pigmentosa. Sensors. 2020;**20**:3454

Chapter 10

OCT-A Choroidal and Retinal Findings in Patients with Retinal Vein Obstruction

Miguel Angel Quiroz-Reyes, Erick Quiroz-Gonzalez and Miguel A. Quiroz-Gonzalez

Abstract

This chapter provides an overview of various retinal abnormalities, pathophysiologies, structural and vascular findings, and therapeutic modalities used to address retinal vein obstruction (RVO) and its associated consequences, which includes vision loss due to macular edema, retinal bleeding, and neovascular glaucoma (NVG). RVO encompasses central retinal vein occlusion (CRVO) and branch retinal vein occlusion (BRVO). Recent research has highlighted the significance of optical coherence tomographic angiography (OCT-A) imaging in managing retinal complications stemming from venous occlusion. Among the primary causes of vision impairment due to RVO complications are perfused and nonperfused macular edema, with the latter being the most prevalent. OCT-A imaging has been instrumental in identifying alterations in vascular blood perfusion and vessel density. Treatment options for macular edema resulting from RVO include laser photocoagulation therapy, which has shown inconsistent results. Additionally, macular edema can be addressed with an implant that releases corticosteroids directly into the eye. Current treatments for RVO involve antivascular endothelial growth factor (anti-VEGF) drugs, such as ranibizumab and aflibercept, as well as the recently approved dual-acting faricimab. Furthermore, the port delivery system with ranibizumab (PDS) can enhance outcomes and compliance in RVO management. RVO treatment plays a critical role in preventing sight-threatening complications.

Keywords: choroidal vascularity index, ischemic index, macular ischemia, nonperfused macular edema, optical coherence tomography angiography, port delivery system, retinal neovascularization, retinal perfusion markers, retinal vein occlusion

1. Introduction

The human retina is one of the most metabolically demanding tissues and requires a rich nutritional arterial supply. When the venous drainage complex is obstructed, capillary hypertension is generated in different venous plexuses, resulting in ischemic tissue suffering, edema, and neovascularization, leading to loss of visual acuity. Research of blood flow in the eyes of primates has provided the groundwork for the knowledge of blood supply to the retina. The visual acuity of primate eyes is notably similar to human eyes [1]. Various investigations have shown that the retina receives blood from four types of capillary plexuses: the superficial, intermediate, deep, and radial peripapillary capillary plexus (RPCP) [1–5]. *Ex vivo* confocal microscopy has validated the presence of these capillary plexuses in the human eye [6, 7]. Optical coherence tomography angiography (OCT-A) imaging has revealed three-dimensional macular and retinal blood vessel features [4].

Proper blood circulation to the macular portion of the retina is crucial for supplying oxygen and nutrients to cells involved in vision, such as photoreceptors and neurons. Reduced retinal blood flow is a risk factor for neovascularization (NV) and macular edema [8]. Systemic cardiovascular diseases, including atherosclerosis and hypertension, can increase the likelihood of developing NV [9, 10].

Chronic conditions such as compression, inflammation, and atherosclerosis can reduce retinal venous blood return with hypertension in the capillary venous plexus and consequently cause retinal vein occlusion (RVO) [11, 12]. The distinction between branch and central RVO is significant. **Figure 1** illustrates obstructions within the retinal branches, while **Figure 2** highlights obstructions within the optic nerve. It is worth noting that central RVO is more prevalent in both types, as investigated by Ip et al. [13].

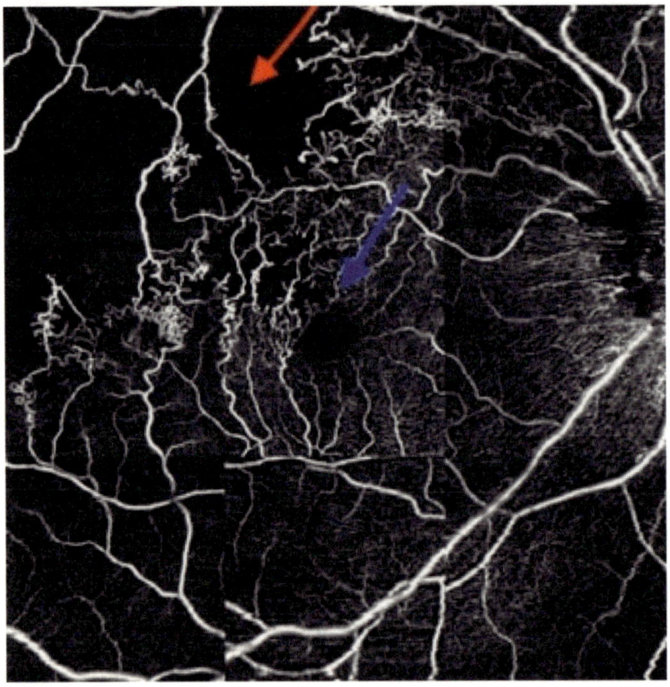

Figure 1.
OCT-A image of superior branch retinal vein occlusion (BRVO) with a red arrowhead pointing to nonperfusion regions and a blue arrowhead pointing to the abnormal FAZ. The Retina Image Bank® website first released this picture. The writer is Manish Nagpal, M.D. Gayathri Mohan who is the photographer. Retinal Vein Occlusion in a Branch Case of OCTA. Retinal image bank. 2019; 34,186. © American Society of Retina Specialists.

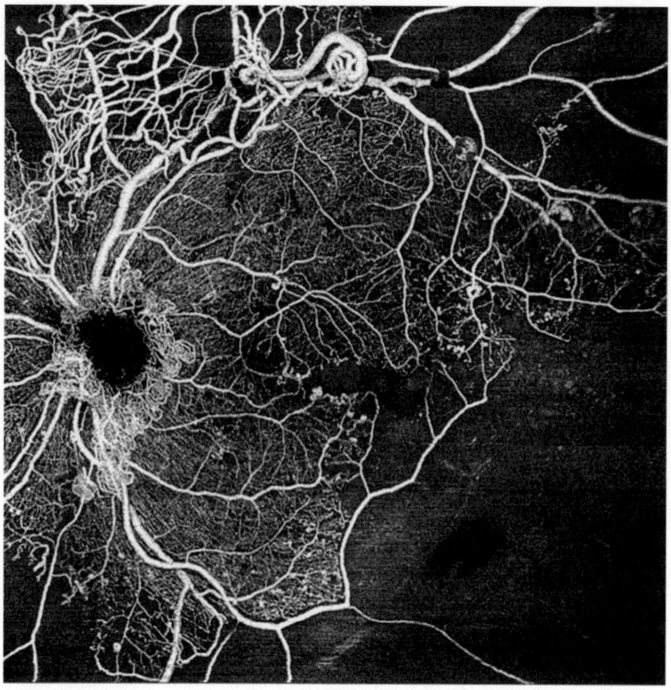

Figure 2.
Ischemic (nonperfused) CRVO using OCT-A imaging. An arteriovenous shunt, neovascularization, and retinal ischemia were observed in a 63-year-old patient with CRVO. The original version of this photo was posted to the Retina Image Bank® website. © American Society of Retina Specialists; Jorge I. Soberanes, M.D. Central Retinal Vein Occlusion by OCT Angiography, Retina Image Bank, 2022, 94,589.

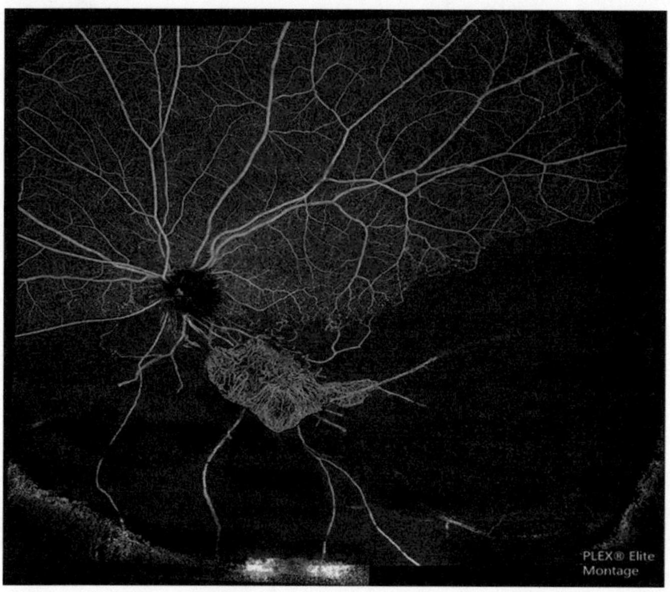

Figure 3.
A sweeping wide-field source of hemi-retinal vein occlusion on OCT-A (HRVO). In the inferior hemi-quadrant, a 59-year-old patient's OCT-A revealed significant artery loss along with a branching out neovascular frond inferior to the disc with terminal loops. The Retina Image Bank® website first released this picture. The Barren Field, Sandeep Kumar, MBBS, Retina Image Bank, 2022; 59,123. © American Society of Retina Specialists.

Hemiretinal RVO (HRVO) is another type of RVO that can occur in large forks (**Figure 3**). Macular edema, ischemia, and neovascularization are complications of RVO [14]. Further complications, such as optic neuropathy, vitreous hemorrhage, and retinal detachment, may occur [13].

Atherosclerosis, diabetes, arterial hypertension, and thrombophilia are among the most prominent risk factors for RVO [13]. Central RVO (CRVO) and branch RVO (BRVO) can be categorized into ischemic and nonischemic types based on the extent of the capillary nonperfusion area (NPA). Notably, up to 30% of eyes initially diagnosed with nonischemic central RVO may eventually develop the ischemic subtype. This is typically accompanied by a subsequent rapid decline in visual acuity and necessitates further evaluation [14–16].

Using OCT-A imaging, we provide a comprehensive overview of blood perfusion in healthy and RVO patients, including its effects on macular perfusion and visual complications. We discuss all possible treatments for RVO and their associated side effects.

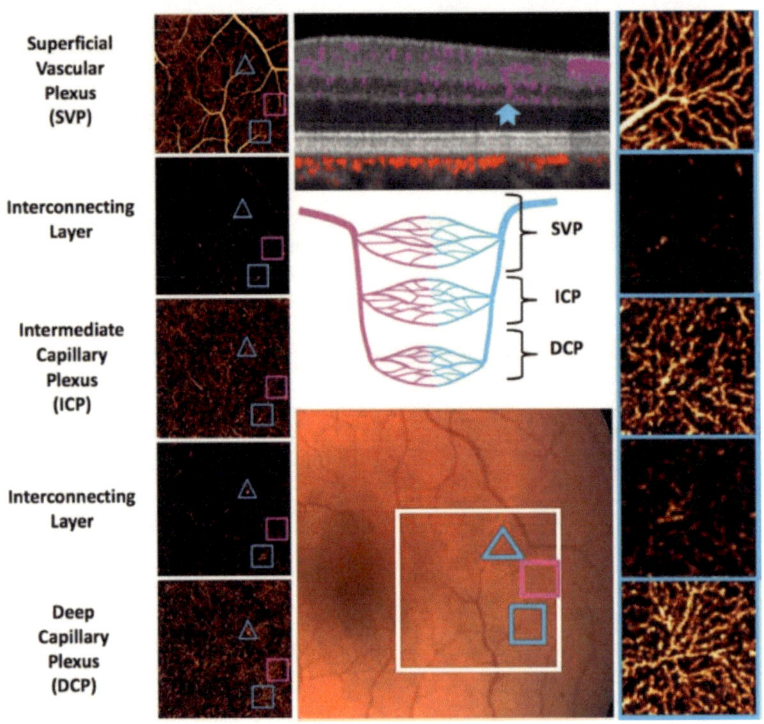

Figure 4.
Images depicting the macular retinal vascular plexuses and the layers that link them. The middle bottom panel displays a color fundus image, with the white square representing a 2 × 2 mm scan area. The entire face can be seen in the left panels. The PR-OCT-A images were ordered from the deepest to the most superficial. In the color fundus image, a dividing venule extends from the SCP to the DCP (solid blue-notched arrow), and the surrounding blue hollow triangles can be observed in the middle top panel of the cross-sectional PR-OCT image. Pink squares with holes surround a dividing arteriole in the SCP, ICP, and DCP and the connecting layer between the ICP and DCP. At every amplification, pink squares with holes surround a separating arteriole. At every magnified en-face PR-OCT-A (right panels) slab, the diving venule is encased in empty blue squares. All three plexuses receive capillary networks from their venules. The central panel of the image shows the interconnected layers of the three vascular plexuses and the anatomical links between the venous and arterial systems. They are copied from Campbell et al. [4] with permission under a CC BY 4.0 license.

2. Macular perfusion in control eyes

The four main capillary plexuses—the superficial capillary plexus (SCP), intermediate capillary plexus (ICP), deep capillary plexus (DCP), and RPCP—are the retinal and choroidal arteries that nourish the optic nerve, photoreceptors, and ancillary cells. Campbell et al. used projection-resolved OCT-A (PR OCT-A) in normal human eyes to study blood flow in different retinal areas [4]. **Figure 4** shows that, compared with two-dimensional (2D) color fundus photos, this method is far better for evaluating the intricate vasculature of the blood supply. Consistent with other primate studies, its results shed light on the SCP, ICP, and DCP structures with an interconnecting layer linking these capillary plexuses.

OCT-A imaging provides a more detailed visualization of the blood vessels in the retina than was previously achievable. It has proven highly effective in diagnosing retinal vascular diseases such as RVO, diabetic retinopathy, and AMD. Compared with fundus fluorescein angiography (FFA), which has been utilized for over five decades, OCT-A can visualize the microvasculature of both the superficial and deep retinal plexus without needing dyes. Only the SCP is observed when FFA is employed for retinal vasculature imaging, while the deeper retinal layers remain unobservable (**Figure 5**). Compared with FFA, OCT-A provides superior delineation of the foveal avascular zone (FAZ). The drawbacks of OCT-A include the absence of standardized patient data, challenges related to projection artifacts, and difficulty in identifying low-flow lesions or pathologies [13, 14].

Figure 6 displays further findings from the OCT-A investigation, which sheds light on the vessel density quantification and binarizing processing to calculate the CVI.

Autoregulation, whether static or dynamic, controls blood flow to the retina. Endothelial cells and the surrounding extraretinal tissue secrete local mediators that allow the retina to self-regulate blood flow. The sympathetic nervous system regulates blood flow to choroidal blood vessels, affecting blood flow to the retina [17]. Dynamic autoregulation allows for more rapid changes in ocular blood flow and pressure than static autoregulation, which takes a long time to alter blood pressure in the retinal arteries [18, 19]. Nitrous oxide, oxygen, carbon dioxide, endothelin-1, adenosine,

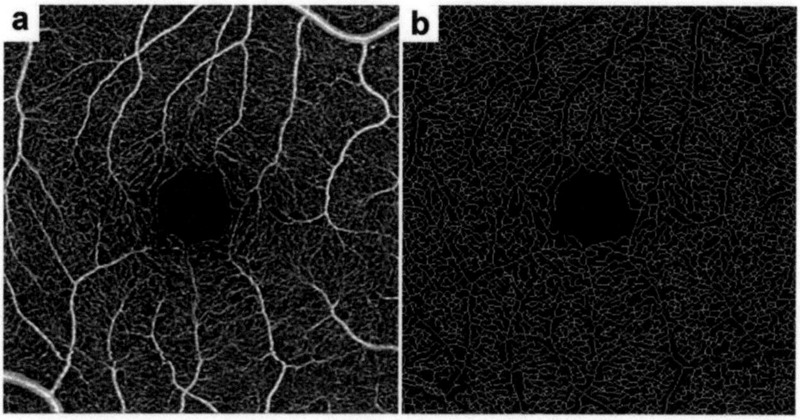

Figure 5.
(a) The FAZ is nicely depicted in the middle. (b) A binarized image displaying the blood vessel skeleton and an OCT-A image of healthy retinal vasculature. Kyle Green, M.D., kindly supplied the picture with permission.

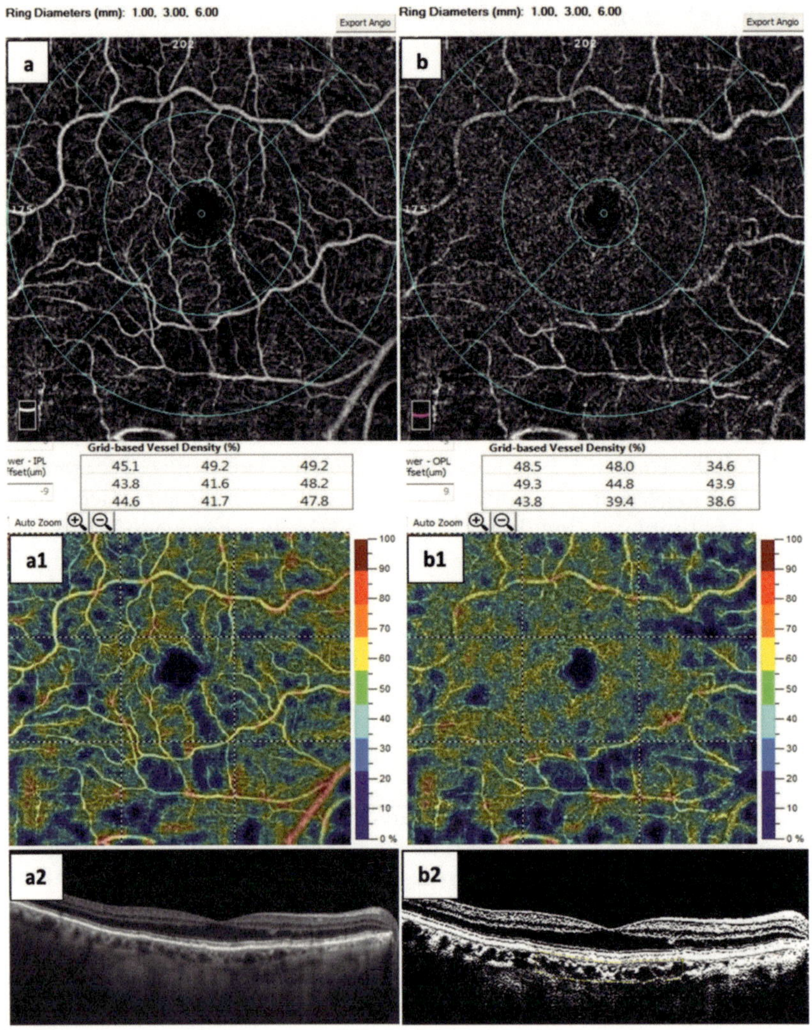

Figure 6.
OCT-A imaging showing vascular plexuses of a healthy eye. (a) SCP and (b1) DCP. (a1) and (b1) show vessel density quantification, with the values displayed at the superior border of the image. (a2) Corresponding 9-mm SD-OCT line, and (b2) binarizing processing to calculate the CVI in a selected subfoveal area of choroidal flow delineated by the white-yellow dotted line. —multipanel pictures from the Authors' collection.

and angiotensin-2 are mediators [20]. In normal eyes, autoregulation is crucial for responding to environmental and internal variables affecting blood perfusion and maintaining a good blood supply to the retina [21].

Even in healthy eyes, there can be significant individual variations in retinal blood flow. Garhofer et al. reported notable variations in retinal blood flow among 64 young and healthy individuals with normal blood pressure (BP) or intraocular pressure (IOP) and a refraction error of less than three diopters [22]. There may be racial differences in ocular perfusion pressure (OPP) and several other risk factors for ocular diseases [23]. A recent meta-analysis included 72 studies examining the relationships between OPP and different patient features to determine the risk of ocular disease. This meta-analysis revealed that a reduced OPP may increase the likelihood of developing eye disorders [24].

Macular thickness has been the subject of substantial research because of its potential link to ocular perfusion. Milani et al. [25] studied the effects of visual diseases, including glaucoma and ocular hypertension, on macular thickness. Compared with healthy eyes, eyes with ocular hypertension/glaucoma presented a linear relationship between increased macular thickness and vessel density in the SCP. Similarly, Ayhan et al. [26] investigated the effects of smoking on macular perfusion in healthy individuals. A possible explanation for the reduced blood flow to the choriocapillary area in the eyes of smokers is the influence of nicotine and other chemicals in cigarettes. Yoga has exciting benefits, such as lowering IOP and increasing average macular thickness in healthy individuals [27]. A Turkish study comparing males and females revealed that the parafoveal vessel density and FAZ area were considerably more significant in females [28].

Overall, the retina's health, visual function, and general well-being depend on adequate blood flow to the area. The network of capillaries branching from the retinal and choroidal arteries supplies blood to the optic nerve, photoreceptors, ganglion cells, and neurons. In response to internal and external stimuli, the OPP is autoregulated through static and dynamic processes to maintain good blood flow. Because there may be significant individual differences in retinal blood flow, and in OPP, macular thickness, smoking status, and lifestyle may affect retinal blood circulation and eye health.

3. Macular perfusion in obstructive venous disease of the retina

Reduced venous return of retinal blood is known as RVO. This ailment affects millions worldwide, and BRVO is five times more common than CRVO [29]. BRVO and CRVO can be further categorized as either nonischemic (using blood perfusion) or ischemic (with no perfusion) (**Figure 7**) [31]. The most common consequence of RVO is macular edema, which can cause visual loss. Visual loss due to vitreous

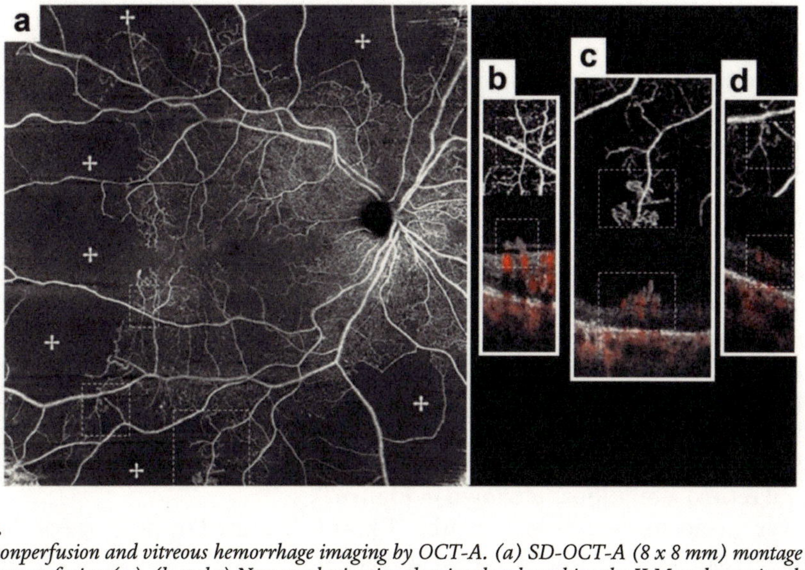

Figure 7.
Retinal nonperfusion and vitreous hemorrhage imaging by OCT-A. (a) SD-OCT-A (8 x 8 mm) montage showing areas of nonperfusion (+). (b and c) Neovascularization that involves breaching the ILM and entering the vitreous. (d) Intraretinal neovascularization within the ILM. The image is unchanged from Ref. [30]. (used under CC BY 4.0 license).

hemorrhage, retinal detachment, or neovascular glaucoma can occur as a result of NV, another common consequence of RVO [31]. A patient's level of vision loss is often proportional to their macular perfusion status, and vision loss typically occurs suddenly and painlessly in patients with RVO [31].

OCT-A has become a prominent noninvasive method for studying macular perfusion in patients with RVO [32]. Vessel density and blood perfusion can help identify and distinguish RVO-affected areas, distinguishing between BRVO and CRVO [33–36]. According to Coscas et al. [37], the DCP is more affected than the SCP, which is especially crucial in assessing qualitative and quantitative changes in RVO. Their study found more grayish lesions that correspond to NPAs of the retina, increased capillary network dilation or disruption, and greater involvement in the DCP than in the SCP. Additionally, cystoid spaces that produce DROL alterations were more commonly found in the outer retinal layer, coinciding with extensive areas of vascular alteration in the DCP. Martinet et al. [38] utilized an experimental retinal microcirculation mouse model to demonstrate that transverse venules establish direct connections between the more prominent retinal veins in the SCP and the DCP. A decrease in perfusion in the retinal tissues supplied by the DCP is likely to occur when hydrostatic pressure in the DCP increases rapidly and significantly due to elevated IOP from RVO in the large veins. The retinal arterioles, characterized by elevated oxygen supply and perfusion pressure, are directly linked to the SCP. This anatomical characteristic may be associated with the superior preservation of the SCP in RVO compared to the DCP.

NPAs, vascular tortuosity, collateral vessels, perifoveal capillary plexus disruption, capillary plexus dilation and venous dilation, microaneurysms, cystoid spaces, intraretinal hemorrhages, nonperfused ghost vessels, optic disc venous collaterals (OVCs), neovascularization of the disc (NVD), and neovascularization elsewhere (NVE) are qualitative changes [33, 34, 37–43]. These changes can be quantified by measuring parameters such as OPP, vessel density, and NPAs according to ETDRS subfields [28, 39, 40, 44].

Koulisis et al. [45] used OCT-A to study capillary plexus alterations caused by RVO by comparing healthy eyes with those with RVO. Vessel density was substantially lower in eyes with CRVO and BRVO than in healthy eyes. Furthermore, the vascular diameter index (VDI) was significantly greater in RVO-affected eyes than in healthy ones. **Figure 8a-d** shows the healthy eye, and **Figure 8e-h** shows the afflicted eye used to compare the OCT-A images.

Additionally, Mousa et al. [33] analyzed a case series of patients with ischemic RVO to determine the best method for grading macular perfusion. They reported that OCT-A was better than FFA was. According to their findings, SCP or DCP ischemia can result in poor visual outcomes. Additionally, macular perfusional consequences and sequelae of impaired vision include an increase in central macular thickness (CMT), disruption of the retinal outer layers (DROL), and a disorganized retinal inner layer (DRIL) [33]. Khodabandeh et al.'s [46] study revealed that OCT-A can accurately differentiate nonperfused from perfused CRVO. The results of this investigation support the idea that OCT-A can be used to study the effects of RVO on retinal perfusion in the different capillary plexuses of the retina, as well as accompanying structural retinal alterations, as shown in **Figure 9**.

Paracentral acute middle maculopathy (PAMM) is caused by blockage of the DCP in the lesion area. Researchers have investigated PAMM *via* OCT-A. [47, 48]. Dansingani et al. published a case study that contrasted OCT-A with near-infrared (nIR) imaging to detect lesions at the location of venous occlusions. OCT-A detected the lesions, changes in retinal layer thicknesses at the occlusion location, and abnormalities in blood flow to the affected area; however, nIR failed to identify the lesion 1 month after the initial detection. The parafoveal region showed a flow void in

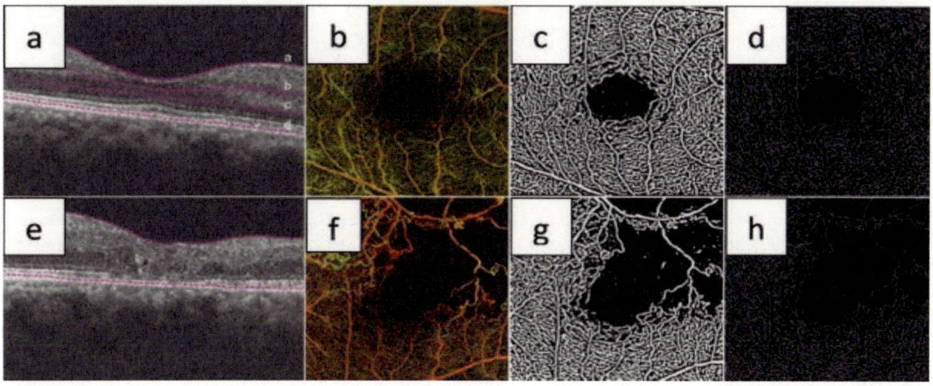

Figure 8.
(a) B-scan of a healthy fellow eye showing purple dotted lines depicting the vascular layers of interest: nonsegmented retina layer (NS-RL) (a-d), superficial retina layer (SRL) (a-b), and deeper retina layer (DRL) (b-c). OCT-A map depth-encoded image (b), binarizing processed image (c), and digitally skeletonized image (d), (e) through (h) Images of the RVO eye analyzed via *NS-RL (copied from [45] Koulisis N. et al. PLOS ONE. 2017;12(4) with permission under CC BY 4.0 license).*

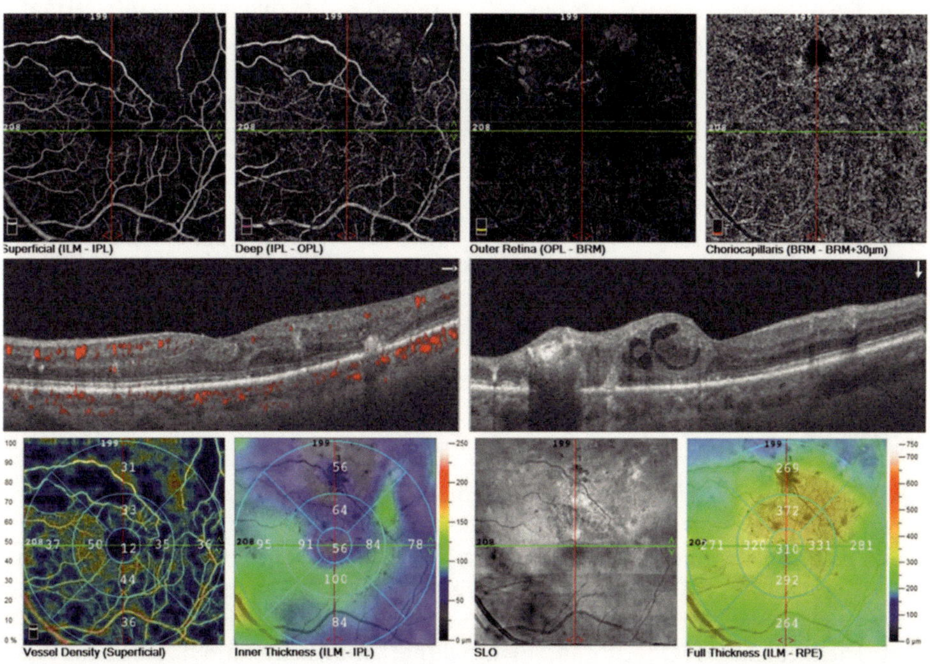

Figure 9.
A patient with superotemporal RVO of 4 months of evolution complained of distortion and vision drop. (a) SCP and DCP showed multiple vascular alterations with NPAs and vascular segment abnormalities. The horizontal OCT showed DROL and foveal thickening. The vertical OCT showed significant macular edema with large cysts and DRIL and DROL structural alterations. OCT-A imaging of the vascular density showed lower than average values in the SCP, and inner and full-retina thickness were abnormally thicker—multipanel pictures from the Authors' collection.

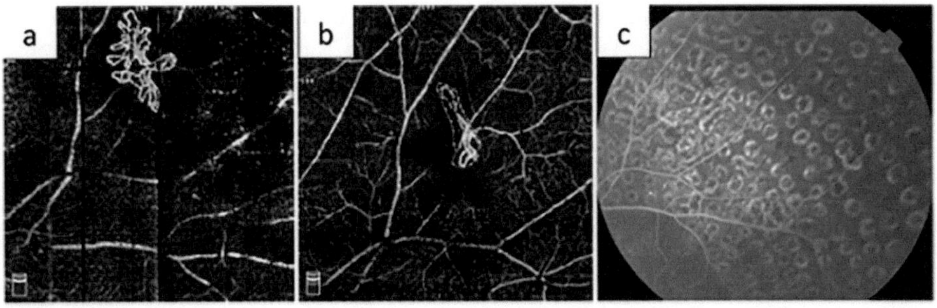

Figure 10.
(a) Initially, neovascularization was observed on OCT-A with an area of 0.653 mm². (b) Even after one year of PRP treatment, OCT-A still revealed an aberrant vascular shape with an area of 0.272 mm². (c) No evidence of fluorescein leakage is observed at the FFA (right) (copied from [49] He F. et al. Eye. 2020 Aug 12;34(8):1413–8 with permission under CC BY 4.0 license).

addition to thinning of the ganglion cell layer (GCL), inner nuclear layer (INL), and inner perivascular layer (IPL) and thickening of the outer nuclear layer (ONL) [48]. He et al. compared FFA with OCT-A to determine whether the retinal vasculature improved after pan-retinal photocoagulation (PRP) treatment [49]. OCT-A helps reveal mild vascular alterations, and the vessel density can be quantitatively evaluated as long as the inner and full thickness of the different retina layers, as depicted in **Figure 10**.

OCT-A assessment of macular blood flow provides valuable insights into retinal perfusion from both qualitative and quantitative perspectives. This method is particularly effective for studying arterial and venous occlusions and determining the severity of perfusion-related consequences and their subsequent developments.

4. Effective treatment strategies

Here, we discuss the various treatment options for RVO complications and their effects on macular perfusion. The most common treatment methods for RVO vary according to the severity of the problem, the degree of ischemia, and the presence or absence of macular edema.

4.1 Laser therapy

Laser treatment is one of the most commonly used options in developing countries to treat macular edema due to RVO, the second most common macular condition after diabetic retinopathy in terms of prevalence [29], selective or focal, and grid pattern photocoagulation or PRP. In the Central Vein Occlusion Study, researchers followed up with 155 patients for up to 3 years after undergoing laser photocoagulation treatment. The results of this study demonstrated that visual acuity did not improve noticeably in these patients after laser treatment [50].

On the other hand, the Branch Vein Occlusion Study Group used laser photocoagulation therapy in 139 eyes and monitored patient outcomes for as long as 3.1 years. According to this study, those who underwent laser treatment had significantly improved visual acuity compared with those with untreated eyes [51]. Researchers in the Branch Vein Occlusion Study Group investigated how laser photocoagulation therapy could help patients with BRVO with less neovascularization and retinal hemorrhage. To assess the efficacy of laser treatment in decreasing neovascularization, 319 eyes were subjected to laser treatment. A comparison of the treated and untreated eyes revealed that neovascularization was significantly lower in the treated eyes than in the untreated eyes. The risk of vitreous hemorrhage was also much lower in eyes that received laser treatment than in those that did not [52]. Laser photocoagulation therapy can help patients with BRVO in the long term; however, better alternatives are more widely used.

4.2 Glucocorticoids

Research on using intravitreal glucocorticoids to alleviate macular edema and enhance visual acuity in patients with RVO is ongoing. Dexamethasone has received the most attention among the glucocorticoids examined for treating BRVO. The SCORE study compared laser therapy with triamcinolone intravitreal injections to enhance visual acuity in patients with BRVO [53]. Patients who received standard treatment (laser therapy) or an intravitreal injection of triamcinolone (1 or 4 mg) were randomly assigned to one of the two groups, and 411 patients were randomly assigned to the other two groups. Twelve months after baseline, there were no statistically significant differences between the groups treated with laser therapy and those treated with triamcinolone *via* intravitreal injection. Patients who received higher doses of triamcinolone were more likely to experience high IOP [53]. Another trial that examined 271 patients with CRVO compared observation (no treatment) with intravitreal triamcinolone injections (1 or 4 mg) [54]; after 12 months of therapy with triamcinolone, patients' visual acuity significantly improved. Although a 1 mg injection of triamcinolone had a better safety profile, there was no discernible difference in effectiveness between 1 and 4 mg of triamcinolone [54].

Owing to the approval of a tiny intravitreal implant that slowly releases dexamethasone over time without the need for repeated injections (Ozurdex®, 0.7 mg dexamethasone), dexamethasone has recently become famous for the treatment of macular edema resulting from RVO. CRVO and BRVO patients can benefit from using this type of implant to treat macular edema [55]. Haller et al. examined dexamethasone implants in 1267 individuals with RVO (CRVO or BRVO) vision loss in two seminal trials. Patients were selected to receive one of three doses of dexamethasone intravitreally implants at random: 0.7 mg, 0.35 mg, or placebo. Compared with the sham group, the group that received dexamethasone contained a significantly greater number of patients with $\geq$15 letters of improvement in BCVA from baseline. After 180 days of monitoring, there were no discernible differences in IOP between the sham and dexamethasone groups [55]. These results support the effectiveness and safety of dexamethasone implants in addressing RVO-related macular edema. After injecting RVO patients with dexamethasone implants, Mastropasqua et al. [41] studied alterations in the macular region and the clearance of edema. The resolution of macular edema led to an improvement in vessel perfusion, as shown in **Figure 11**, which, in turn, led to a decrease in vascular density following dexamethasone treatment.

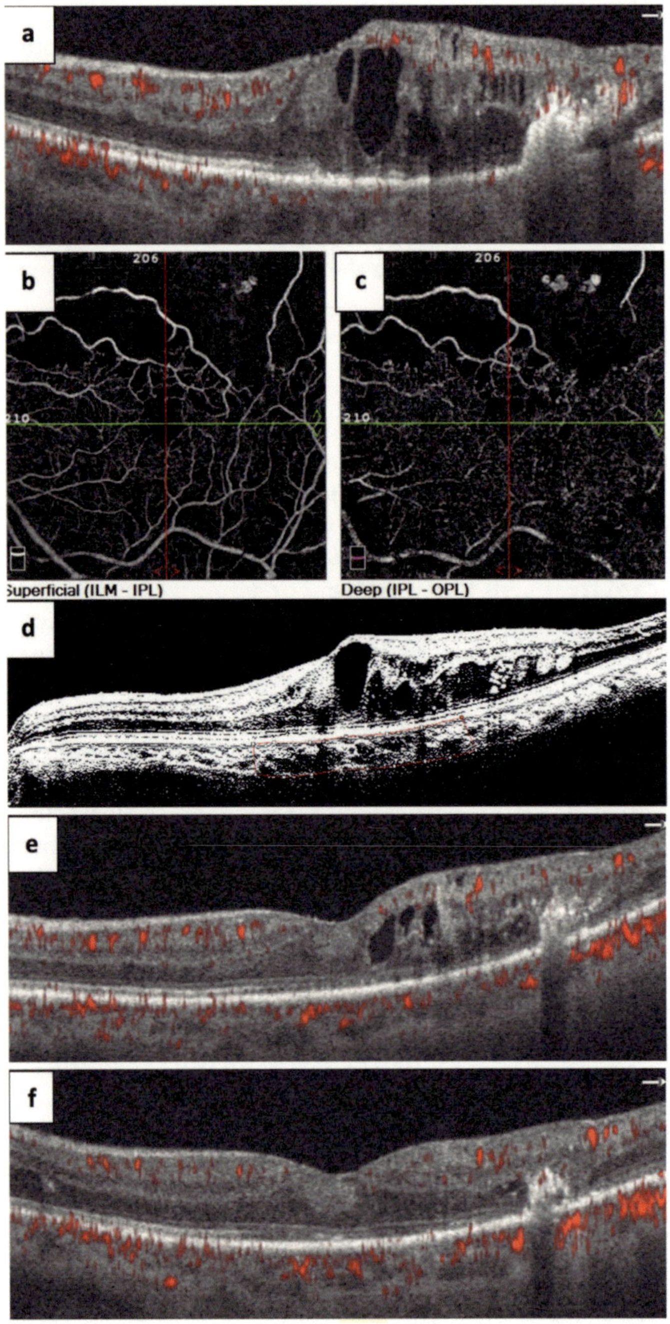

Figure 11.
(a) SD-OCT structural aspect of a 72-year-old female patient with sudden loss of vision to 20/200, suffering from RVO with ischemic macular edema and large intraretinal cystic spaces, along with DRIL and DROL retinal abnormalities. (b) The SCP shows extensive areas of capillary dropout. (c) The DCP reveals an irregular and enlarged FAZ. (d) Binarizing processing of the subfoveal choroidal vasculature (red-dotted square), where the CVI is calculated at 54.3%. (e) The structural aspect of the macula after three anti-VEGF injections. (f) Final OCT evaluation after 8 months of evolution and eight injections of anti-VEGF, with resolution of macular edema, a decrease in vascular density, and improvement in perfusion. The last BCVA was 20/50. —multipanel pictures from the Authors' collection.

5. Intravitreal injectable approach

Currently, anti-VEGF drugs are utilized to treat RVO-related disorders such as nonperfused and perfused macular edema. Qian et al.'s recent meta-analysis highlights their use in enhancing patients' visual acuity and addressing other issues [56]. In terms of enhancing BCVA and decreasing CMT, injectable interventions such as anti-VEGF treatment appear to outperform laser therapy or corticosteroids. Furthermore, anti-VEGF drugs are considered safer because of their reduced likelihood of increasing IOP. According to the same meta-analysis, anti-VEGF drugs had a more significant and longer-lasting effect on improving BCVA and reducing central retinal thickness (CRT) than corticosteroid and laser treatment in eyes with RVO. Anti-VEGF drugs are associated with a reduced likelihood of IOP. Moreover, anti-VEGF drugs have greater efficacy in treating BRVO than CRVO [56]. An increase in the VEFG signaling after RVO could contribute to macular edema by increasing the vascular permeability in the macular region and causing pathological neovascularization [57, 58].

Ranibizumab (Lucentis®) was the first anti-VEGF drug approved for treating perfused and nonperfused macular edema caused by venous obstructive disease. Intravitreal ranibizumab was the subject of two seminal investigations that examined its potential for treating BRVO and CRVO [59, 60]. Three hundred ninety-seven patients with BRVO-related macular edema were included in the BRAVO study, whereas 392 patients with CRVO-related macular edema were included in the CRUISE study. Both trials used a random assignment system to determine whether the patients would receive sham treatment, ranibizumab (0.3 mg) or 0.5 mg. Within 6 months of starting treatment, patients treated with ranibizumab (at a dosage of 0.5 mg) showed a marked improvement in BCVA and decreased CMT [59, 60]. The results from the 12-month follow-up showed that ranibizumab was safe and effective for patients with CRVO and BRVO in the long term [61, 62]. In addition to BRAVO and CRUISE, HORIZON is a follow-up trial that offers more evidence and recommendations for the use of ranibizumab to treat RVO. After 12 months of treatment, patients with CRVO should be customized according to the study's advice, which further supports the utility of ranibizumab in treating BRVO and CRVO [63].

Lida-Miwa et al. recently investigated how macular edema improved in patients treated with ranibizumab after BRVO. Interestingly, neovascularization was also observed as a problem following BRVO. The results of this prospective study indicated that older age, lower initial visual acuity, and greater central subfield thickness (CST) are linked to a poorer final BCVA in eyes with macular edema associated with BRVO treated with ranibizumab (administered with 3+ pro re nata injections). However, the macular NPA or the total NPA may not correlate with functional outcomes or the treatment burden. Hence, the clinical BRVO subtype may be linked to an increased likelihood of neovascular alterations, irrespective of the administration of ranibizumab injections for macular edema. Gaining knowledge about the correlation in the size of the NPA will aid in creating a more efficient treatment plan for each case of BRVO [64], and **Figure 12** shows the presence of ischemic macula edema despite ranibizumab treatment in a patient with extensive areas of NPA not shown in the image.

Additional uses of bevacizumab (Avastin®) beyond its approved label include the treatment of macular edema. Zhang et al. reported that compared with sham surgery, bevacizumab improved visual acuity over 18 months by increasing BCVA and

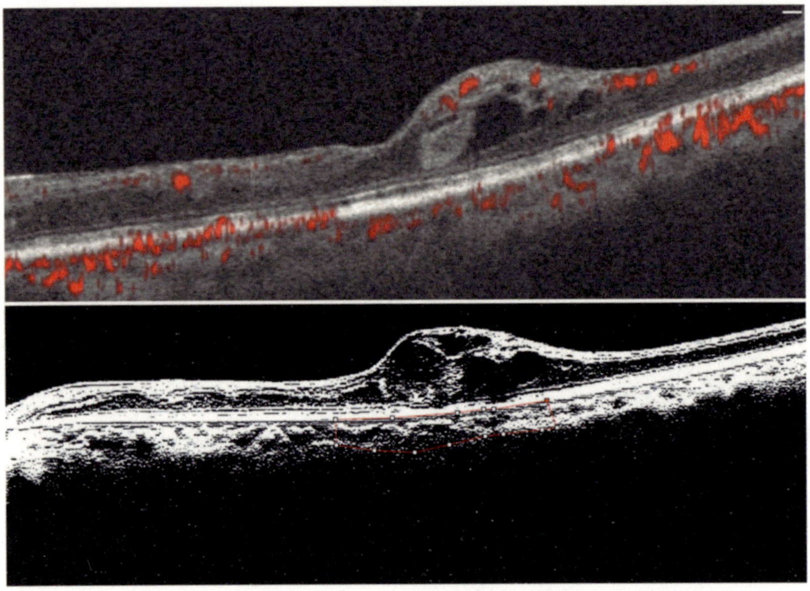

Figure 12.
Sixty-four-year-old uncontrolled hypertensive male patient who developed a sudden drop in vision in his right eye. This image corresponded to his first examination, which showed a vision of 20/300; the SD-OCT revealed the presence of DRIL and DROL with severe ischemic macular edema due to superotemporal BRVO with macular involvement. Extensive capillary abnormalities and NPA areas were found (not shown in the image). The bottom picture shows the binarizing processing of the choroidal vasculature to calculate the CVI in the subfoveal choroid. The CVI was 56.4%, lower than the 63.4% estimated in the fellow eye. —multipanel pictures from the Authors' collection.

decreasing CMT [65]. Choi et al. investigated whether bevacizumab reduces retinal edema in patients with BRVO. This study highlights the effectiveness of OCT-A in measuring vascular irregularities, particularly the NPAs in two capillary networks in eyes with macular edema recurrence due to BRVO. These findings indicated a clear correlation between the NPAs and the recurrence of macular edema, particularly in the central foveal and parafoveal areas. **Figure 13** shows that the macular region recovered in a 56-year-old patient with no recurrence of ischemic macular edema (non-perfused macular edema). As Choi et al. reported, off-label use of bevacizumab injections benefits OCT-A visual outcomes in BRVO [66]. **Figure 13** shows sequential OCT and OCT-A improvement after the serial anti-VEGF injection approach.

In 2014, for the treatment of macular edema and other RVO consequences, the COPERNICUS trial was a pioneering investigation of the safety and effectiveness of aflibercept (Eylea®) in patients with CRVO and randomized 189 patients to receive 2 mg of intravitreal aflibercept or placebo. After the first 6 months of treatment, visual acuity improved significantly in the aflibercept treatment group compared with the sham group. Additionally, this trial confirmed that aflibercept is safe and well tolerated [67]. Another seminal trial that investigated the use of aflibercept for treating macular edema after BRVO was the VIBRANT study. The participants in this trial were randomly assigned to receive laser photocoagulation therapy or 2 mg of intravitreal aflibercept. None of the patients had previously undergone treatment. The enhanced visual acuity and decreased CMT results showed that aflibercept was noticeably better than laser photocoagulation therapy [68]. Ghashut et al. used OCT-A to study macular edema in patients with CRVO-related macular edema.

DOI: http://dx.doi.org/10.5772/intechopen.1007952

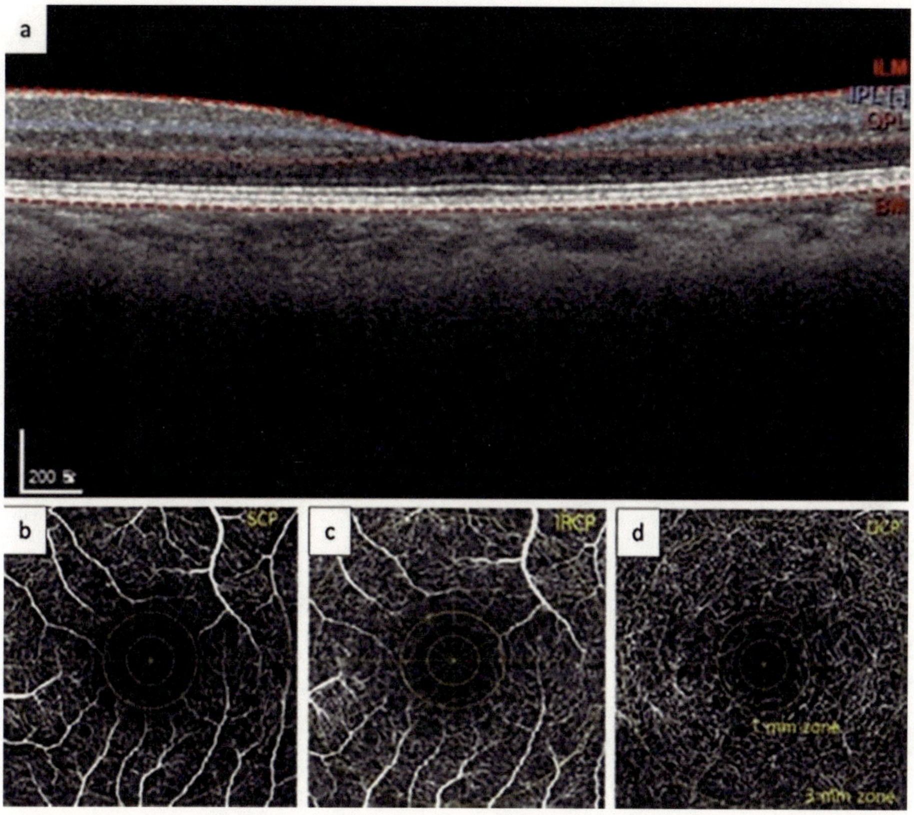

Figure 13.
(a) OCT image and (b–d) OCT-A images of the fellow eye in a 69-year-old male patient in the nonrecurrence group. OCT-A image of (d) the DCP showing a more prominent FAZ than in (b) the SCP. Single-layered capillaries were shown to adhere to the FAZ within (c) the inner retinal capillary plexus layer (IRCP) and (d) the DCP but not (b) the SVP (copied from [66] Choi KE. et al. Scientific Reports. 2019 Dec 2;9(1):14153 with permission under CC BY 4.0 license).

Aflibercept treatment restored macular area alterations and increased visual acuity in individuals without foveal photoreceptor impairment and with minor NPAs. Although aflibercept effectively reduces macular edema, it does not enhance visual acuity in individuals with moderate foveal photoreceptor impairment or relatively large NPAs [69]. Amer et al. [70] reported a significant reduction in the CST after investigating improvements in macular edema secondary to CRVO following aflibercept treatment. **Figure 14** shows retinal sequels of severe RVO with profound ischemic abnormalities due to extensive capillary dropouts and abnormal thick CST.

Two phase 3 clinical trials, BALATON and COMINO, have investigated the use of faricimab (Vabysmo®), the most recently approved anti-VEGF and anti-angiopoietin-2 (anti-Ang2) drugs, respectively, to treat macular edema resulting from BRVO and CRVO [71, 72]. It appears that patients with RVO have higher levels of Ang-2 in their retinas, according to a recent literature analysis by Heier et al. [73], which examined the angiopoietin-tie route and the possible use of faricimab to treat RVO. As faricimab is a combination of anti-VEGF and anti-Ang-2 drugs, it is anticipated to improve RVO treatment significantly.

Finally, the US FDA recently approved the Port Delivery System with ranibizumab (PDS) (commercially available as Susvimo®). This new device can deliver

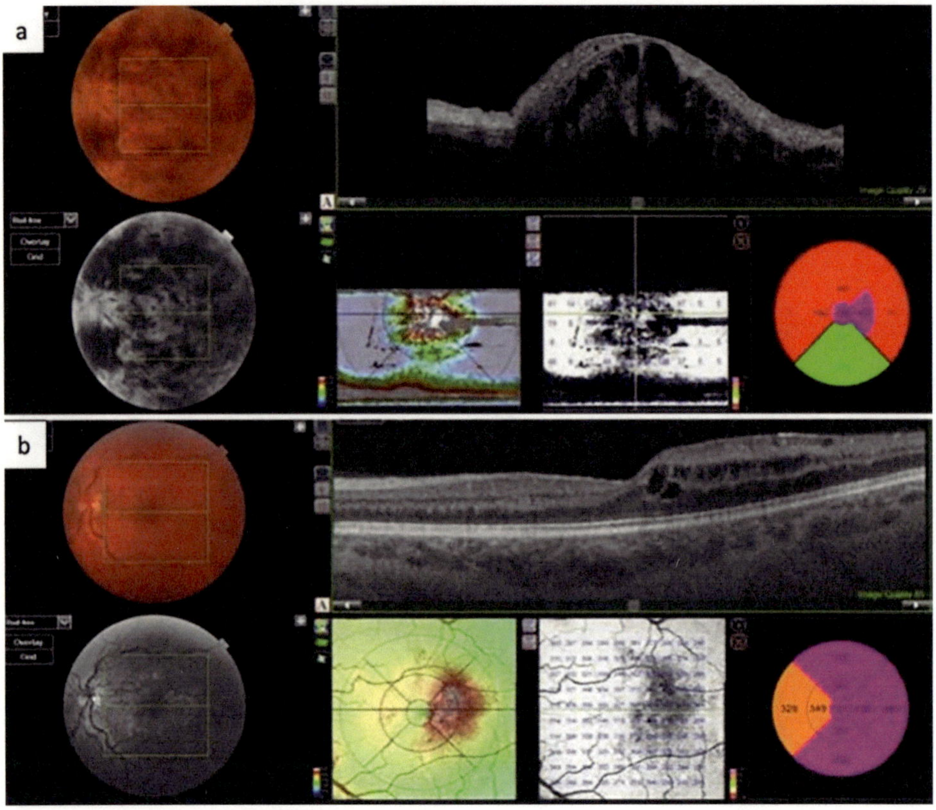

Figure 14.
(a) CST significantly decreased over time (at baseline [570.7 ± 59 Um], six months [388.5 ± 80 Um], and (b) 12 months [328.2 ± 72 Um], p < 0.001) (copied from [70] Amer AA et al.30 March 2022 with permission under CC BY 4.0 license).

ranibizumab to the retina for an extended period (6 months or more) [74, 75]. As it offers sustained delivery of anti-VEGF drugs, this groundbreaking drug delivery system can treat macular edema and other consequences of RVO in addition to neovascular AMD. Recent literature reviews have focused on intravitreal dexamethasone-slow tiny implants for approval and usage OZURDEX®, suggesting that PDS could treat RVO by continuously delivering anti-VEGF drugs [75]. To further explore the potential benefits of targeting the VEGF and Ang-2 pathways and prolonging the delivery of medications, PDS was also used for the sustained administration of faricimab [76].

The authors included a selected group of RVO patients treated with anti-VEGF and analyzed the structural and quantitative outcomes. All statistical analyses were performed using GraphPad Prism version 9.2.0 software and R environment version 4.1.1, with statistical significance set at $p < 0.05$. The Kruskal-Wallis test with Benjamini and Hochberg correction was used to determine the differences in BCVA after injection, postinjection CVI, and CFA between the study and control groups. The two-tailed Wilcoxon matched-pairs signed-rank test assessed BCVA changes after injection at the final visit. No significant difference in age was found among the two study groups ($p = 0.642$). Perfused and nonperfused groups had significantly worse baseline BCVA than the control group ($p < 0.0001$); however, no difference in BCVA was identified between the two study groups ($p = 0.53$). Patients in the nonperfused group had approximately 1 week less time with an ischemic macula before anti-VEGF therapy, and this difference was statistically significant ($p = 0.005$). No difference in the postoperative follow-up time was found between the two study groups ($p = 0.912$). In both study groups, the post-operative BCVA was significantly better than the preoperative BCVA ($p < 0.0001$). The logMAR BCVA improved by an average of −0.76 in the nonperfused group and − 0.62 in the perfused group. However, the final BCVA remained worse than

SD-OCT and OCT-A findings BRVO with macular involvement	**Perfused RVO eyes**	**Nonperfused RVO eyes**	**Fellow eye (control)**
Number of patients (eyes)	18	12	30
Mean age	62.72 ± 7.6	64.06 ± 8.2	63.39 ± 7.9
Mean baseline BCVA	1.05 ($p = 0.644$)	1.22 ($p = 0.346$)	0.00
Mean time before anti-VEFG	6.6 ± 1.5 weeks	5.7 ± weeks	N/A
Mean final BCVA (logMAR)	−0.62 ($p < 0.001$)	−0.76 ($p < 0.001$)	N/A
Mean follow-up (months)	8.4 ($p = 0.912$)	7.4 ($p = 0.822$)	N/A
SD-OCT marker	n (%)		
CST abnormalities	9 (75%)	11(91,6%)	none
DRIL	10 (55.6%)	10 (83.3%)	none
DROL	14 (77.8%)	12 (100%)	none
Final OCT-A outcomes			
Whole vessel density in SCP	16.22 ± 2.47 ($p = 0.036^{\#}$)	17.22 ± 2.04 ($p = 0.036^{\#}$)	17.52 ± 2.30
Whole vessel density in DCP	14.48 ± 2.47 ($p = 0.044^{\#}$)	15.20 ± 2.41 ($p = 0.044^{\#}$)	18.21 ± 1.56
Whole PD in SCP (%)	0.39 ± 0.07 ($p = 0.039^{\#}$)	0.40 ± 0.12 ($p = 0.039^{\#}$)	0.43 ± 0.04
Whole PD in DCP (%)	0.39 ± 0.07 ($p = 0.032^{\#}$)	0.41 ± 0.12 ($p = 0.032^{\#}$)	0.43 ± 0.04
Mean macular CVI (%)	53.16% ($p < 0.001$)	51.32% ($p < 0.001$)	63.35%
CVI, 95% CI (%)	64.07,67.44	62.10,64.44	55.61,59.08
Mean macular CFA (mm^2)	1.38 ($p < 0.001$)	1.48 ($p < 0.001$)	2.28
Correlation coefficients between BCVA and choroidal perfusion markers			
CVI	−0.117	−0.120	−0.124
CFA	−0.355	−0.378	−0.211

Note. BRVO, branch retinal vein occlusion; CFA, choriocapillaris flow area; CST, central subfield thickness; CVI, choroidal vascularity index; CI, coefficient interval; DCP, deep capillary plexus; DRIL, disorganization of the retinal inner layers; DROL, disruption of retinal outer layers; OCT-A, optical coherence tomography angiography; PD, perfusion density; SD-OCT, spectral-domain optical coherence tomography; RVO, retinal vein occlusion; SCP, superficial capillary plexus; VD, vessel density. Bold values indicate statistical significance: $p < 0.05$.[#]*Wilcoxon test.*

Table 1.
Demographic data and macular structural and quantitative perfusion outcomes.

the control eyes in both study groups ($p < 0.0001$). The final binarized OCT images were analyzed to obtain LA and TCA values, which were used to calculate the CVI values in percentages. The average CVI was 59.35% in the control group, 53.66% in the perfused group, and 54.32% in the nonperfused group. The differences in the CVI between the control and study groups were statistically significant ($p = 0.002$ for the control and nonperfused groups, $p = 0.049$ for the control and perfused groups). Between the study groups, a negative correlation was found between the last CVI and final BCVA (Pearson's correlation = −0.292); eyes with a higher CVI tended to have a lower logMAR (i.e., better vision) and vice versa. This negative correlation was observed in the perfused and nonperfused groups (Pearson's correlation = −0.265 for the perfused group and − 0.232 for the nonperfused group). The CFA was significantly lower in both patient groups than in the control group. Patient demographic data, macular structural, and perfused clinical characteristics are summarized in **Table 1**.

6. Discussion

Concerning choroidal perfusion in patients with CRVO and BRVO, the choriocapillaris becomes more permeable because of soluble VEGF and inflammatory mediators [77, 78]. VEGF increases the permeability of blood vessels in the choroid, leading to an increase in choroidal thickness.

Additionally, the thickening of the choroid is caused by the formation of nitric oxide, which is stimulated by VEGF [78]. In eyes with macular edema due to RVO, the absence or reduction of the inflammatory response may prevent choroidal thickening [79]. Previous investigations have validated this notion *via* binarized enhanced depth imaging (EDI) SD-OCT images, which revealed only an elevated choroidal vascularity index (CVI) in eyes with significant macular edema. The CVI has been widely debated and internationally acknowledged as a dependable and encouraging instrument for examining choroidal perfusion. A certain level of proficiency in the program is necessary to binarize the EDI SD-OCT slabs. The CVI could offer valuable insights as a predictive measure for effectively managing eyes with RVO [77].

To summarize, recent advancements in intravitreal pharmacological treatments have demonstrated the effectiveness of VEGF inhibitors and intravitreal corticosteroids in treating macular edema associated with RVO. The treatment options for different types of macular edema due to RVO have been significantly widened and improved by the intravitreal administration of the FDA-approved ranibizumab and a sustained-release dexamethasone implant (**Figure 15**), as well as the off-label use of bevacizumab, preservative-free triamcinolone, and the newly developed PDS with ranibizumab and faricimab. Aflibercept combined with ranibizumab significantly improved the BCVA and reduced the CRT. Therefore, aflibercept might be more effective than ranibizumab. These treatments have replaced the previous standard of care for RVO-associated macular edema. Although anti-VEGF agents can lead to rapid regression of neovascularization, scattered laser photocoagulation remains an established treatment for preventing neovascular complications. Intravitreal pharmacotherapy has revolutionized the treatment of retinal vascular diseases such as RVO. Although intravitreal agents demonstrate efficacy, our understanding of their precise indications and long-term functions is still evolving.

Moreover, while the fundamental occlusive pathophysiology of RVO remains unresolved, our treatment options are restricted to temporary measures for

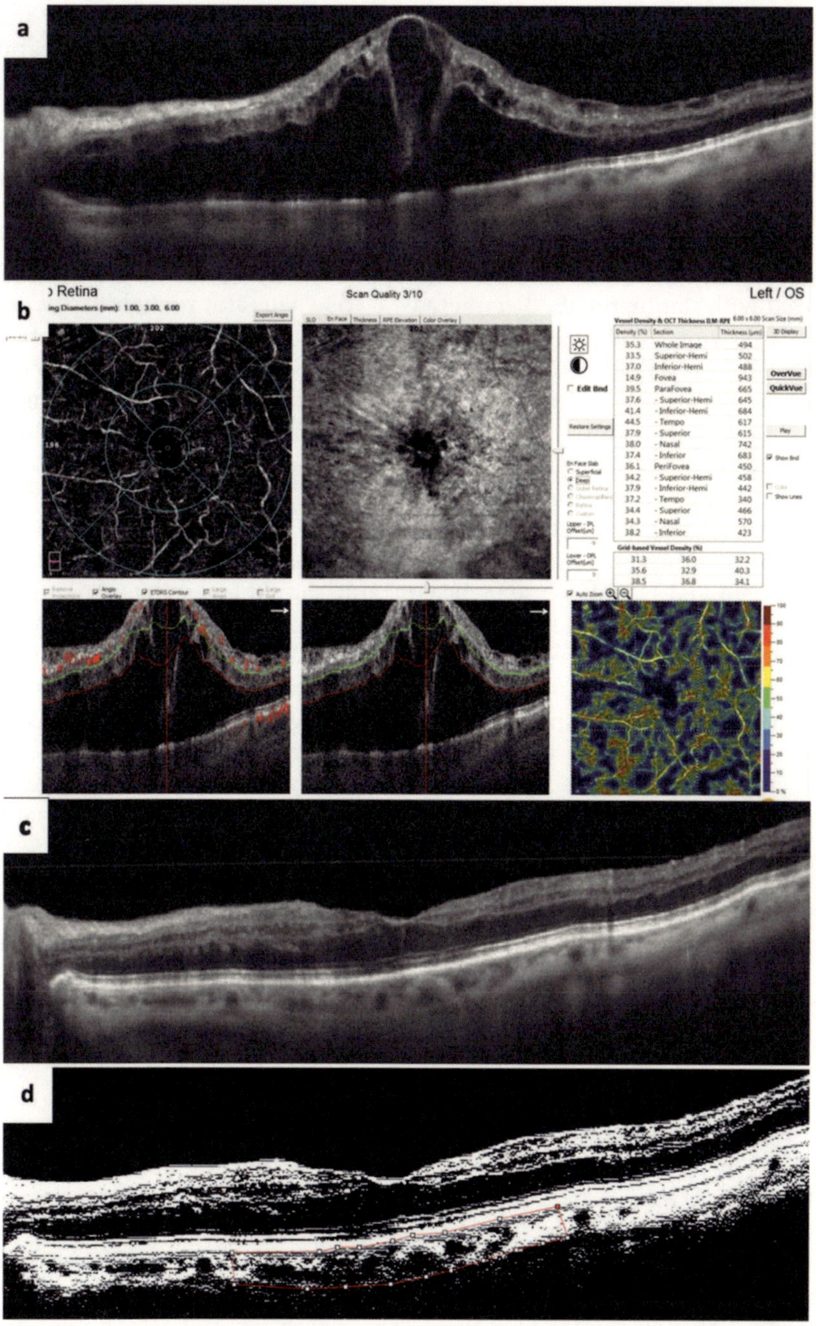

Figure 15.
(a) Image that shows severe macular edema due to CRVO. (b) Multipanel picture showing the SCP with capillary dropouts in the different ETDRS subfields, cystoid macular edema on the en face image, and other values of quantified vessel densities in the SCP. Horizontal and vertical crossline OCT showing large cystic spaces and binarized images of the SCP on the left with reduced vessel density values. (c) After three monthly intravitreal injections of aflibercept and Ozurdex implant, the macular edema has resolved, and the disruption of retinal outer layers (DROL) and disorganized inner retinal layers (DRIL) defects have recovered, as did the ellipsoid zone (EZ) biomarker. (d) The high-resolution B scan through the center of the fovea, and choroidal vascularity index (CVI) obtained after binarizing processing revealed 68.3%. —multipanel pictures from the Authors' collection.

managing persistent conditions. Current investigations have verified that anti-VEGF drugs offer more significant benefits than corticosteroids in the treatment of retinal edema resulting from CRVO. A more substantial percentage of patients who were administered intravitreal anti-VEGF injections experienced an improvement of at least 15 letters compared with those who received corticosteroid treatment at 6-month and 12-month intervals. Among these anti-VEGF medicines, aflibercept and ranibizumab have shown better efficacy in improving BCVA and reducing CRT. A network meta-analysis revealed that, compared with aflibercept and ranibizumab, dexamethasone was more likely to cause increased IOP. Compared with ranibizumab, dexamethasone had a greater probability of causing cataract formation. Aflibercept was superior in reducing the occurrence of significant vitreous hemorrhage. Aflibercept demonstrated marginal superiority over ranibizumab regarding benefit risk, but no statistically significant difference was detected. Every patient must have an individual evaluation to determine the most suitable treatment regimen [75, 76, 80, 81].

Finally, another essential retinal perfusion marker used to evaluate patients with RVOs is the ischemic index (ISI), which is the ratio of the area of the nonperfused retina to the total fundus retina area for evaluating perfusion status. Traditionally, ultrawide field FFA (UWFFA) sequence imaging should be used in patients with RVOs to assess and quantify ISIs, which represents another potential way to treat and prevent abnormal neovascularization. This method compares a single image that best illustrates retinal nonperfusion to a summarized UWFFA image generated by the computerized superimposition of angiograms. Then, nonperfused and ungradable retinal areas are outlined, and the ISIs between the single and summarized images are compared. The computer-generated summarized images are similar to single images for grading the ISI in BRVO and CRVO, thus facilitating surveillance and management [82].

Patients with an association between RVO and glaucoma have been reported previously. Recent studies in patients with unilateral RVO have shown that the peripapillary retinal nerve fiber layer (pRNFL) is thinner than in healthy patients. This finding indicates the possible existence of shared systemic risk factors for RVO and glaucoma [83]. Additional well-designed RCTs should be conducted to elucidate the causes of functional and structural alterations in the pRNFL and GCC in patients with unilateral BRVO and unaffected and affected eyes [84].

Extensive research has been dedicated to identifying potential treatments that could affect NPAs because of their importance in evaluating RVO progression and determining appropriate therapies based on the importance of biomarkers. This is crucial for preventing retinal complications such as bleeding, macular edema, and rubeosis iridis. These efforts involve the use of anti-VEGF therapy to slow the progression of NPA. Consistent and frequent dosing of anti-VEGF therapy may be effective for achieving this outcome in certain patients. However, it is essential to note that reperfusion, a phenomenon not usually observed with anti-VEGF treatment, is the desired outcome. Furthermore, several different molecular entities that employ novel modes of action, such as the modulation of the semaphorin-3 pathway, are currently being investigated in ongoing clinical trials [85, 86].

The utilization of artificial intelligence (AI) has significantly expanded and deepened, particularly in the domain of retinal vascular disorders. AI-based research studies offer significant potential for the early detection and treatment of retinal vascular illnesses [87].

7. Goals for the future

Continuous research on choroidal perfusion in patients with RVO is required to provide crucial insights into novel pharmacological molecules for treating this condition. Additionally, further exploration is necessary to address knowledge gaps and enhance patient care.

Developing animal models that can assess choroidal perfusion through the CVI, CFA, and other perfusion markers to simulate and better comprehend the pathophysiology of retinal venous obstructive disease could lead to developing new drugs to treat or prevent the disease process and reduce vision loss.

The natural history of vascular obstructive disease and the potential risk factors for its progression can be better understood through longitudinal investigations that track the evolution of the disease and its correlation with perfusion changes over time.

Emerging imaging methods, including enhanced indocyanine green angiography (ICGA), ultrawide-field OCT-A, and CVI assessment through binarizing processes, offer promising avenues for studying choroidal and retinal perfusion, as well as their relationship with vision rehabilitation and recovery.

Collaborative large-scale studies that combine multiple sites and patient cohorts could produce larger sample sizes, greater statistical significance, and more generalizable results.

More research is required to create methods that can speed up the restoration of blood flow to RVOs occurring in areas where blood vessels are obstructed. This is important for preventing the pathological development of new blood vessels on the retina's surface. Pharmacological inhibition of the semaphorin-3 pathway produced by neurons may aid in encouraging the natural regrowth of blood vessels in the retina.

The development and utilization of artificial intelligence (AI) programs with deep learning models should continue to be explored to recognize RVOs early and reduce vision damage.

8. Concluding remarks

Proper circulation in the retina, particularly in the macular area, is crucial for good eye health. We used nIR, FFA, and OCT-A, among other methods, to learn about and evaluate changes in retinal blood flow mechanisms. Researchers have utilized OCT-A to determine the retinal blood vasculature and look for racial, age-, sex-, and lifestyle-related variations. The ability of OCT-A to noninvasively produce a detailed image of retinal blood vessels and perfusion makes it a valuable tool for the noninvasive diagnosis of illnesses affecting retinal blood flow, such as RVO. The current focus of RVO studies includes the quantitative assessment of the ISI, the FAZ and NPA areas, vascular density, perfusion in the SCP and DCP, CVI, and CFA, and their correlation with macular function and response to treatment. The use of OCT-A will not only enhance our understanding of alterations in the intricate microvasculature of the macula following vein occlusion but also undoubtedly play a crucial role in the treatment of patients with RVO in the future.

According to the current studies, compared with other imaging and visualization techniques, such as nIR or FFA, OCT-A can offer a clearer picture of the consequences and effects of RVO on blood perfusion. This is because no other imaging technique can match the depth and resolution of OCT-A. This chapter discusses cases where other methods fail to detect the retinal blood vasculature specific to OCT-A. Furthermore, OCT-A does not cause cataracts, unlike nIR, which harms eyesight in another way. Additionally, unlike OCT-A, FFA requires fluorescein dye. By mapping and measuring the retinal vascular network and blood flow, OCT-A has dramatically enhanced our understanding of RVO processes. OCT-A allows the visualization and investigation of various qualitative and quantitative changes in retinal blood flow. Studying and quantifying any increase in retinal blood flow can also help determine therapeutic outcomes in addition to diagnosis. Glucocorticoids and anti-VEGF drugs have been approved for RVO treatment. Dexamethasone implants are a standard glucocorticoid option for treating RVO and improving visual acuity. Anti-VEGF medications are the most effective treatments for RVO. Currently, the most common first-line treatments for RVO are aflibercept and ranibizumab.

Future therapeutic alternatives, such as the recently approved dual-acting faricimab, may offer further benefits for RVO treatment. Furthermore, PDSs can improve treatment outcomes and patient compliance when used to treat RVO. Advances in our knowledge and ability to treat RVO may result in a general increase in patient's visual acuity and the prevention of blindness.

Acknowledgements

We sincerely appreciate the technical staff of the Retina Specialists Unit at Oftalmologia Integral ABC, which is affiliated with the Postgraduate Division of Studies at the National Autonomous University of Mexico.

Conflict of interests

The authors declare that they have no conflict of interests.

Third-party financial contributions

The authors declare that they received no third-party financial contributions.

List of abbreviations

AI	artificial intelligence
AMD	age-related macular degeneration
Ang2	angiopoietin-2
BCVA	best-corrected visual acuity
BP	blood pressure
BRVO	branch retinal vein occlusion
CFA	choriocapillaris foveal area
CMT	central macular thickness
CRVO	central retinal vein occlusion
CRT	central retinal thickness
CST	central subfield thickness

CVI	choroidal vascularity index
DCP	deep capillary plexus
DRIL	disorganized inner retinal layers
DROL	disruption of retinal outer layers
DRL	deep retinal layer
EDI-CVI	enhanced depth imaging-choroidal vascularity index
EZ	ellipsoid zone
FAZ	foveal avascular zone
FA	fluorescein angiography
FFA	fundus fluorescein angiography
GCC	ganglion cell complex
GCL	ganglion cell layer
HRVO	hemiretinal vein occlusion
ICP	inner capillary plexus
ICGA	indocyanine green angiography
INL	inner nuclear layer
IPL	inner perivascular layer
IOP	intraocular pressure
IPL	inner plexiform layer
ISI	ischemic index
ME	macular edema
NFL	nerve fiber layer
nIR	near-infrared
NS-RL	nonsegmented retina layer
NPAs	nonperfused areas
NV	neovascularization
NVD	neovascularization of the disc
NVE	neovascularization elsewhere
OCT-A	optical coherence tomography angiography
ONL	outer nuclear layer
OPP	ocular perfusion pressure
OVCs	optic disc venous collaterals
PAMM	paracentral acute middle maculopathy
PDS	the port delivery system with ranibizumab
PRP	panretinal photocoagulation
PR-OCT	projection resolved OCT
pRNFL	peripapillary retinal nerve fiber layer
RPCP	radial peripapillary capillary plexus
RNFL	retinal nerve fiber layer
RVO	retinal vein occlusion
SCP	superficial capillary plexus
SRL	superficial retina layer
UWFFA	ultrawide field FFA
2D	two-dimensional
3D	three-dimensional
US-FDA	United States-food and drug administration
VD	vessel density
VDI	vascular diameter index

Author details

Miguel Angel Quiroz-Reyes*, Erick Quiroz-Gonzalez and Miguel A. Quiroz-Gonzalez
Oftalmologia Integral ABC, Retina Specialist Unit, The Medical and Surgical Assistance Institution (Nonprofit Organization) is affiliated with the Postgraduate Studies Division at the National Autonomous University of Mexico, Lomas de Chapultepec, Mexico City, Mexico

*Address all correspondence to: drquiroz@prodigy.net.mx

References

[1] Provis J. Development of the primate retinal vasculature. Progress in Retinal and Eye Research. 2001;**20**(6):799-821

[2] Alterman M, Henkind P. Radial peripapillary capillaries of the retina. II. Possible role in Bjerrum scotoma. The British Journal of Ophthalmology. 1968;**52**(1):26-31

[3] Henkind P. Radial peripapillary capillaries of the retina. I. Anatomy: Human and comparative. The British Journal of Ophthalmology. 1967;**51**(2):115-123

[4] Campbell JP, Zhang M, Hwang TS, Bailey ST, Wilson DJ, Jia Y, et al. Detailed vascular anatomy of the human retina by projection-resolved optical coherence tomography angiography. Scientific Reports. 2017;7:42201

[5] Snodderly D, Weinhaus R, Choi J. Neural-vascular relationships in central retina of macaque monkeys (*Macaca fascicularis*). The Journal of Neuroscience. 1992;**12**(4):1169-1193

[6] Chan G, Balaratnasingam C, Yu PK, Morgan WH, McAllister IL, Cringle SJ, et al. Quantitative morphometry of perifoveal capillary networks in the human retina. Investigative Ophthalmology & Visual Science. 2012;**53**(9):5502

[7] Tan PEZ, Yu PK, Balaratnasingam C, Cringle SJ, Morgan WH, McAllister IL, et al. Quantitative confocal imaging of the retinal microvasculature in the human retina. Investigative Ophthalmology & Visual Science. 2012;**53**(9):5728

[8] Boltz A, Luksch A, Wimpissinger B, Maar N, Weigert G, Frantal S, et al. Choroidal blood flow and progression of age-related macular degeneration in the fellow eye in patients with unilateral choroidal neovascularization. Investigative Ophthalmology & Visual Science. 2010;**51**(8):4220

[9] Vingerling JR, Dielemans I, Bots ML, Hofman A, Grobbee DE, de Jong PTVM. Age-related macular degeneration is associated with atherosclerosis. American Journal of Epidemiology. 1995;**142**(4):404-409

[10] Hyman L. Hypertension, cardiovascular disease, and age-related macular degeneration. Archives of Ophthalmology. 2000;**118**(3):351

[11] Yen YC, Weng SF, Chen HA, Lin YS. Risk of retinal vein occlusion in patients with systemic lupus erythematosus: A population-based cohort study. The British Journal of Ophthalmology. 2013;**97**(9):1192-1196

[12] O'Mahoney PRA, Wong DT, Ray JG. Retinal vein occlusion and traditional risk factors for atherosclerosis. Archives of Ophthalmology. 2008;**126**(5):692-699

[13] Ip M, Hendrick A. Retinal vein occlusion review. Asia-Pacific Journal of Ophthalmology. 2018;**7**(1):40-45

[14] Sivaprasad S, Amoaku WM, Hykin P. The Royal College of ophthalmologists guidelines on retinal vein occlusions: Executive summary. Eye. 2015;**29**(12):1633-1638

[15] Singer M, Cohen S, Groth S, Porbandarwalla S. Comparing bevacizumab and ranibizumab for initial reduction of central macular thickness in patients with retinal vein occlusions. Clinical Ophthalmology. 2013;**1377**

[16] Onda E, Cioffi GA, Bacon DR, van Buskirk EM. Microvasculature of the human optic nerve. American Journal of Ophthalmology. 1995;**120**(1):92-102

[17] Delaney C, van de Voorde J. Regulatory mechanisms in the retinal and choroidal circulation. Ophthalmic Research. 2000;**32**(6):249-256

[18] Iester M, Torre PG, Bricola G, Bagnis A, Calabria G. Retinal blood flow autoregulation after dynamic exercise in healthy young subjects. Ophthalmologica. 2007;**221**(3):180-185

[19] Liang Y, Fortune B, Cull G, Cioffi GA, Wang L. Quantification of dynamic blood flow autoregulation in optic nerve head of rhesus monkeys. Experimental Eye Research. 2010;**90**(2):203-209

[20] Lesk MR, Wajszilber M, Deschenes MC. The effects of systemic medications on ocular blood flow. Canadian Journal of Ophthalmology. 2008;**43**(3):351-355

[21] Pournaras C. Autoregulation of ocular blood flow. In: Kaiser HJ, Flammer J, Hendrickson P, editors. Ocular Blood Flow: Glaucoma Meeting 1995. Basel, Switzerland: Karger Basel Publications; 1996. pp. 40-50

[22] Garhofer G, Werkmeister R, Dragostinoff N, Schmetterer L. Retinal blood flow in healthy young subjects. Investigative Opthalmology & Visual Science. 2012;**53**(2):698

[23] Siesky B, Harris A, Verticchio Vercellin AC, Guidoboni G, Tsai JC. Ocular blood flow as it relates to race and disease on glaucoma. Advances in Ophthalmology and Optometry. 2021;**6**:245-262

[24] Kim KE, Oh S, Baek SU, Ahn SJ, Park KH, Jeoung JW. Ocular perfusion pressure and the risk of open-angle glaucoma: Systematic review and meta-analysis. Scientific Reports. 2020;**10**(1):10056

[25] Milani P, Bochicchio S, Urbini LE, Bulone E, Callegarin S, Pisano L, et al. Diurnal measurements of macular thickness and vessel density on OCT angiography in healthy eyes and those with ocular hypertension and glaucoma. Journal of Glaucoma. 2020;**29**(10):918-925

[26] Ayhan Z, Kaya M, Ozturk T, Karti O, Hakan OF. Evaluation of macular perfusion in healthy smokers by using optical coherence tomography angiography. Ophthalmic Surgery, Lasers and Imaging Retina. 2017;**48**(8):617-622

[27] Galina D, Etsuo C, Takuhei S, Kanno J, Antonela L, Olivera L, et al. Immediate effect of yoga exercises for eyes on the macular thickness. International Journal of Yoga. 2020;**13**(3):223

[28] Kaya M, Ayhan Z, Ozturk AT, Kocak N, Arikan G, Kaynak S. Evaluation of the macular and choroidal perfusion in healthy Turkish population using optical coherence tomography angiography. Korean Journal of Ophthalmology. 2021;**35**(5):360-367

[29] Rogers S, McIntosh RL, Cheung N, Lim L, Wang JJ, Mitchell P, et al. The prevalence of retinal vein occlusion: Pooled data from population studies from the United States, Europe, Asia, and Australia. Ophthalmology. 2010;**117**(2):313-319.e1

[30] Vaz-Pereira S et al. International Journal of Retina and Vitreous. 2020;**6**:26

[31] Wong TY, Scott IU. Retinal-vein occlusion. New England Journal of Medicine. 2010;**363**(22):2135-2144

[32] Bonini Filho MA, Adhi M, de Carlo TE, Ferrara D, Baumal CR, Witkin AJ, et al. Optical coherence tomography angiography in retinal artery occlusion. Retina. 2015;**35**(11):2339-2346

[33] Glacet-Bernard A, Sellam A, Coscas F, Coscas G, Souied EH. Optical coherence tomography angiography in retinal vein occlusion treated with dexamethasone implant: A new test for follow-up evaluation. European Journal of Ophthalmology. 2016;**26**(5):460-468

[34] Adhi M, Filho MAB, Louzada RN, Kuehlewein L, de Carlo TE, Baumal CR, et al. Retinal capillary network and Foveal avascular zone in eyes with vein occlusion and fellow eyes analyzed with optical coherence tomography angiography. Investigative Ophthalmology & Visual Science. 2016;**57**(9):OCT486

[35] Suzuki N, Hirano Y, Yoshida M, Tomiyasu T, Uemura A, Yasukawa T, et al. Microvascular abnormalities on optical coherence tomography angiography in macular Edema associated with branch retinal vein occlusion. American Journal of Ophthalmology. 2016;**161**:126-132.e1

[36] Moussa M, Leila M, Bessa AS, Lolah M, Abou Shousha M, el Hennawi HM, et al. Grading of macular perfusion in retinal vein occlusion using en-face swept-source optical coherence tomography angiography: A retrospective observational case series. BMC Ophthalmology. 2019;**19**(1):127

[37] Coscas F, Glacet-Bernard A, Miere A, Caillaux V, Uzzan J, Lupidi M, et al. Optical coherence tomography angiography in retinal vein occlusion: Evaluation of superficial and deep capillary Plexa. American Journal of Ophthalmology. 2016;**161**:160-171.e2

[38] Martinet V, Guigui B, Glacet-Bernard A, Zourdani A, Coscas G, Soubrane G, et al. Macular edema in central retinal vein occlusion: Correlation between optical coherence tomography, angiography, and visual acuity. International Ophthalmology. 2012;**32**(4):369-377. DOI: 10.1007/s10792-012-9578-5. Epub 2012 May 6

[39] Tsai G, Banaee T, Conti F, Singh R. Optical coherence tomography angiography in eyes with retinal vein occlusion. Journal of Ophthalmic and Vision Research. 2018;**13**(3):315

[40] Rispoli M, Savastano MC, Lumbroso B. Capillary network anomalies in branch retinal vein occlusion on optical coherence tomography angiography. Retina. 2015;**35**(11):2332-2338

[41] Mastropasqua R, Toto L, di Antonio L, Borrelli E, Senatore A, di Nicola M, et al. Optical coherence tomography angiography microvascular findings in macular edema due to central and branch retinal vein occlusions. Scientific Reports. 2017;**7**(1):40763

[42] Kashani AH, Lee SY, Moshfeghi A, Durbin MK, Puliafito CA. Optical coherence tomography angiography of retinal venous occlusion. Retina. 2015;**35**(11):2323-2331

[43] Sogawa K, Nagaoka T, Ishibazawa A, Takahashi A, Tani T, Yoshida A. En-face optical coherence tomography angiography of neovascularization elsewhere in hemicentral retinal vein occlusion. International Medical Case Reports Journal. 2015;**8**:263

[44] Kadomoto S, Muraoka Y, Ooto S, Miwa Y, Iida Y, Suzuma K, et al. Evaluation of macular ischemia in eyes with branch retinal vein occlusion. Retina. 2018 Feb;**38**(2):272-282

[45] Koulisis N, Kim AY, Chu Z, Shahidzadeh A, Burkemper B, Olmos de Koo LC, et al. Quantitative microvascular analysis of retinal venous occlusions by spectral domain optical coherence tomography angiography. PLoS One. 2017;**12**(4):e0176404

[46] Khodabandeh A, Shahraki K, Roohipoor R, Riazi-Esfahani H, Yaseri M, Faghihi H, et al. Quantitative vascular density and flow measurement using optical coherence tomography angiography (OCTA) in patients with central retinal vein occlusion: Can OCTA help distinguish ischemic from nonischemic type? International Journal of Retina and Vitreous. 2018;**4**(1):47

[47] Casalino G, Williams M, McAvoy C, Bandello F, Chakravarthy U. Optical coherence tomography angiography in paracentral acute middle maculopathy secondary to central retinal vein occlusion. Eye. 2016;**30**(6):888-893

[48] Dansingani KK, Inoue M, Engelbert M, Freund KB. Optical coherence tomographic angiography shows reduced deep capillary flow in paracentral acute middle maculopathy. Eye. 2015;**29**(12):1620-1624

[49] He F, Yu W. Longitudinal neovascular changes on optical coherence tomography angiography in proliferative diabetic retinopathy treated with pan-retinal photocoagulation alone versus with intravitreal concept plus pan-retinal photocoagulation: A pilot study. Eye. 2020;**34**(8):1413-1418

[50] Clarkson JG, Chuang E, Gass D, Pedroso M, Cubillas T, Duria ES, et al. Evaluation of grid pattern photocoagulation for macular Edema in central vein occlusion. Ophthalmology. 1995;**102**(10):1425-1433

[51] The Branch Vein Occlusion Study Group. Argon laser photocoagulation for macular Edema in branch vein occlusion. American Journal of Ophthalmology. 1984;**98**(3):271-282

[52] The Branch Vein Occlusion Study Group. Argon laser scatter photocoagulation for prevention of neovascularization and vitreous hemorrhage in branch vein occlusion. Archives of Ophthalmology. 1986;**104**(1):34

[53] Scott IU, Ip MS, VanVeldhuisen PC, Oden NL, Blodi BA, Fisher M, et al. A randomized trial comparing the efficacy and safety of intravitreal triamcinolone with standard care to treat vision loss associated with macular edema secondary to branch retinal vein occlusion. Archives of Ophthalmology. 2009;**127**(9):1115

[54] Scott IU, Ip MS, VanVeldhuisen PC, Oden NL, Blodi BA, Fisher M, et al. A randomized trial comparing the efficacy and safety of intravitreal triamcinolone with observation to treat vision loss associated with macular edema secondary to central retinal vein occlusion. Archives of Ophthalmology. 2009;**127**(9):1101

[55] Haller JA, Bandello F, Belfort R, Blumenkranz MS, Gillies M, Heier J, et al. Randomized, sham-controlled trial of dexamethasone intravitreal implant in patients with macular edema due to retinal vein occlusion. Ophthalmology. 2010;**117**(6):1134-1146.e3

[56] Qian T, Zhao M, Xu X. Comparison between anti-VEGF therapy and corticosteroid or laser therapy for macular edema secondary to retinal vein occlusion: A meta-analysis. Journal of Clinical Pharmacy and Therapeutics. 2017;**42**(5):519-529

[57] Campochiaro PA, Akhlaq A. Sustained suppression of VEGF for

retinal/choroidal vascular disease treatment. Progress in Retinal and Eye Research. 2021;**83**:100921

[58] Stahl A, Buchwald A, Martin G, Junker B, Chen J, Hansen LL, et al. Vitreal levels of erythropoietin are increased in patients with retinal vein occlusion and correlate with vitreal VEGF and the extent of macular edema. Retina. 2010;**30**(9):1524-1529

[59] Brown DM, Campochiaro PA, Singh RP, Li Z, Gray S, Saroj N, et al. Ranibizumab for macular Edema following central retinal vein occlusion. Ophthalmology. 2010;**117**(6):1124-1133.e1

[60] Campochiaro PA, Heier JS, Feiner L, Gray S, Saroj N, Rundle AC, et al. Ranibizumab for macular Edema following branch retinal vein occlusion. Ophthalmology. 2010;**117**(6):1102-1112.e1

[61] Brown DM, Campochiaro PA, Bhisitkul RB, Ho AC, Gray S, Saroj N, et al. Sustained benefits from ranibizumab for macular edema following branch retinal vein occlusion: 12-month outcomes of a phase III study. Ophthalmology. 2011;**118**(8):1594-1602

[62] Campochiaro PA, Brown DM, Awh CC, Lee SY, Gray S, Saroj N, et al. Sustained benefits from ranibizumab for macular edema following central retinal vein occlusion: Twelve-month outcomes of a phase III study. Ophthalmology. 2011;**118**(10):2041-2049

[63] Heier JS, Campochiaro PA, Yau L, Li Z, Saroj N, Rubio RG, et al. Ranibizumab for macular edema due to retinal vein occlusions. Ophthalmology. 2012;**119**(4):802-809

[64] Iida-Miwa Y, Muraoka Y, Iida Y, Ooto S, Murakami T, Suzuma K, et al. Branch retinal vein occlusion: Treatment outcomes according to the retinal nonperfusion area, clinical subtype, and crossing pattern. Scientific Reports. 2019;**9**(1):6569

[65] Zhang H, Liu ZL, Sun P, Gu F. Intravitreal bevacizumab for treatment of macular edema secondary to central retinal vein occlusion: Eighteen-month results of a prospective trial. Journal of Ocular Pharmacology and Therapeutics. 2011;**27**(6):615-621

[66] Choi KE, Yun C, Cha J, Kim SW. OCT angiography features associated with macular edema recurrence after intravitreal bevacizumab treatment in branch retinal vein occlusion. Scientific Reports. 2019;**9**(1):14153

[67] Brown DM, Heier JS, Clark WL, Boyer DS, Vitti R, Berliner AJ, et al. Intravitreal aflibercept injection for macular edema secondary to central retinal vein occlusion: 1-year results from the phase 3 COPERNICUS study. American Journal of Ophthalmology. 2013;**155**(3):429-437.e7

[68] Campochiaro PA, Clark WL, Boyer DS, Heier JS, Brown DM, Vitti R, et al. Intravitreal aflibercept for macular edema following branch retinal vein occlusion. Ophthalmology. 2015;**122**(3):538-544

[69] Ghashut R, Muraoka Y, Ooto S, Iida Y, Miwa Y, Suzuma K, et al. Evaluation of macular ischemia in eyes with central retinal vein occlusion. Retina. 2018;**38**(8):1571-1580

[70] Amer AA, Aldghaimy AH, Abdellah MM et al. Ranibizumab versus aflibercept for macular edema secondary to nonischemic central retinal vein occlusion in young adult patients, 30 March 2022, Preprint (Version 1) available at research square. DOI: 10.21203/rs.3.rs-1490565/v1

[71] A study to evaluate the efficacy and safety of faricimab in participants with macular edema secondary to branch retinal vein occlusion (Balaton). Available from: https://clinicaltrials.gov/ct2/show/NCT04740905

[72] A study to evaluate the efficacy and safety of faricimab in participants with macular edema secondary to central retinal or hemiretinal vein occlusion (COMINO). Available from: https://clinicaltrials.gov/ct2/show/NCT04740931.

[73] Heier JS, Singh RP, Wykoff CC, Csaky KG, Lai TYY, Loewenstein A, et al. The angiopoietin/tie pathway in retinal vascular diseases. Retina. 2021;**41**(1):1-19

[74] FDA approves Genentech's Susvimo, a first-of-its-kind therapeutic approach for wet age-related macular degeneration (AMD). Available from: https://www.gene.com/media/press-releases/14935/2021-10-22/fda-approves-genentechs-susvimo-a-first-

[75] Ranade SV, Wieland MR, Tam T, Rea JC, Horvath J, Hieb AR, et al. The port delivery system with ranibizumab: A new paradigm for long-acting retinal drug delivery. Drug Delivery. 2022;**29**(1):1326-1334

[76] Ghanchi F, Bourne R, Downes SM, Gale R, Rennie C, Tapply I, et al. An update on long-acting therapies in chronic sight-threatening eye diseases of the posterior segment: AMD, DMO, RVO, uveitis, and glaucoma. Eye. 2022;**36**(6):1154-1167

[77] Loiudice P, Covello G, Figus M, Posarelli C, Sartini MS, Casini G. Choroidal vascularity index in central and branch retinal vein occlusion. Journal of Clinical Medicine. 2022;**11**(16):4756. DOI: 10.3390/jcm11164756

[78] Mrejen S, Spaide RF. Optical coherence tomography: Imaging of the choroid and beyond. Survey of Ophthalmology. 2013;**58**(5):387-429. DOI: 10.1016/j.survophthal.2012.12.001. Epub 2013. Aug 2

[79] Tsuiki E, Suzuma K, Ueki R, Maekawa Y, Kitaoka T. Enhanced depth imaging optical coherence tomography of the choroid in central retinal vein occlusion. American Journal of Ophthalmology. 2013;**156**(3):543-547.e1. DOI: 10.1016/j.ajo.2013.04.008 Epub 2013 May 17

[80] Hahn P, Fekrat S. Best practices for treatment of retinal vein occlusion. Current Opinion in Ophthalmology. 2012;**23**(3):175-181. DOI: 10.1097/ICU.0b013e3283524148

[81] Qian T, Zhao M, Wan Y, et al. Comparison of the efficacy and safety of drug therapies for macular edema secondary to central retinal vein occlusion. BMJ Open. 2018;**8**:e022700. DOI: 10.1136/bmjopen-2018-022700

[82] Tsui I, Kaines A, Havunjian Margaret A, Hubschman S, Heilweil G, Prasad PS, et al. Ischemic index and neovascularization in central retinal vein occlusion. Retina. 2011;**31**(1):105-110. DOI: 10.1097/IAE.0b013e3181e36c6d

[83] Goda I, Saliem EA, Mostafa SM, Amin AM, Omran MY, Eltantawy B, et al. Longitudinal changes in peripapillary retinal nerve fiber layer thickness in patients with unilateral branch retinal vein occlusion. Medical Hypothesis, Discovery and Innovation Ophthalmology Journal. 2023;**12**(2):62-69. DOI: 10.51329/mehdiophthal1471

[84] Sorour OA, Mehta N, Baumal CR, Ishibazawa A, Liu K, Konstantinou EK, et al. Morphological changes in

intraretinal microvascular abnormalities after anti-VEGF therapy visualized on optical coherence tomography angiography. Eye and vision (London, England). 2020;7:29

[85] Joyal JS, Sitaras N, Binet F, Rivera JC, Stahl A, Zaniolo K, et al. Ischemic neurons prevent vascular regeneration of neural tissue by secreting semaphorin 3A. Blood. 2011;**117**:6024-6035

[86] Zippel N, Kenny CH, Wu H, Garneau M, Kroe-Barrett R, Gupta P, et al. Sema3A antibody BI-X prevents cell permeability and cytoskeletal collapse in HRMECs and increases tip cell density in mouse oxygen-induced retinopathy. Translational Vision Science & Technology. 2022;**11**:17

[87] Ji Y, Ji Y, Liu Y, Zhao Y, Zhang L. Research progress on diagnosing retinal vascular diseases based on artificial intelligence and fundus images. Frontiers in Cell and Development Biology. 2023;**11**:1168327. DOI: 10.3389/fcell.2023.1168327

Chapter 11

Optical Coherence Tomography and Optical Coherence Tomography Angiography Biomarkers in Diabetic Retinopathy

Ceren Durmaz Engin

Abstract

Optical Coherence Tomography (OCT) and Optical Coherence Tomography Angiography (OCTA) are essential tools for the diagnosis, treatment, and prognosis of diabetic retinopathy (DR) and diabetic macular edema (DME). OCT biomarkers, such as retinal thickness, intraretinal cystoid spaces, hyperreflective retinal foci, and disorganization of retinal inner layers, provide critical insights into disease severity and treatment response. OCTA offers a detailed understanding of retinal microvascular alterations, utilizing metrics like vessel density and choriocapillaris flow deficits. This chapter emphasizes the predictive value of these biomarkers, highlighting their role in early detection, precise monitoring, and selecting appropriate therapeutic strategies. By integrating OCT and OCTA, clinicians can enhance visual outcomes and optimize the management of DR and DME.

Keywords: diabetic retinopathy, diabetic macular edema, optical coherence tomography, optical coherence tomography angiography, biomarkers

1. Introduction

Diabetes mellitus (DM), a disease marked by elevated blood glucose levels due to metabolic dysfunction, affects 537 million adults aged 20–79 years globally, a figure projected to rise to 643 million by 2030 and 783 million by 2045 [1]. Diabetic retinopathy (DR), a vascular complication of DM, is the leading cause of blindness among adults of working age. A recent meta-analysis revealed a global prevalence of 22.27% for DR, 6.17% for vision-threatening DR, and 4.07% for clinically significant diabetic macular edema (CS-DME) among diabetic individuals [2].

The pathophysiology of DR involves capillary endothelial cell proliferation, basement membrane thickening, and pericyte loss, leading to microaneurysms (MAs), increased vessel permeability, blood-retinal barrier (BRB) destruction, and neurodegeneration due to chronic hyperglycemia [3]. This results in diabetic macular edema

(DME), the primary cause of vision loss among diabetic patients. Without treatment, about 50% of DME patients lose more than two lines of visual acuity (VA) within two years [4]. In advanced stages, capillary blockage and ischemia lead to new blood vessel formation, resulting in proliferative diabetic retinopathy (PDR).

Clinically, DR is identified by the presence of MAs, intraretinal hemorrhages, cotton wool spots, and venous beading. Advanced stages may exhibit neovascularization (NV), vitreous hemorrhage (VH), and tractional retinal detachment (TRD). Diagnostic modalities for detecting DR include fundus fluorescein angiography (FFA), which is essential for visualizing retinal microvascular abnormalities, NVs, and areas of retinal non-perfusion. Fundus autofluorescence (FAF) aids in diagnosing DR by detecting changes in the retinal pigment epithelium (RPE) and providing information on metabolic stress within the retina. Ultra-widefield (UWF) imaging captures a comprehensive view of the peripheral retina, detecting lesions that conventional methods might miss. However, in contemporary practice, Optical Coherence Tomography (OCT) and Optical Coherence Tomography Angiography (OCTA) play a more significant role in the screening and diagnosis of DR, offering high-resolution images and detailed views of retinochoroidal vasculature without any dye injection [5].

OCT has become essential in assessing DR due to its non-invasive, reproducible, high-resolution, cross-sectional retinal imaging capability. It does not require skilled operation or pupil dilation and can detect subtle retinal changes not visible during clinical examination [6]. OCT is valuable for both the quantitative and qualitative assessment of structural changes in DR, specifically DME. Various imaging biomarkers have been identified to determine severity, prognosticate, assess treatment response, and detect disease recurrence [7–9].

OCTA is an advanced imaging modality that provides detailed visualization of the retinochoroidal circulation. It separates capillaries at three different levels, identifying MAs, capillary non-perfusion areas (NPAs), and neovascularization before they are clinically apparent [10]. Morphological and qualitative assessment of vascular changes via OCTA aids in understanding the pathophysiological processes, treatment, and follow-up of DR.

This chapter will discuss OCT and OCTA-related biomarkers in the diagnosis, treatment, and prognosis of DR.

2. OCT biomarkers of diabetic retinopathy

2.1 Retinal biomarkers

2.1.1 Retinal thickness

In DME, increased retinal thickness can be present secondary to a breakdown of the BRB and extravasation of fluid into and beneath the retina. The most common terms indicating retinal thickness measurements in OCT are given in **Table 1**.

Numerous studies have examined retinal thickness measurements using OCT. Markan et al. [11] showed that central subfield thickness (CST) might not be reliable for prognosis in DR patients, as the location, extent, and pattern of DME, along with other OCT-related parameters, should be considered. Contrarily, Saxena et al. [12] identified three OCT biomarkers, mean CST, cube volume (CV), and central area thickness (CAT), as valid diagnostic and predictive factors for DME. Their study

Retinal thickness	Definition
Central retinal thickness (CRT)/ Central subfield thickness (CST)	The mean retinal thickness within the circular field of 1-mm diameter surrounding the foveola
Central foveal thickness (CFT) / Center point thickness (CPT)	The retinal thickness at the intersection of the six radial OCT scans
Macular volume (MV)	The sum of all volumes of all nine sections defined by the ETDRS grid
Cube average thickness (CAT)	The average thickness for the tissue layers between ILM and RPE over the entire 6 x 6 mm square area
Cube volume (CV)	The average volume of the tissue layers between ILM and RPE over the entire 6 × 6 mm square area

ETDRS, Early Treatment Diabetic Retinopathy Study; ILM, internal limiting membrane; OCT, optical coherence tomography; RPE, retinal pigment epithelium.

Table 1.
Definitions of retinal thickness measurements in optical coherence tomography.

found that significant increases in CST, CAT, and CV were correlated with the severity of DR. Despite these controversial results, failure to achieve a CST of <300 μm or a reduction of ≤10% in CST is generally seen as a suboptimal anatomical response to anti-vascular endothelial growth factor (anti-VEGF) therapy [13, 14].

Although retinal thickness is a major follow-up criterion in most of the studies, evidence has shown differing correlation between retinal thickness values and both initial and final VA. A subanalysis of the Study of Ranibizumab Injection in Subjects with CD-DME with Center Involvement Secondary to DM (RIDE and RISE) trials revealed that patients with non-significant changes in central foveal thickness (CFT) after anti-VEGF therapy showed similar VA gains and DR improvement as those with early retinal thinning [14]. Similarly, in the Protocol T study, people with 20/40 or better vision who were given bevacizumab (BVZ) treatment had the same functional improvements as those who were given other anti-VEGF drugs, even though they had thicker retina [15]. The study also indicated that while a single CST measurement might modestly correlate with VA, CST fluctuation between visits could be a prognostic indicator. On the other hand, Zhang et al. [7] used machine learning to predict DME patient outcomes after anti-VEGF treatment, identifying CST as a critical predictive factor for VA prognosis. The reason for these contradictory results could be due to the fact that edema can stretch the retina beyond its capacity, causing damage to bipolar axons and permanent changes to the RPE. This, in turn, can lead to VA recovery that does not align with edema resolution. Also, a decrease in CST is not always desirable, as central foveal atrophy, defined as CST below 200 μm, can occur in about 4% of treated DR eyes. In a study by Karst et al. [16], the patients who developed atrophy initially had higher CST and lower VA and received both intravitreal injections and laser treatments for DME.

Macular volume (MV), though strongly correlated with CST, is unlikely to be a reliable prognostic marker due to conflicting results of its relationship with vision in eyes with DRP. Hannouche et al. [17] found that MV is correlated with VA, while Maheswary et al. [18] found no significant correlation. The poor correlation between MV and VA may be due to MV considering extra-foveal thickness, whereas VA reflects foveal function.

2.1.2 Intraretinal cystoid spaces

Intraretinal cystoid spaces (ICS) around the fovea stem from inner BRB disruption due to elevated VEGF levels and Müller cell dysfunction. The prognostic significance of ICS depends on their location, size, and the presence of hyperreflective material within. ICS are classified as small (<100 μm), large (101–200 μm), and giant (>200 μm) according to their size. Larger cysts are shown to be related to macular ischemia, which is an unfavorable prognostic factor for VA [19]. Large as well as giant intraretinal cysts may lead to irreversible visual loss by affecting the outer nuclear layer (ONL) and damage the inner segment/outer segment (IS/OS) junction. In long-standing cases, large coalescent macrocysts may indicate retinal cystoid degeneration (RCD), an end-stage result linked with Müller cell dysfunction or death [20]. A representative OCT image of a large retinal cyst is shown in **Figure 1**.

VEGF levels are crucial in ICS formation, and anti-VEGF therapy effectively reduces vessel permeability and ICS size and number. The location and size of ICS, as well as presence of hyperreflective material—likely fibrin and inflammatory by-products—within the cysts correlate with baseline VA, and improvement in macular anatomy as well as function during intravitreal anti-VEGF therapy [21]. ICS in the inner nuclear layer (INL) respond better to anti-VEGF or corticosteroids than those in the ONL. The inflammatory nature of ICS involves cytokines like Intercellular adhesion molecule 1 (ICAM-1), Interleukin-6 (IL-6), Interleukin-8 (IL-8), and Monocyte chemoattractant protein-1 (MCP-1) [22]. Improvement in ICS after dexamethasone (DEX) implant, related to inflammation reduction, has been reported in previous studies [9, 23].

2.1.3 Subretinal fluid

Subretinal fluid (SRF), resulting from outer retinal layer disruption and RPE dysfunction, leads to extracellular fluid accumulation. SRF is generally considered associated with worse VA than ICS at baseline. Although SRF usually responds quickly to treatment in DME cases, it is generally indicative of more severe disease [24].

There are contradictory results about the significance of SRF in DR. A recent study by Park et al. [25] found that the baseline SRF is both a valuable marker for a greater reduction in CST and an indicator of improvement in VA in DME cases. In the post hoc analysis of the Bevacizumab and Ranibizumab in Diabetic Macular Edema (BRDME) trial, eyes with SRF exhibited greater letter gains at 6 months compared

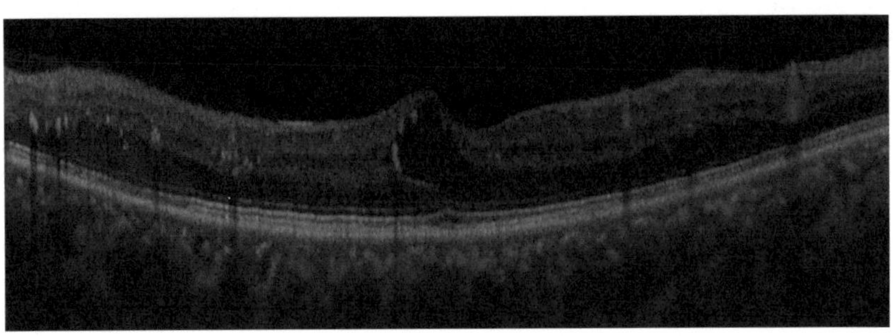

Figure 1.
The presence of a central large retinal cyst with hyperreflective retinal foci on its wall (Courtesy of Mahmut Kaya, MD).

to eyes without SRF, despite no significant difference in the reduction of CST [26]. On the other hand, in the Study of Intravitreal Aflibercept Injection in Patients With DME (VISTA) and Intravitreal Aflibercept Injection in Vision Impairment due to DME (VIVID) studies, although patients with baseline SRF had a greater treatment effect from aflibercept (AFL), SRF status did not significantly impact overall treatment outcomes with AFL [27]. In the Diabetic Retinopathy Clinical Research Network (DRCR) Protocol T, eyes with centrally located fluid had a mean of 23-μm greater reduction in CST, although no significant VA change was observed [28]. The morphology of retina in terms of edema type may affect the visual and anatomical results. The cystoid macular edema (CME) morphology was found to be favorable in achieving at least a 20% reduction in CST, followed by serous retinal detachment (SRD) and diffuse retinal thickening (DRT) in eyes treated with ranibizumab (RBZ) or AFL; however, morphology was not associated with visual outcome [29]. Similarly, a retrospective study reported that the CME subtype showed the greatest improvement in VA and reduction in CST in eyes treated with intravitreal triamcinolone acetonide (TA) compared to DRT and SRD subtypes [30].

The exact reasons for the association between SRF and improved outcomes are unclear. One hypothesis is that SRF acts as a physical barrier, protecting retinal structures from further damage. Additionally, SRF may contain protective substances, with anti-VEGF injections enhancing this effect. This is supported by studies indicating that eyes with SRF have a lower risk of developing geographic atrophy (GA) [31].

2.1.4 Disorganization of the retinal inner layers

Disorganization of the retinal inner layers (DRIL) is marked by the loss of clear boundaries between the ganglion cell complex (GCC), INL, and outer plexiform layer (OPL). This novel biomarker appears in various retinal diseases as a response to retinal stress and may represent disruptions in the neural transmission pathway involving bipolar, amacrine, and horizontal cells [32]. These disruptions impair the transmission of visual signals from photoreceptors to ganglion cells and the nerve fiber layer. Therefore, it's not surprising that DRIL has been associated with abnormalities in multiple measures of visual function, such as VA, contrast sensitivity, multifocal electroretinography (mfERG), and standard automated perimetry (SAP), even in the absence of DME [32, 33].

The exact pathophysiology of DRIL remains unclear, but it is proposed that mechanical stretching of bipolar axons due to chronic retinal thickening may cause damage, as Pelosini et al. [34] found that the neurosensory retina (NSR) has a degree of elasticity that if exceeded, leads to snapping of bipolar neurons. Also, macular ischemia may contribute to DRIL formation, as studies have found a correlation between DRIL and capillary non-perfusion on both FFA and OCTA [35].

DRIL is more frequently identified in eyes with increasing DR severity and is associated with worse visual outcomes. It is more likely to occur in mild to moderate non-proliferative diabetic retinopathy (NPDR) compared to diabetic patients without retinopathy, with the risk increasing with the duration of diabetes [32]. According to the study by Nadri et al. [36], there was a significant positive correlation between DRIL and CAT, CST, and the level of ellipsoid zone (EZ) disruption, while there was a negative correlation between DRIL and retinal nerve fiber layer (RNFL) thickness. Correlation has also been made between DRIL and other OCT findings, including enlargement of the FAZ and disruption of the external limiting membrane (ELM) [37, 38]. Moreover, DRIL can have a VA-predictive value independent of macular thickness [29, 39].

The change in DRIL extent is an important predictor of vision change after intravitreal anti-VEGF and steroid treatment. A greater baseline DRIL extent in the 1-mm foveal area and an early worsening in DRIL were predictive of worse VA at long-term follow-up after anti-VEGF treatment [40]. In a study by Vujosevic et al. [41] comparing the response of OCT signs to RBZ and DEX implant in eyes with DME, a greater reduction in DRIL extent was observed in eyes treated with DEX implant. Several other studies also reported better outcomes with steroid and proposed that in case DRIL does not adequately improve, an early switch from anti-VEGF treatment to intravitreal steroids may be preferred [29, 42]. These observations may be explained by the neuroprotective effect of corticosteroids, as they may promote neuronal survival via Müller cells and by suppressing microglial reactivity. **Figure 2** shows the presence of disorganization of the retinal inner layers in a patient with DR, which is observed during the first week of anti-VEGF treatment.

2.1.5 Hyperreflective retinal foci

Hyperreflective foci (HFs) in DME are small, well-circumscribed dots not visible on biomicroscopy or fundus photography, often appearing before clinically detectable DR or DME [43]. HF is not specific to DR; it is also observed in conditions like age-related macular degeneration, central serous chorioretinopathy (CSC), retinal vein occlusions (RVOs), and Coats disease, and occasionally in normal individuals [44]. Initially, HF is detected in the inner retinal layers on OCT and may later move to the outer layers. Vujosevic et al. [43] identified three types of HFs based on the appearance and location:

- HF ≤30 μm in diameter, reflecting like the nerve fiber layer and located in both the inner and outer retina, likely represents activated microglial cells

- HF >30 μm in diameter, reflecting like the RPE-Bruch membrane complex with back shadowing, located in the outer retina, likely represents hard exudates

- HF >30 μm in diameter, similar reflectivity to the RPE-Bruch membrane complex with back shadowing, located in the inner retina, may indicate MAs.

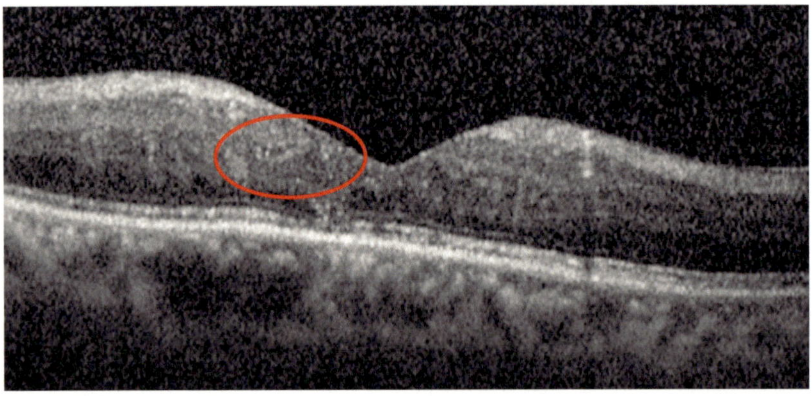

Figure 2.
The presence of disorganization of the retinal inner layers (red circle).

Initial descriptions suggested that HFs could be lipid-laden macrophages or extravasated lipoproteins, early indicators of subclinical BRB breakdown, but later evidence proposed that HFs could be markers of chronic inflammation and activated microglia in DR [45]. A significant correlation between small HF numbers and subclinical neurodegeneration supports the inflammatory hypothesis [46].

Studies show that DEX implants reduce HFs more effectively than anti-VEGF treatments, though some studies found similar reductions with both treatments [47, 48]. While some studies found a correlation between HF and better VA after treatment, others show no such association or even poorer outcomes [49, 50].

2.1.6 Pearl necklace sign

First defined by Gelman et al. [51], the pearl necklace sign refers to HF forming a continuous ring around the inner wall of cystoid spaces in the retina. These dots often become hard exudates as the edema resolves, suggesting the pearl necklace sign is a precursor to hard exudates. Generally, the presence of this sign does not affect the visual prognosis or the response to intravitreal treatment, except when located subfoveally. In such cases, irreversible photoreceptor damage can lead to poor visual outcomes [52]. **Figure 3** shows the presence of a pearl necklace sign in a patient with poorly controlled DM.

2.1.7 Bridging retinal processes

Bridging retinal processes are vertical remnants of neuroretinal tissue, primarily composed of Müller and bipolar cells, stretched between cystic cavities, connecting the inner and outer retinal layers. Their presence helps in transmitting visual impulses to the optic nerve axons; therefore, it is associated with better visual outcomes post-treatment, serving as a reliable biomarker for visual prognosis. Moreover, Markan et al. [11] showed that the lack of bridging processes leads to retinal thinning and atrophy. **Figure 4** illustrates the presence of bridging retinal processes.

2.1.8 Integrity of external retina

The cone outer segment tip (COST), also known as the interdigitation zone (IZ), appears as a hyperreflective band between the EZ and RPE on OCT. It is a marker of

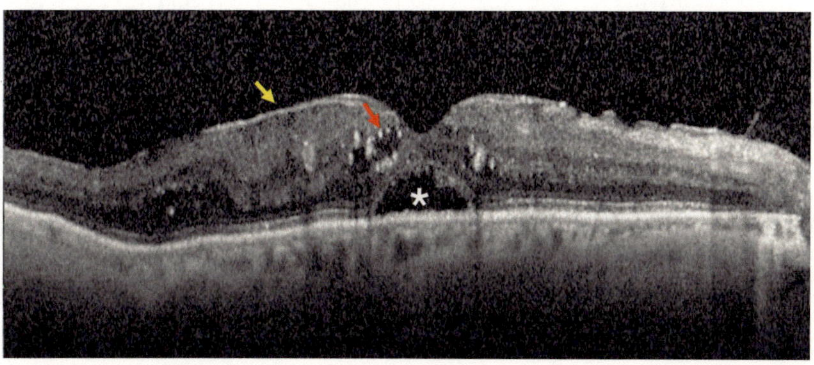

Figure 3.
The presence of pearl necklace sign (red arrow), epiretinal membrane (yellow arrow), and subretinal fluid (white asterisk) in a patient with poorly controlled DM.

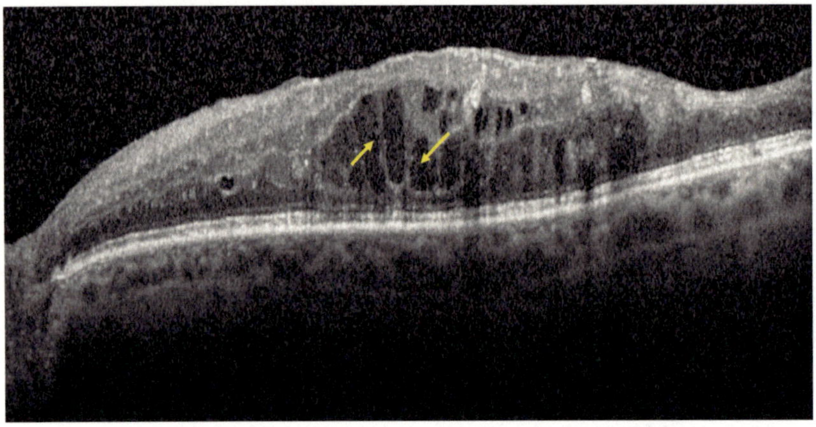

Figure 4.
The bridging retinal processes (yellow arrows) between intraretinal cystic cavities.

photoreceptor integrity. The EZ, previously termed the inner segment/outer segment (IS/OS) junction, represents the photoreceptors' mitochondria-rich zone, essential for their high-energy consumption. The ELM comprises zonula adherens connecting photoreceptor inner segments and Müller cell apical processes, acting as a barrier for macromolecule movement between these cells. In diabetic eyes, elevated VEGF levels can decrease occludin, a tight junction protein, compromising the ELM's barrier and increasing vascular permeability [53]. The mechanism of photoreceptor dysfunction in DME is multifactorial and involves impaired energy metabolism, inflammation, and microvascular ischemia [54].

Damage or disruption of photoreceptors is commonly visualized on OCT as a loss of integrity in the ELM, EZ, and IZ bands. Although the correlation between photoreceptor damage stages and OCT findings is not yet clearly established histopathologically, OCT studies of retinal degenerative diseases show that the lengths of the ELM, EZ, and IZ bands are highly correlated [55]. Disorganization appears to occur sequentially: first in the IZ, then in the EZ, and finally in the ELM. Qualitatively, each outer retinal layer is classified as absent (not visible), disrupted (partially visible), or intact (fully visible) in the foveal region [20]. A more recent approach involves a quantitative assessment of the EZ's relative intensity. This method expresses the EZ's relative intensity as a ratio compared to the ELM on OCT [56]. On the other hand, Borrelli et al. [57] developed an algorithm using the vitreous and RNFL intensities as references to normalize EZ intensity to better evaluate its status. The photoreceptor outer segment (PROS) is defined as the distance between the RPE and the junction of the photoreceptor IS/OS. In patients with DR, the PROS length is shorter compared to those without DR and correlates better with VA than macular thickness, serving as a more reliable prognostic marker [58].

Achiron et al. [59] first reported the association between treatment and EZ/COST integrity, demonstrating that the recovery of EZ/COST defects correlated with VA improvement following intravitreal BVZ injections in treatment-naive DME patients over a 3-month follow-up. Similarly, Serizawa et al. [60] found that in 41 DME eyes treated with laser therapy, anti-VEGF, and/or vitrectomy, the restoration of retinal outer layers, especially the COST, was a sensitive marker of treatment outcome. On the other hand, Koc et al. [61] proposed that EZ and ELM integrity may be more reliable than COST, as COST fragmentation artifacts are not uncommon in healthy eyes. Longitudinal studies show that disrupted foveal EZ, ELM, and COST predict worse subsequent VA and less VA gain in eyes treated with anti-VEGF and DEX implants, with this association observable up to 24 months [29, 62]. Post hoc analysis of the VISTA study showed that AFL treatment improved EZ integrity, which was maintained through week 100 follow-up [63].

2.1.9 Retinal pigment epithelium thickness

RPE thickness is a biomarker for predicting the functionality of the outer BRB. Eyes with PDR and DME exhibit decreased RPE thickness, indicating degenerative changes, likely due to ischemia disrupting the RPE-photoreceptor complex [64]. Boynton et al. [65] found that untreated patients with PDR had diffusely thinned RPE layers compared with healthy controls. On the other hand, Tavares Ferreira et al. [66] reported no significant change of RPE in subjects with or without diabetes.

2.1.10 Foveal eversion

A completely convex central fovea, known as foveal eversion, is linked to a higher rate of persistent DME compared to a normal foveal profile, regardless of treatment with intravitreal anti-VEGF or corticosteroids. It is also associated with higher retreatment rates in eyes treated with intravitreal steroids and a higher frequency of persistent DME. The underlying cause may involve Müller cell impairment, although the precise mechanism is not yet understood [67].

Figure 5 illustrates various OCT biomarkers observed in a patient undergoing anti-VEGF therapy.

2.1.11 Parallelism

SD-OCT introduced the parameter "parallelism," which refers to the integrity of retinal layers and serves as a potential biomarker for predicting visual outcomes in DME [68]. This parameter encompasses the continuity of the ELM, the EZ of the

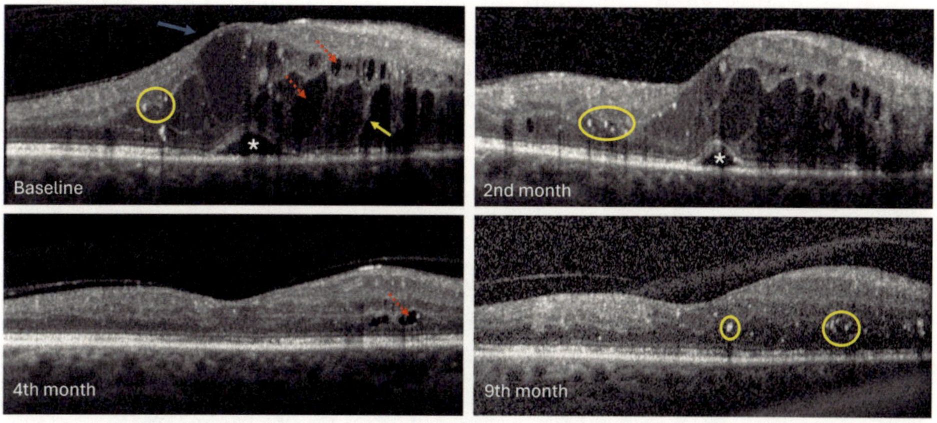

Figure 5.
The initial OCT image displays subretinal fluid (white asterisks), intraretinal cystoid spaces (red dashed arrows), hyperreflective dots (yellow circle), bridging retinal processes (yellow arrow), and foveal eversion (blue arrow). Follow-up OCT images at 2, 4, and 9 months post anti-VEGF treatment show a reduction in retinal thickness and improvement in subretinal fluid and intraretinal cystoid spaces. The 9-month OCT image reveals a few hyperreflective dots and disruption in the integrity of the outer retinal layers. (Courtesy of Taylan Ozturk, MD).

inner segment, as well as the presence of HF in the outer retinal layers. Parallelism is notably reduced in eyes with DME compared to normal eyes and shows a positive correlation with VA. A lack of HF in the outer retinal layers is significantly linked to increased parallelism and improved VA.

2.2 Vitreomacular interface biomarkers

The vitreomacular interface biomarker is crucial in the pathogenesis and progression of DR. Metabolic factors in diabetes can cause early vitreous liquefaction and cross-linking, leading to incomplete posterior vitreous detachment (PVD) and vitreoschisis. This can result in vitreous instability and macular traction. Studies have shown elevated levels of inflammatory and angiogenic factors, such as VEGF, IL-6, IL-8, ICAM-1, and MCP-1, in the vitreous fluid of patients with DME and PDR, implicating these molecules in retinal vascular permeability and macular edema [69].

Early studies, such as those by Nasrallah et al. [70], highlighted the importance of the vitreous in DME. A significant relationship between PVD and the absence of macular edema was found, suggesting that vitreous detachment plays a key role in DME resolution. Further research indicated that spontaneous resolution of macular edema occurred in a higher percentage of eyes with PVD compared to those without PVD. However, in eyes requiring anti-VEGF treatment, those with vitreomacular adhesion (VMA) showed greater VA improvements than those with complete PVD, possibly due to prolonged clearance of anti-VEGF molecules in eyes with VMA [71]. The posterior hyaloid's separation from the macula during PVD formation improves retinal oxygenation and reduces the reservoir of cytokines and angiogenic mediators near the macula.

The posterior hyaloid acts as a scaffold for neovascular growth due to its tight adhesions with retinal blood vessels, while the internal limiting membrane (ILM) supports glial proliferation, contributing to persistent macular edema and recurrent epiretinal membrane (ERM). According to Kang et al. [50], the incidence of new ERM formation is approximately 9.5% in DR. Significant vitreomacular traction (VMT) may necessitate pars plana vitrectomy (PPV) and ERM removal for eyes with suboptimal response to anti-VEGF or DEX implants, as recommended by the European Society of Retina Specialists (EURETINA) guidelines for DME eyes with anteroposterior traction [72]. Vitrectomy has been shown to reduce central subfield thickness and improve VA in such cases. The DRCR Protocol D offered vitrectomy to patients with DME and VMT, achieving a reduction of central subfield thickness to less than 250 μm in almost half of the eyes and a mean gain of 5 letters in visual acuity at 6 months [73]. **Figure 6** shows the thick posterior hyaloid and ERM formation in diabetic eyes.

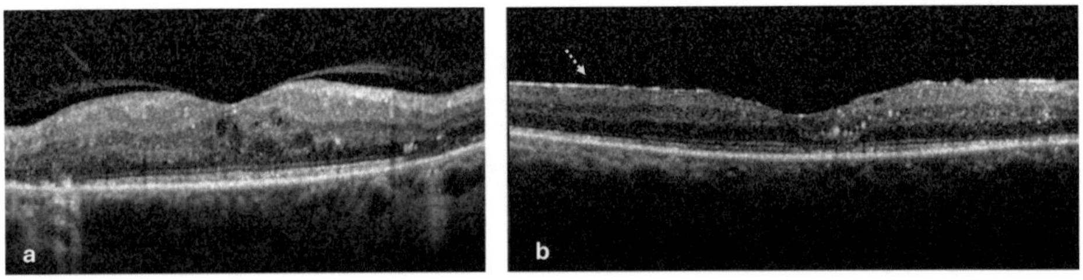

Figure 6.
(a) The presence of a thickened posterior hyaloid (red arrow) and (b) the formation of an epiretinal membrane (yellow dashed arrow) in patients with diabetic retinopathy.

2.3 Choroidal biomarkers

The choroid plays a critical role in supplying blood to the photoreceptor cells and the RPE, receiving approximately 95% of ocular blood flow and serving as the primary source of oxygen and nutrients for the outer retina. The involvement of the choroid in DR was first evidenced through histopathological studies, which revealed increased arteriosclerosis and periodic-acid Schiff (PAS) positive material within the arterial and capillary walls of diabetic eyes [74]. The term "diabetic choroidopathy" was later introduced by Hidayat et al. [75] in 1985, based on their description of histopathological findings in seven enucleated eyes suffering from late complications of diabetes. Choroidal impairment in DR can lead to photoreceptor dysfunction and death, as well as damage to the choriocapillaris (CC), which impairs the clearance of waste products from the RPE cells, resulting in their accumulation at Bruch's membrane.

The advent of advanced imaging technologies, such as enhanced depth imaging (EDI)-OCT and swept-source (SS)-OCT, has significantly improved the visualization and measurement of the choroidal vasculature. These technologies enable detailed examination of choroidal structure and provide reproducible measurements of choroidal thickness. Recently, investigations have focused on the subfoveal choroidal thickness (SFCT), choroidal vascularity index (CVI), and hyperreflective choroidal foci (HCF) as potential biomarkers for DR. These biomarkers offer new insights into the pathophysiology of DR and could contribute to the development of more effective diagnostic and therapeutic strategies.

2.3.1 Subfoveal choroidal thickness

Subfoveal choroidal thickness (SFCT), measured from the outer edge of the RPE to the inner sclera on EDI-OCT, may serve as a potential marker for choroidal vascularity. However, there is consensus about the SFCT findings in DR. While some studies found thicker SFCT in diabetic patients compared to controls, regardless of DR or DME severity, others linked thicker SFCT with increased DR severity and DME presence [76]. Conversely, some studies noted reduced SFCT associated with DME and DR severity [77, 78]. The relationship between choroidal thinning and DR is unclear, as it is not known whether choroidal thinning occurs before the onset of DR or is a consequence of DR-related alterations. Choroidal vasculature alterations may precede DR in diabetes [79, 80]. Choroidal thickening in diabetic eyes may result from vascular hyperpermeability due to elevated nitric oxide (NO) and VEGF levels [81]. SFCT reduction following anti-VEGF therapy supports VEGF's role in choroidal thickening [82]. These discrepancies between the studies may stem from differences in study design, patient demographics, and racial backgrounds. Various confounding factors, including age, sex, axial length (AL), and treatment history, influence choroidal thickness [83]. Standardizing measurement times in future studies is crucial due to significant diurnal variation [84].

The predictive value of SFCT for treatment response in DME is inconclusive. A thicker baseline SFCT was shown to be correlated with favorable functional and anatomical results with DEX implant and anti-VEGF treatment [85]. On the other hand, Campos et al. [86] showed that baseline SFCT decreased with anti-VEGF treatment but did not predict DME outcome. Moon et al. [85] reported that greater SFCT reduction with DEX implant was associated with greater VA gain and CST reduction. Several other studies also showed that anti-VEGF and DEX treatments consistently reduce choroidal thickness, though the extent of reduction does not correlate with treatment outcomes [87, 88].

2.3.2 Choroidal vascularity index

Given the numerous confounding factors and diurnal variations affecting SFCT, a reproducible quantitative analysis of choroidal vascularity is necessary. CVI is a newly developed metric in OCT that quantifies the vascular condition of the choroid and has been recently presented as a novel biomarker for monitoring the course of DR [89]. Studies have shown that while choroidal thickness is unaltered in DR, CVI correlates with progressing DR [90]. Comparing diabetic eyes and healthy ones, a study by Keskin et al. [91] found that CVI tends to be lower in diabetic patients with or without DR compared to healthy controls. CVI can be affected by the severity of DR. According to Kim et al. [92], CVI declined as DR advanced to PDR. In the mild/moderate NPDR group, SFCT was higher, and CVI was significantly lower compared to the no DR group. The status of CVI also affects the treatment response, as DME eyes with higher baseline CVI are more likely to achieve at least a 5-letter gain in VA with anti-VEGF treatment [93].

2.3.3 Hyperreflective choroidal foci

Hyperreflective choroidal foci (HCF) are typically dot-like or round, regular lesions in the choroid. According to a study by Roy et al. [94], the first to define HCF, these lesions are likely composed of migrated hyperreflective retinal foci (HRF), as all eyes with HCF also had HRF. In that study, eyes with HCF had significantly worse VA and higher mean CFT compared to those without HCF, indicating that HCF is associated with greater severity of DR and poorer visual outcomes. Another study by Saurabh et al. [95] found that the presence of HCF is associated with poorer initial VA and may also be indicative of worse final visual outcomes. In a retrospective longitudinal study, Szeto et al. [29] found that nearly half of the eyes with baseline HCF experienced a decrease in HCF numbers following treatment, with greater improvements in VA compared to those without a reduction in HCF.

3. OCT angiography biomarkers of diabetic retinopathy

OCTA functions by monitoring the movement of red blood cells (RBCs) over time through volumetric OCT scans. Repeated scans at each B-scan position enable the detection of motion contrast, which corresponds to blood flow, the primary expected motion in retinal vessels [5]. Unlike FFA, OCTA does not reveal vascular leakage. Also, the limited field of view restricts OCTA's utility as a screening tool. On the other hand, it has several advantages, such as being non-invasive, having more rapid data acquisition, and thus facilitating more frequent and faster monitoring. Furthermore, OCTA can generate three-dimensional (3D) images that reveal the depth of structures, allowing for the observation of specific capillary networks. This capability provides important quantitative information about the microvasculature of the retina. Enhanced software algorithms generate images of the superficial capillary plexus (SCP) and deep capillary plexus (DCP), and users can further refine segmentation to visualize additional layers, such as the intermediate capillary plexuses (ICPs), thus revealing pathologies not detectable with traditional dye-based angiography.

Various OCTA scan protocols cater to different clinical and research needs, utilizing a consistent 304 × 304 B-scan framework. The 3 × 3 mm scan, due to its increased density in comparison to the 6 × 6 mm and 12 x 12 mm scans, provides enhanced resolution, leading to a more accurate identification of findings. Hirano et al. [96] conducted a study in which they analyzed three different scan sizes (3 × 3 mm, 6 × 6 mm, and 12 × 12 mm) to compare retinal parameters between patients with DR and individuals without the disease. DR patients exhibited markedly reduced perfusion density (PD), vascular length density (VLD), and fractal dimensions (FDs) across all scan sizes and retinal layers. The swept source (SS)-OCTA images, sized 3 x 3 mm, clearly showed notable variations in these measurements between NPDR eyes with and without DME in the deeper layers of the retina. The discrepancies were not detected in the 6 × 6 mm and 12 × 12 mm SS-OCTA images. Another study comparing 3 × 3 mm and 6 × 6 mm OCTA scans for evaluating NPDR found that 3 × 3 mm scans better delineated the FAZ and detected vascular remodeling due to higher scan density [97]. Conversely, 6 × 6 mm scans were more sensitive in detecting MAs due to their larger scan area (**Table 2**).

3.1 Foveal avascular zone

The human foveola, characterized by its absence of rods and maximum density of cone photoreceptors, is crucial for central vision. This region, known as foveal avascular zone (FAZ), lacks vasculature and overlying inner retinal tissue, which minimizes light scattering and enhances optical quality. In healthy eyes, the FAZ area varies widely, ranging from 0.071 mm^2 to 0.527 mm^2 [98].

In DR, the FAZ is shown to be enlarged due to capillary loss in adjacent vessels, with a larger FAZ linked to thinner SFCT, lower body mass index (BMI), shorter AL, and more severe DR [99]. In addition to the FAZ area, metrics, such as FAZ perimetry, radius, and circularity, are employed for the evaluation of FAZ. FAZ circularity,

OCTA metric	Description
Foveal Avascular Zone (FAZ) area	Measurement of the FAZ size in mm^2
Foveal Avascular Zone (FAZ) circularity	A quantitative representation of the extent to which the FAZ resembles a perfect circle
Non-perfusion Area (NPA)	Area of absent blood flow
Vessel Density (VD)	Total area of perfused vasculature per unit area indicating the extent of blood flow within a given area. Similar to perfusion density
Vessel Length Density (VLD)	Percentage of the total vascular length divided by the total area
Vessel Skeleton Density (VSD)	Density of binarized vessel network evaluating the density of the simplified, skeletonized representation of the vessel network
Vessel Diameter Index (VDI)	The average vessel caliber of blood vessels is represented by the area occupied by a blood vessel from the binarized picture throughout the entire length of the vessel from the skeletonized image
Fractal Dimensions (FDs)	A mathematical parameter used to describe the complexity of blood vessels
Intercapillary Spaces	Space between adjacent capillaries

Table 2.
The detailed explanation of the metrics used in Optical Coherence Tomography Angiography for evaluating retinal vascular health.

which refers to its similarity to a perfect circle, can provide more informative insights into disease-induced microvascular changes compared to merely considering the FAZ area. Obstruction of the innermost capillaries around the fovea causes the FAZ to become irregular, making FAZ circularity a marker for capillary dropout and macular ischemia. A study by Tang et al. [99] found that worsening DR is significantly associated with an enlarged FAZ area, decreased FAZ circularity, lower vessel density (VD), and reduced FD in the SCP, as well as an enlarged FAZ area and lower VD in the DCP. A larger FAZ correlates with the presence of DRIL and poorer visual outcomes [100]. Furthermore, abnormalities in the FAZ have been observed in diabetic patients without clinical DR. De Carlo et al. [101] demonstrated significant FAZ enlargement in these patients compared to non-diabetic individuals. Nevertheless, the evidence remains equivocal, since several studies validate the FAZ enlargement as a biomarker in DR, while others indicate no significant correlation between FAZ and the severity of DR [102, 103]. **Figure 7** shows the enlarged FAZ area with decreased FAZ circularity as well as presence of MAs.

3.2 Non-perfusion areas

Non-perfusion areas (NPAs) are markers of vascular damage and retinal ischemia, and although not currently included in the grading of DR, they hold predictive potential for the progression from NPDR to PDR [104]. As DR advances, the extent of NPA increases. OCTA appears to outperform FFA in visualization of these regions, frequently detecting non-perfusion in areas that FFA identifies as perfused, probably attributed to slow blood flow.

NPA in all three retinal plexuses, including SCP, ICP, and DCP, has a correlation with intraretinal microvascular abnormalities (IRMAs) and neovascularization [105]. A study involving 122 individuals with NPDR from type 2 DM (T2DM) found

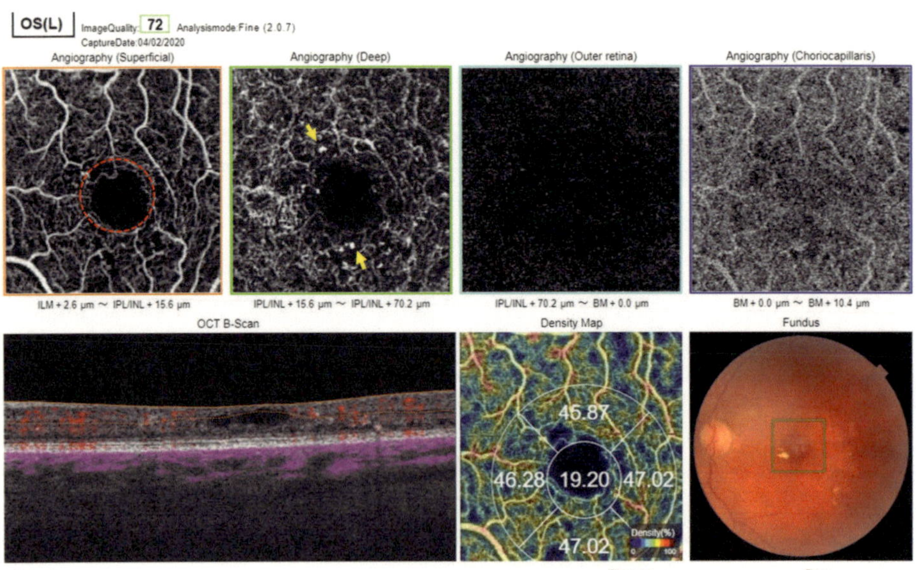

Figure 7.
Enlarged FAZ area with decreased FAZ circularity (red dashed circle) and the presence of MAs (yellow arrows) (Courtesy of Ali Osman Saatci, MD).

a significant association between retinal neurodegeneration, thinning of the retinal GCC, and increased retinal NPA [106]. This highlights the clinical value of NPA as a marker for tracking DR progression.

3.3 Vessel density

Vessel density (VD) is a measure of retinal microvasculature perfusion, calculated by dividing the area of blood vessels by the total measured area in binarized images. VD is influenced by age, gender, retinal layer thickness, and is highly correlated with signal strength [107, 108].

Notably, diabetic patients without DR exhibit a decrease in VD in both SCP and the DCP. Santos et al. [109] reported that eyes with preclinical retinopathy show early retinal capillary closure, predominantly within the SCP, resulting in decreased VD. These findings suggest that initial retinal microvascular changes in type 2 DM are characterized by capillary closure or reduced blood flow, primarily within the SCP, corroborating the results of de Carlo et al. [101] Conversely, some studies emphasize a significant decrease in VD in the DCP more than in the SCP. Veiby et al. [110] found that lower VD in the DCP was the only significant OCTA factor associated with the progression of NPDR. The susceptibility of DCP to ischemic damage, due to its location in a watershed zone adjacent to the high oxygen demands of the OPL, is supported by histologic studies indicating its vulnerability to injury [111]. Tang et al. [99] observed that lower VD was associated with shorter AL, worse VA, and more severe DR, with decreased VD in the DCP correlating with VA deterioration, implying that DCP VD reflects capillary loss in patients with DME. Additionally, the ICP VD and flow index decrease, and the area of non-perfusion increases with DR progression, paralleling changes in the DCP [112].

The extent of DCP loss and OPL disruption in DME can predict responsiveness to anti-VEGF treatment, with decreased VD in the DCP indicating worse VA and reflecting capillary loss in patients with visual impairment due to DME [113].

3.4 Choriocapillaris

Choroidal circulation supplies oxygen and nutrients crucial for the choroid and outer retina. Traditional dye-based angiography has limitations in measuring choroidal blood flow. OCTA offers promise in visualizing and quantifying choroidal vasculature, particularly the CC. Nevertheless, commercial OCTA systems frequently do not possess adequate resolution to quantify the highly packed CC in the posterior pole, where the distances between capillaries (5–20 μm) are greater than the lateral resolution of OCT (15–20 μm). To address this, researchers propose using flow deficit analysis to assess CC perfusion, where flow deficits indicate areas with inadequate or below-detectable CC flow by OCT systems [114]. Studies, such as by Dai et al. [103], have noted increased CC flow deficits in diabetic eyes without retinopathy compared to age-matched healthy controls. This reduction in CC flow may precede macular flow changes, suggesting it could serve as an early marker for microvascular dysfunction in diabetes. Histopathological studies have similarly observed more pronounced CC dropouts postmortem in diabetic individuals compared to non-diabetic subjects [115].

3.5 Vessel length density

Vessel length density (VLD), also known as skeleton density (SD), enhances VD by quantifying the total length of vessels without regard to their diameters [116].

Unlike VD, which assesses vessel presence per unit area, VLD assigns equal weight to large vessels and small capillaries, each represented as single-pixel lines. Therefore, VLD is particularly sensitive to changes in capillary-level perfusion compared to VD. Therefore, VLD is considered a more refined metric for evaluating microvascular perfusion dynamics [96].

3.6 Vessel tortuosity

Retinal vessel tortuosity quantifies the curvature integral normalized by the vessel's total path length. Initially assessed via computer-assisted programs on fundus photographs, increased vessel tortuosity has been observed in diabetic patients compared to healthy controls [117].

3.7 Microaneurysms, intraretinal microvascular abnormalities, and neovascularization

Microaneurysms, clinically identified as deep-red dots ranging from 25 to 100 μm in diameter on ophthalmoscopy, are often the earliest visible signs of DR. Studies have linked increased MA count and turnover with higher risks of DR progression and DME [118]. Using OCTA, Thompson et al. [119] demonstrated superior detection of MAs compared to dilated clinical examination alone, highlighting OCTA's depth-resolved capability in precisely localizing these lesions. However, OCTA may not detect all MAs seen on FFA, possibly due to slow blood flow rates or turbulence within MAs [120]. Parravano et al. [121] integrated OCT and OCTA parameters to study MA progression and its impact on retinal extracellular fluid accumulation over one year in NPDR patients. They found that hyperreflective MAs at baseline were significantly associated with increased fluid accumulation, emphasizing OCTA's potential for predicting disease progression and guiding treatment timing in DME. Studies, including those by Park et al. [122], have identified MAs across all retinal plexuses, with a predilection for originating from the DCP over the SCP. This suggests that initial DR changes may originate more frequently from the DCP [121].

In severe NPDR, IRMA is a hallmark according to the Early Treatment Diabetic Retinopathy Study (ETDRS). OCTA, combined with conventional OCT B-scan, provides both en face and cross-sectional views, aiding in the differentiation of IRMA from NV [123]. IRMAs appear on OCTA as anomalous, branched, dilated retinal vessels that remain confined within the retina without protruding into the vitreous [124]. On the other hand, NV typically shows supraretinal flow crossing membranes and extending into the posterior hyaloid, thereby enhancing diagnostic accuracy. Recent studies demonstrate OCTA's capability to detect early NVs, classify lesions, and understand their morphological patterns in PDR [123, 125]. Longitudinal studies using OCTA, such as by Motulsky et al. [126], monitor NV progression and treatment response in PDR, noting decreased flow within NV post-treatment with anti-VEGF and/or panretinal photocoagulation (PRP). Comparisons with FFA, as seen in a study by Russell et al. [127], reveal OCTA's superior visualization of NV dynamics pre- and post-PRP treatment [128, 129]. These findings suggest OCTA could become the primary imaging tool for managing NV in PDR, showcasing its potential in assessing treatment outcomes following PRP. **Figure 8** presents an OCTA image of the optic disk, revealing severe NV in a patient with PDR.

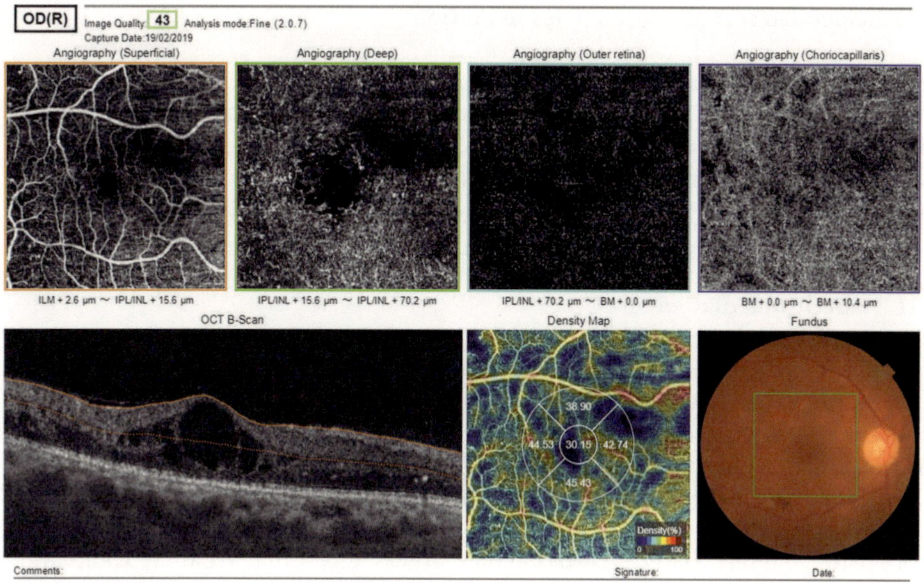

Figure 8.
OCTA image of the optic disk in a patient with PDR demonstrating the presence of an extensive NV (Courtesy of Ali Osman Saatci, MD).

3.8 Fractal dimension and lacunarity

Fractal dimension (FD) quantifies vascular complexity by analyzing skeletonized images through the box-counting method. Studies by Bhardwaj et al. [130] and Kim et al. [131] reveal significantly lower FD values in DR eyes compared to healthy controls, particularly in the SCP, with FD decreasing as DR severity worsens. Serra et al. [132] demonstrate that eyes with peripheral NPAs exhibit lower FD and higher lacunarity (LAC) in both SCP and DCP, correlating with the extent of NPAs.

Reduced FD values are associated with increased LAC, suggesting compromised perfusion in the peripheral retina. This condition may contribute to diabetic microangiopathy, promoting NPAs and triggering inflammatory responses via cytokine release and VEGF activity. Higher LAC values indicate larger and more irregularly distributed lacunae, characteristic of severe DME observed on OCTA [133]. Fan et al. [134] found that FD of the entire retina correlates strongly with the extent of peripheral retinal ischemia in DR. These findings underscore the utility of fractal analysis in objectively assessing microvascular changes and their systemic implications in diabetic retinal diseases.

3.9 Intercapillary spacing

Intercapillary spacing has emerged as a sensitive indicator for early capillary dropouts and ischemic regions in DR. Bhanushali et al. [135] showed intercapillary spacing as more sensitive parameter than VD and FAZ to detect NPA. Mendes et al. [136] demonstrated that abnormal intercapillary spaces effectively distinguished eyes with DR from controls across different ETDRS severity stages. However, the reliability of this metric is influenced by the quality of binarized en face slab images, exhibiting greater variability compared to measures such as VD and FAZ.

3.10 Suspended scattering particles in motion

Suspended scattering particles in motion (SSPiM) are OCTA detected signals found within retinal fluid pockets near vascular-avascular junctions, predominantly in the Henle fiber layer [137]. These signals are not exclusive to DME but are also present in other exudative maculopathies. Their formation is attributed to extravasated lipids, and their presence may decrease as hard exudates develop in some patients [138].

3.11 Diabetic macular edema

OCTA metrics associated with DME include lower VD in the SCP, diminished perfusion in the DCP, increased flow deficit in the CC, as well as altered FAZ characteristics, such as increased area and decreased circularity [139]. ICS, visualized as round black flow voids on OCTA, are more prominent in the DCP than in the SCP. These cystic areas, often surrounded by NPA in chronic DME, suggest underlying ischemia preceding the development of edema. MAs within the DCP are also implicated in DME pathogenesis [140]. OCTA-based biomarkers, including FAZ dimensions and VD across multiple capillary plexuses, aid in diagnosis, prognosis, and monitoring of VA in response to treatment. Studies indicate that a higher number of MAs within the DCP and a larger FAZ area correlate with poorer response to anti-VEGF treatment in DME cases [141].

OCTA has practical limitations in evaluating DME, such as segmentation errors due to retinal edema and signal intensity reduction due to fluid accumulation in deeper retinal layers [142]. Furthermore, discrepancies between OCTA flow voids and actual cystic spaces are noted, as fluid may compress vessels, reducing flow below

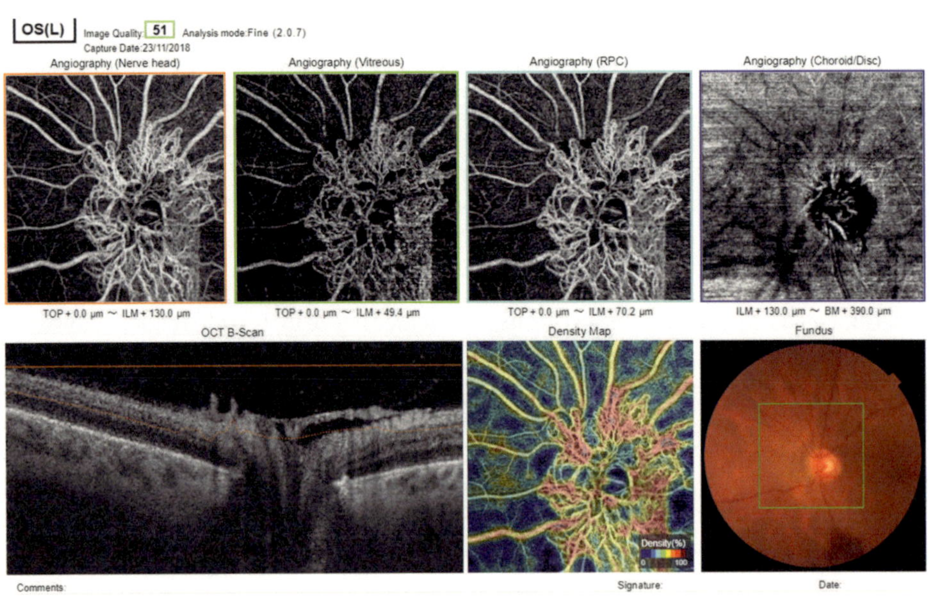

Figure 9.
OCTA image of a patient with severe diabetic macular edema (DME) showing intraretinal cysts (ICS) in both the superficial capillary plexus (SCP) and the deep capillary plexus (DCP) (Courtesy of Ali Osman Saatci, MD).

OCTA detection limits [143]. Lee et al. [144] addressed segmentation challenges by manually adjusting the SCP/DCP boundary in severe DME cases, revealing significant DCP damage, particularly in poor responders to anti-VEGF therapy. This underscores the critical role of DCP integrity as a biomarker for treatment response prediction in DME. Longitudinal studies, such as those by Sun et al. [139], highlight the predictive value of SCP VD in identifying individuals at risk of developing DME over time. As OCTA technology advances and more studies are conducted, its role in the comprehensive management of DME is expected to expand significantly. **Figure 9** shows the OCTA image of a patient with severe DME.

4. Conclusions

In conclusion, OCT and OCTA provide valuable insights into the pathophysiology, diagnosis, and management of DR and DME. OCT biomarkers offer critical information on disease severity, prognosis, and treatment response. Similarly, OCTA metrics enhance our understanding of microvascular changes in DR. These biomarkers facilitate early detection, precise monitoring, and tailored therapeutic strategies, ultimately improving visual outcomes for patients with DR and DME. The integration of OCT and OCTA in clinical practice underscores their indispensable role in advancing diabetic eye care, offering non-invasive, high-resolution imaging that supports comprehensive disease management. Future research should continue to refine these biomarkers, address current limitations, and explore their full potential in enhancing patient care and outcomes.

Author details

Ceren Durmaz Engin[1,2]

1 Department of Ophthalmology, Izmir Democracy University Buca Seyfi Demirsoy Education and Research Hospital, Izmir, Turkey

2 Department of Biomedical Technologies, The Graduate School of Natural and Applied Sciences, Dokuz Eylul University, Izmir, Turkey

*Address all correspondence to: cerendurmaz@gmail.com

References

[1] Kumar A, Gangwar R, Zargar AA, Kumar R, Sharma A. Prevalence of diabetes in India: A review of IDF diabetes atlas 10th edition. Current Diabetes Reviews. 2024;**20**(1):e130423215752

[2] Teo ZL et al. Global prevalence of diabetic retinopathy and projection of burden through 2045: Systematic review and meta-analysis. Ophthalmology. 2021;**128**(11):1580-1591

[3] Wang W, Lo ACY. Diabetic retinopathy: Pathophysiology and treatments. International Journal of Molecular Sciences. 2018;**19**(6):1816. DOI: 10.3390/ijms19061816

[4] Sabanayagam C, Yip W, Ting DSW, Tan G, Wong TY. Ten emerging trends in the epidemiology of diabetic retinopathy. Ophthalmic Epidemiology. 2016;**23**(4):209-222

[5] Spaide RF, Fujimoto JG, Waheed NK, Sadda SR, Staurenghi G. Optical coherence tomography angiography. Progress in Retinal and Eye Research. 2018;**64**:1-55

[6] Virgili G et al. Optical coherence tomography (OCT) for detection of macular oedema in patients with diabetic retinopathy. Cochrane Database of Systematic Reviews. 2015;**1**(1):CD008081

[7] Zhang Y et al. Prediction of visual acuity after anti-VEGF therapy in diabetic macular edema by machine learning. Journal Diabetes Research. 2022;**2022**:5779210

[8] Zhou J, Song S, Zhang Y, Jin K, Ye J. OCT-based biomarkers are associated with systemic inflammation in patients with treatment-Naïve diabetic macular edema. Ophthalmology and. Therapy. 2022;**11**(6):2153-2167

[9] Visioli G et al. OCT biomarkers as predictors of visual improvement in diabetic macular edema eyes receiving dexamethasone implants. International Journal of Retina and Vitreous. 2023;**9**(1):35

[10] Sun Z, Yang D, Tang Z, Ng DS, Cheung CY. Optical coherence tomography angiography in diabetic retinopathy: An updated review. Eye (London). 2021;**35**(1):149-161

[11] Markan A, Agarwal A, Arora A, Bazgain K, Rana V, Gupta V. Novel imaging biomarkers in diabetic retinopathy and diabetic macular edema. Therapeutic Advances in Ophthalmology. 2020;**12**:2515841420950513

[12] Saxena S et al. Spectral domain optical coherence tomography based imaging biomarkers for diabetic retinopathy. Endocrine. 2019;**66**(3):509-516

[13] Bressler NM et al. Persistent macular thickening following intravitreous aflibercept, bevacizumab, or ranibizumab for central-involved diabetic macular edema with vision impairment: A secondary analysis of a randomized clinical trial. JAMA Ophthalmology. 2018;**136**(3):257-269

[14] Pieramici DJ, Wang P-W, Ding B, Gune S. Visual and anatomic outcomes in patients with diabetic macular edema with limited initial anatomic response to ranibizumab in RIDE and RISE. Ophthalmology. 2016;**123**(6):1345-1350

[15] Wells JA et al. Aflibercept, bevacizumab, or ranibizumab for diabetic macular edema. The New England Journal of Medicine. 2015;**372**(13):1193-1203

[16] Karst SG et al. Atrophy of the central neuroretina in patients treated for diabetic macular edema. Acta Ophthalmologica. 2019;**97**(8): e1054-e1061

[17] Hannouche RZ, de Avila MP, Isaac DLC, e Silva RSC, Rassi AR. Correlation between central subfield thickness, visual acuity and structural changes in diabetic macular edema. Arquivos Brasileiros de Oftalmologia. 2012;**75**(3):183-187

[18] Maheshwary AS, Oster SF, Yuson RMS, Cheng L, Mojana F, Freeman WR. The association between percent disruption of the photoreceptor inner segment-outer segment junction and visual acuity in diabetic macular edema. American Journal of Ophthalmology. 2010;**150**(1):63-67.e1

[19] Yalçın NG, Özdek Ş. The relationship between macular cyst formation and ischemia in diabetic macular edema. Turkish Journal of Ophthalmology. 2019;**49**(4):194-200

[20] Panozzo G et al. An optical coherence tomography-based grading of diabetic maculopathy proposed by an international expert panel: The European school for advanced studies in ophthalmology classification. European Journal of Ophthalmology. 2020;**30**(1):8-18

[21] Reznicek L et al. Functional and morphological changes in diabetic macular edema over the course of anti-vascular endothelial growth factor treatment. Acta Ophthalmologica. 2013;**91**(7):e529-e536

[22] Karst SG et al. Detailed analysis of retinal morphology in patients with diabetic macular edema (DME) randomized to ranibizumab or triamcinolone treatment. Graefe's Archive for Clinical and Experimental Ophthalmology = Albrecht von Graefes Archiv fur Klinische und Experimentelle Ophthalmologie. 2018;**256**(1):49-58

[23] Huang Y-T et al. Optical coherence tomography biomarkers in predicting treatment outcomes of diabetic macular edema after dexamethasone implants. Frontiers in Medicine. 2022;**9**:852022

[24] Khoramnia R et al. Exploring the role of retinal fluid as a biomarker for the management of diabetic macular oedema. Eye (London). 2024;**38**(1):54-60

[25] Park J, Felfeli T, Kherani IZ, Altomare F, Chow DR, Wong DT. Prevalence and clinical implications of subretinal fluid in retinal diseases: A real-world cohort study. BMJ Open Ophthalmology. 2023;**8**(1):e001214. DOI: 10.1136/bmjophth-2022-001214

[26] Fickweiler W, Schauwvlieghe A-SME, Schlingemann RO, Maria Hooymans JM, Los LI, Verbraak FD. Predictive value of optical coherence tomographic features In the bevacizumab and ranibizumab In patients with diabetic macular edema (BRDME) study. Retina. 2018;**38**(4):812-819

[27] Korobelnik J-F et al. Effect of baseline subretinal fluid on treatment outcomes in VIVID-DME and VISTA-DME studies. Ophthalmology Retina. 2019;**3**(8):663-669

[28] Bressler SB et al. Factors associated with visual acuity and central subfield thickness changes when treating diabetic macular edema with anti-vascular endothelial growth factor therapy: An exploratory analysis of the protocol T randomized clinical trial. JAMA Ophthalmology. 2019;**137**(4):382-389

[29] Szeto SK et al. OCT-based biomarkers for predicting treatment response in eyes

with centre-involved diabetic macular oedema treated with anti-VEGF injections: A real-life retina clinic-based study. The British Journal of Ophthalmology. 2023;**107**(4):525-533

[30] Shimura M et al. Visual outcome after intravitreal triamcinolone acetonide depends on optical coherence tomographic patterns in patients with diffuse diabetic macular edema. Retina. 2011;**31**(4):748-754

[31] Grunwald JE et al. Risk of geographic atrophy in the comparison of age-related macular degeneration treatments trials. Ophthalmology. 2014;**121**(1):150-161

[32] Joltikov KA et al. Disorganization of retinal inner layers (DRIL) and neuroretinal dysfunction in early diabetic retinopathy. Investigative Ophthalmology & Visual Science. 2018;**59**(13):5481-5486

[33] Khojasteh H et al. Multifocal electroretinogram in diabetic macular edema and its correlation with different optical coherence tomography features. International Ophthalmology. 2020;**40**(3):571-581

[34] Pelosini L, Hull CC, Boyce JF, McHugh D, Stanford MR, Marshall J. Optical coherence tomography may be used to predict visual acuity in patients with macular edema. Investigative Ophthalmology & Visual Science. 2011;**52**(5):2741-2748

[35] Tsai W-S et al. Characterization of the structural and functional alteration in eyes with diabetic macular ischemia. Ophthalmology Retina. 2023;7(2):142-152

[36] Nadri G et al. Disorganization of retinal inner layers correlates with ellipsoid zone disruption and retinal nerve fiber layer thinning in diabetic retinopathy. Journal of Diabetes and its Complications. 2019;**33**(8):550-553

[37] Das R, Spence G, Hogg RE, Stevenson M, Chakravarthy U. Disorganization of inner retina and outer retinal morphology in diabetic macular edema. JAMA Ophthalmology. 2018;**136**(2):202-208

[38] Balaratnasingam C et al. Visual acuity is correlated with the area of the foveal avascular zone in diabetic retinopathy and retinal vein occlusion. Ophthalmology. 2016;**123**(11):2352-2367

[39] Zur D et al. Disorganization of retinal inner layers as a biomarker in patients with diabetic macular oedema treated with dexamethasone implant. Acta Ophthalmologica. 2020;**98**(2):e217-e223

[40] Sun JK et al. Disorganization of the retinal inner layers as a predictor of visual acuity in eyes with center-involved diabetic macular edema. JAMA Ophthalmology. 2014;**132**(11):1309-1316

[41] Vujosevic S et al. Diabetic macular edema with neuroretinal detachment: OCT and OCT-angiography biomarkers of treatment response to anti-VEGF and steroids. Acta Diabetologica. 2020;**57**(3):287-296

[42] Munk MR, Somfai GM, de Smet MD, et al. The role of intravitreal corticosteroids in the treatment of DME: predictive OCT biomarkers. International Journal of Molecular Sciences. 2022;**23**(14):7585. Published 2022 Jul 8. DOI: 10.3390/ijms23147585

[43] Vujosevic S, Bini S, Midena G, Berton M, Pilotto E, Midena E. Hyperreflective intraretinal spots in diabetics without and with nonproliferative diabetic retinopathy: An in vivo study using spectral domain OCT.

Journal Diabetes Research. 2013;**2013**:491835

[44] Szeto SK et al. Optical coherence tomography in the management of diabetic macular oedema. Progress in Retinal and Eye Research. 2024;**98**:101220

[45] Bolz M, Schmidt-Erfurth U, Deak G, Mylonas G, Kriechbaum K, Scholda C. Optical coherence tomographic hyperreflective foci: A morphologic sign of lipid extravasation in diabetic macular edema. Ophthalmology. 2009;**116**(5):914-920

[46] Vujosevic S, Torresin T, Berton M, Bini S, Convento E, Midena E. Diabetic macular edema with and without subfoveal neuroretinal detachment: Two different morphologic and functional entities. American Journal of Ophthalmology. 2017;**181**:149-155

[47] Vujosevic S et al. Imaging retinal inflammatory biomarkers after intravitreal steroid and anti-VEGF treatment in diabetic macular oedema. Acta Ophthalmologica. 2017;**95**(5):464-471

[48] Chatziralli IP, Sergentanis TN, Sivaprasad S. Hyperreflective foci as an independent visual outcome predictor In macular edema due to retinal vascular diseases treated with intravitreal dexamethasone or ranibizumab. Retina. 2016;**36**(12):2319-2328

[49] Huang C-H, Yang C-H, Hsieh Y-T, Yang C-M, Ho T-C, Lai T-T. Hyperreflective foci in predicting the treatment outcomes of diabetic macular oedema after anti-vascular endothelial growth factor therapy. Scientific Reports. 2021;**11**(1):5103

[50] Kang J-W, Chung H, Chan Kim H. Correlation of optical coherence tomographic hyperreflective foci with visual outcomes in different patterns of diabetic macular edema. Retina. 2016;**36**(9):1630-1639

[51] Gelman SK, Freund KB, Shah VP, Sarraf D. The pearl necklace sign: A novel spectral domain optical coherence tomography finding in exudative macular disease. Retina. 2014;**34**(10):2088-2095

[52] Ajay K, Mason F, Gonglore B, Bhatnagar A. Pearl necklace sign in diabetic macular edema: Evaluation and significance. Indian Journal of Ophthalmology. 2016;**64**(11):829-834

[53] Omri S et al. The outer limiting membrane (OLM) revisited: Clinical implications. Clinical Ophthalmology. 2010;**4**:183-195

[54] Becker S, Carroll LS, Vinberg F. Diabetic photoreceptors: Mechanisms underlying changes in structure and function. Visual Neuroscience. 2020;**37**:E008

[55] Saxena S, Srivastav K, Cheung CM, Ng JY, Lai TY. Photoreceptor inner segment ellipsoid band integrity on spectral domain optical coherence tomography. Clinical Ophthalmology. 2014;**8**:2507-2522

[56] Wu Z, Ayton LN, Guymer RH, Luu CD. Second reflective band intensity in age-related macular degeneration. Ophthalmology. 2013;**120**(6):1307-8.e1

[57] Borrelli E, Palmieri M, Viggiano P, Ferro G, Mastropasqua R. Photoreceptor damage in diabetic choroidopathy. Retina. 2020;**40**(6):1062-1069

[58] Forooghian F et al. Relationship between photoreceptor outer segment length and visual acuity in diabetic macular edema. Retina. 2010;**30**(1):63-70

[59] Achiron A et al. Photoreceptor integrity predicts response to anti-VEGF treatment. Ophthalmic Research. 2017;**57**(1):37-41

[60] Serizawa S, Ohkoshi K, Minowa Y, Soejima K. Interdigitation zone band restoration after treatment of diabetic macular edema. Current Eye Research. 2016;**41**(9):1229-1234

[61] Koc F, Güven YZ, Egrilmez D, Aydın E. Optical coherence tomography biomarkers in bilateral diabetic macular edema patients with asymmetric anti-VEGF response. Seminars in Ophthalmology. 2021;**36**(5-6):444-451

[62] Zur D, Iglicki M, Busch C, Invernizzi A, Mariussi M, Loewenstein A. OCT biomarkers as functional outcome predictors in diabetic macular edema treated with dexamethasone implant. Ophthalmology. 2018;**125**(2):267-275

[63] Ehlers JP et al. Higher-order assessment of OCT in diabetic macular edema from the VISTA study: Ellipsoid zone dynamics and the retinal fluid index. Ophthalmology Retina. 2019;**3**(12):1056-1066

[64] Damian I, Nicoara SD. Optical coherence tomography biomarkers of the outer blood-retina barrier in patients with diabetic macular oedema. Journal Diabetes Research. 2020;**2020**:8880586

[65] Boynton GE, Stem MS, Kwark L, Jackson GR, Farsiu S, Gardner TW. Multimodal characterization of proliferative diabetic retinopathy reveals alterations in outer retinal function and structure. Ophthalmology. 2015;**122**(5):957-967

[66] Tavares Ferreira J et al. Retinal neurodegeneration in diabetic patients without diabetic retinopathy. Investigative Ophthalmology & Visual Science. 2016;**57**(14):6455-6460

[67] Arrigo A et al. Foveal eversion patterns in diabetic macular edema. Scientific Reports. 2022;**12**(1):13097

[68] Uji A et al. Parallelism for quantitative image analysis of photoreceptor-retinal pigment epithelium complex alterations in diabetic macular edema. Investigative Ophthalmology & Visual Science. 2014;**55**(5):3361-3367

[69] Noma H, Yasuda K, Shimura M. Involvement of cytokines in the pathogenesis of diabetic macular edema. International Journal of Molecular Sciences. Mar 2021;**22**(7):3427. DOI: 10.3390/ijms22073427

[70] Nasrallah FP et al. The role of the vitreous in diabetic macular edema. Ophthalmology. 1988;**95**(10):1335-1339

[71] Hikichi T, Fujio N, Akiba J, Azuma Y, Takahashi M, Yoshida A. Association between the short-term natural history of diabetic macular edema and the vitreomacular relationship in type II diabetes mellitus. Ophthalmology. 1997;**104**(3):473-478

[72] Schmidt-Erfurth U et al. Guidelines for the Management of Diabetic Macular Edema by the European Society of Retina Specialists (EURETINA). Ophthalmologica Journal International d'ophtalmologie. International Journal Ophthalmology Zeitschrift fur Augenheilkde. 2017;**237**(4):185-222

[73] Sadiq MA et al. Effect of vitreomacular adhesion on treatment outcomes in the ranibizumab for edema of the macula in diabetes (READ-3) study. Ophthalmology. 2016;**123**(2):324-329

[74] Yanoff M. Ocular pathology of diabetes mellitus. American Journal of Ophthalmology. 1969;**67**(1):21-38

[75] Hidayat AA, Fine BS. Diabetic choroidopathy. Light and electron microscopic observations of seven cases. Ophthalmology. 1985;**92**(4):512-522

[76] Kim JT, Lee DH, Joe SG, Kim J-G, Yoon YH. Changes in choroidal thickness in relation to the severity of retinopathy and macular edema in type 2 diabetic patients. Investigative Ophthalmology & Visual Science. 2013;**54**(5):3378-3384

[77] Eliwa TF, Hegazy OS, Mahmoud SS, Almaamon T. Choroidal thickness change in patients with diabetic macular edema. Ophthalmic Surgery, Lasers & Imaging Retina. 2017;**48**(12):970-977

[78] Querques G et al. Enhanced depth imaging optical coherence tomography in type 2 diabetes. Investigative Ophthalmology & Visual Science. 2012;**53**(10):6017-6024

[79] Choi W et al. Ultrahigh speed swept source optical coherence tomography angiography of retinal and choriocapillaris alterations In diabetic patients with and without retinopathy. Retina. 2017;**37**(1):11-21

[80] Nesper PL et al. Quantifying microvascular abnormalities with increasing severity of diabetic retinopathy using optical coherence tomography angiography. Investigative Ophthalmology & Visual Science. 2017;**58**(6):BIO307-BIO315

[81] Wang W et al. Choroidal thickness in diabetes and diabetic retinopathy: A swept source OCT study. Investigative Ophthalmology & Visual Science. 2020;**61**(4):29

[82] Sakanishi Y, Morita S, Mashimo K, Tamaki K, Ebihara N. Subfoveal choroidal thickness and treatment outcomes of intravitreal aflibercept for branch retinal vein occlusion. Life (Basel). Jun 2021;**11**(6):572. DOI: 10.3390/life11060572

[83] Xu J et al. Subfoveal choroidal thickness in diabetes and diabetic retinopathy. Ophthalmology. 2013;**120**(10):2023-2028

[84] Tan CS, Ouyang Y, Ruiz H, Sadda SR. Diurnal variation of choroidal thickness in normal, healthy subjects measured by spectral domain optical coherence tomography. Investigative Ophthalmology & Visual Science. 2012;**53**(1):261-266

[85] Moon KY, Choi SY, Song JH. Changes in subfoveal choroidal thickness after intravitreal dexamethasone implant therapy for diabetic macular edema. Retina. 2021;**41**(6):1283-1292

[86] Campos A et al. Choroidal thickness changes stratified by outcome in real-world treatment of diabetic macular edema. Graefe's Archive for Clinical and Experimental Ophthalmology = Albrecht von Graefes Archiv fur Klinische und Experimentelle Ophthalmologie. 2018;**256**(10):1857-1865

[87] Wang X-N, Cai X, He S, Zhang X, Wu Q. Subfoveal choroidal thickness changes after intravitreal ranibizumab injections in different patterns of diabetic macular edema using a deep learning-based auto-segmentation. International Ophthalmology. 2023;**43**(12):4399-4407

[88] Yiu G, Manjunath V, Chiu SJ, Farsiu S, Mahmoud TH. Effect of anti-vascular endothelial growth factor therapy on choroidal thickness in diabetic macular edema. American

Journal of Ophthalmology. 2014;**158**(4):745-751.e2

[89] Sonoda S et al. Choroidal structure in normal eyes and after photodynamic therapy determined by binarization of optical coherence tomographic images. Investigative Ophthalmology & Visual Science. 2014;**55**(6):3893-3899

[90] Unsal E, Eltutar K, Zirtiloğlu S, Dinçer N, Ozdoğan Erkul S, Güngel H. Choroidal thickness in patients with diabetic retinopathy. Clinical Ophthalmology. 2014;**8**:637-642

[91] Keskin Ç, Dilekçi ENA, Üçgül AY, Üçgül RK, Toprak G, Cengiz D. Choroidal vascularity index as a predictor for the development of retinopathy in diabetic patients. Journal of Endocrinological Investigation. 2024;**47**(5):1175-1180

[92] Kim M, Ha MJ, Choi SY, Park Y-H. Choroidal vascularity index in type-2 diabetes analyzed by swept-source optical coherence tomography. Scientific Reports. 2018;**8**(1):70

[93] Dou N et al. Choroidal vascularity index as a biomarker for visual response to antivascular endothelial growth factor treatment in diabetic macular edema. Journal Diabetes Research. 2021;**2021**:3033219

[94] Roy R, Saurabh K, Shah D, Chowdhury M, Goel S. Choroidal hyperreflective foci: A novel spectral domain optical coherence tomography biomarker in eyes with diabetic macular edema. Asia-Pacific Journal of Ophthalmology (Philadelphia, Pa.). 2019;**8**(4):314-318

[95] Saurabh K, Roy R, Herekar S, Mistry S, Choudhari S. Validation of choroidal hyperreflective foci in diabetic macular edema through a retrospective pilot study. Indian Journal of Ophthalmology. 2021;**69**(11):3203-3206

[96] Hirano T, Kitahara J, Toriyama Y, Kasamatsu H, Murata T, Sadda S. Quantifying vascular density and morphology using different swept-source optical coherence tomography angiographic scan patterns in diabetic retinopathy. The British Journal of Ophthalmology. 2019;**103**(2):216-221

[97] Ho J, Dans K, You Q, Nudleman ED, Freeman WR. Comparison of 3 mm × 3 mm versus 6 mm × 6 mm optical coherence tomography angiography scan sizes In the evaluation of non-proliferative diabetic retinopathy. Retina. 2019;**39**(2):259-264

[98] Samara WA et al. Correlation of foveal avascular zone size with foveal morphology in normal eyes using optical coherence tomography angiography. Retina. 2015;**35**(11):2188-2195

[99] Tang FY et al. Clinically relevant factors associated with quantitative optical coherence tomography angiography metrics in deep capillary plexus in patients with diabetes. Eye and Vision (London, England). 2020;7:7

[100] Cennamo G, Montorio D, Fossataro F, Fossataro C, Tranfa F. Evaluation of vessel density in disorganization of retinal inner layers after resolved diabetic macular edema using optical coherence tomography angiography. PLoS One. 2021;**16**(1):e0244789

[101] de Carlo TE et al. Detection of microvascular changes in eyes of patients with diabetes but not clinical diabetic retinopathy using optical coherence tomography angiography. Retina. 2015;**35**(11):2364-2370

[102] Takase N, Nozaki M, Kato A, Ozeki H, Yoshida M, Ogura Y. Enlargement of foveal avascular zone in diabetic eyes evaluated by en face optical coherence tomography angiography. Retina. 2015;**35**(11):2377-2383

[103] Dai Y et al. Microvascular changes in the choriocapillaris of diabetic patients without retinopathy investigated by swept-source OCT angiography. Investigative Ophthalmology & Visual Science. 2020;**61**(3):50

[104] Wang F, Saraf SS, Zhang Q, Wang RK, Rezaei KA. Ultra-widefield protocol enhances automated classification of diabetic retinopathy severity with OCT angiography. Ophthalmology Retina. 2020;**4**(4):415-424

[105] Lee J, Rosen R. Optical coherence tomography angiography in diabetes. Current Diabetes Reports. 2016;**16**(12):123

[106] Reste-Ferreira D et al. Retinal neurodegeneration in eyes with NPDR risk phenotypes: A two-year longitudinal study. Acta Ophthalmologica. 2024;**102**(4):e539-e547

[107] Durbin MK et al. Quantification of retinal microvascular density in optical coherence tomographic angiography images in diabetic retinopathy. JAMA Ophthalmology. 2017;**135**(4):370-376

[108] Bin Lim H, Kim YW, Kim JM, Jo YJ, Kim JY. The importance of signal strength in quantitative assessment of retinal vessel density using optical coherence tomography angiography. Scientific Reports. 2018;**8**(1):12897

[109] Santos T et al. Swept-source OCTA quantification of capillary closure predicts ETDRS severity staging of NPDR. The British Journal of Ophthalmology. 2022;**106**(5):712-718

[110] Veiby NCBB et al. Associations between macular OCT angiography and nonproliferative diabetic retinopathy in young patients with type 1 diabetes mellitus. Journal Diabetes Research. 2020;**2020**:8849116

[111] Bek T. Transretinal histopathological changes in capillary-free areas of diabetic retinopathy. Acta Ophthalmologica. 1994;**72**(4):409-415

[112] Onishi AC et al. Importance of considering the middle capillary plexus on OCT angiography in diabetic retinopathy. Investigative Ophthalmology & Visual Science. 2018;**59**(5):2167-2176

[113] Chouhan S, Kalluri Bharat RP, Surya J, et al. Preliminary report on optical coherence tomography angiography biomarkers in non-responders and responders to intravitreal anti-VEGF injection for diabetic macular oedema. Diagnostics (Basel). 2023;**13**(10):1735. Published 2023 May 13. DOI: 10.3390/diagnostics13101735

[114] Zheng F et al. Age-dependent changes in the macular choriocapillaris of normal eyes imaged with swept-source optical coherence tomography angiography. American Journal of Ophthalmology. 2019;**200**:110-122

[115] McLeod DS, Lutty GA. High-resolution histologic analysis of the human choroidal vasculature. Investigative Ophthalmology & Visual Science. 1994;**35**(11):3799-3811

[116] Chu Z et al. Quantitative assessment of the retinal microvasculature using optical coherence tomography angiography. Journal of Biomedical Optics. 2016;**21**(6):66008

[117] Sasongko MB, Wong TY, Nguyen TT, Cheung CY, Shaw JE,

Wang JJ. Retinal vascular tortuosity in persons with diabetes and diabetic retinopathy. Diabetologia. 2011;**54**(9):2409-2416

[118] Klein R, Meuer SM, Moss SE, Klein BE. Retinal microaneurysm counts and 10-year progression of diabetic retinopathy. Archives of Ophthalmology (Chicago, Ill. 1960). 1995;**113**(11):1386-1391

[119] Thompson IA, Durrani AK, Patel S. Optical coherence tomography angiography characteristics in diabetic patients without clinical diabetic retinopathy. Eye (London). 2019;**33**(4):648-652

[120] Couturier A et al. Capillary plexus anomalies in diabetic retinopathy on optical coherence tomography angiography. Retina. 2015;**35**(11):2384-2391

[121] Parravano M et al. Diabetic microaneurysms internal reflectivity on spectral-domain optical coherence tomography and optical coherence tomography angiography detection. American Journal of Ophthalmology. 2017;**179**:90-96

[122] Park JJ, Soetikno BT, Fawzi AA. Characterization of the middle capillary plexus using optical coherence tomography angiography in healthy and diabetic eyes. Retina. 2016;**36**(11):2039-2050

[123] Pan J et al. Characteristics of neovascularization in early stages of proliferative diabetic retinopathy by optical coherence tomography angiography. American Journal of Ophthalmology. 2018;**192**:146-156

[124] Arya M et al. Distinguishing intraretinal microvascular abnormalities from retinal neovascularization using optical coherence tomography angiography. Retina. 2020;**40**(9):1686-1695

[125] Hwang TS et al. Optical coherence tomography angiography features of diabetic retinopathy. Retina. 2015;**35**(11):2371-2376

[126] Motulsky EH et al. Widefield swept-source optical coherence tomography angiography of proliferative diabetic retinopathy. Ophthalmic Surgery, Lasers & Imaging Retina. 2019;**50**(8):474-484

[127] Russell JF et al. Longitudinal wide-field swept-source OCT angiography of neovascularization in proliferative diabetic retinopathy after panretinal photocoagulation. Ophthalmology Retina. 2019;**3**(4):350-361

[128] Faghihi H et al. Effect of panretinal photocoagulation on macular vasculature using optical coherence tomography angiography. European Journal of Ophthalmology. 2021;**31**(4):1877-1884

[129] Acar OPA, Onur IU. Effect of panretinal photocoagulation on retina and choroid in diabetic retinopathy: An optical coherence tomography angiography study. Photodiagnosis and Photodynamic Therapy. 2022;**40**:103166

[130] Bhardwaj S et al. Value of fractal analysis of optical coherence tomography angiography in various stages of diabetic retinopathy. Retina. 2018;**38**(9):1816-1823

[131] Kim AY, Chu Z, Shahidzadeh A, Wang RK, Puliafito CA, Kashani AH. Quantifying microvascular density and morphology in diabetic retinopathy using spectral-domain optical coherence tomography angiography. Investigative

Ophthalmology & Visual Science. 2016;**57**(9):OCT362-OCT370

[132] Serra R et al. Optical coherence tomography angiography macular biomarkers of peripheral retinal ischemia in diabetic macular edema: Secondary endpoints from the clinical study 'FOVEA'. Graefe's Archive for Clinical and Experimental Ophthalmology = Albrecht von Graefes Archiv fur Klinische und Experimentelle Ophthalmologie. 2024;**262**(6):1777-1783

[133] Barot M, Gokulgandhi MR, Patel S, Mitra AK. Microvascular complications and diabetic retinopathy: Recent advances and future implications. Future Medicinal Chemistry. 2013;**5**(3):301-314

[134] Fan W et al. Relationship between retinal fractal dimension and nonperfusion in diabetic retinopathy on ultrawide-field fluorescein angiography. American Journal of Ophthalmology. 2020;**209**:99-106

[135] Bhanushali D et al. Linking retinal microvasculature features with severity of diabetic retinopathy using optical coherence tomography angiography. Investigative Ophthalmology & Visual Science. 2016;**57**(9):OCT519-OCT525

[136] Mendes L, Marques IP, Cunha-Vaz J. Comparison of different metrics for the identification of vascular changes in diabetic retinopathy using OCTA. Frontiers in Neuroscience. 2021;**15**:755730

[137] Kashani AH et al. Optical coherence tomography angiography: A comprehensive review of current methods and clinical applications. Progress in Retinal and Eye Research. 2017;**60**:66-100

[138] Kashani AH et al. Suspended scattering particles in motion: A novel feature of OCT angiography in exudative maculopathies. Ophthalmology Retina. 2018;**2**(7):694-702

[139] Sun Z et al. OCT angiography metrics predict progression of diabetic retinopathy and development of diabetic macular edema: A prospective study. Ophthalmology. 2019;**126**(12):1675-1684

[140] Hasegawa N, Nozaki M, Takase N, Yoshida M, Ogura Y. New insights into microaneurysms in the deep capillary plexus detected by optical coherence tomography angiography in diabetic macular edema. Investigative Ophthalmology & Visual Science. 2016;**57**(9):OCT348-OCT355

[141] Nanegrungsunk O, Patikulsila D, Sadda SR. Ophthalmic imaging in diabetic retinopathy: A review. Clinical & Experimental Ophthalmology. 2022;**50**(9):1082-1096

[142] Suciu C-I, Suciu V-I, Nicoara S-D. Optical coherence tomography (angiography) biomarkers in the assessment and monitoring of diabetic macular edema. Journal Diabetes Research. 2020;**2020**:6655021

[143] de Carlo TE et al. Distinguishing diabetic macular edema from capillary nonperfusion using optical coherence tomography angiography. Ophthalmic Surgery, Lasers & Imaging Retina. 2016;**47**(2):108-114

[144] Lee J, Moon BG, Cho AR, Yoon YH. Optical coherence tomography angiography of DME and its association with anti-VEGF treatment response. Ophthalmology. 2016;**123**(11):2368-2375